Havana Syndrome

Havana Syndrome

A Threat to National Security

Armin Krishnan

BLOOMSBURY ACADEMIC
NEW YORK • LONDON • OXFORD • NEW DELHI • SYDNEY

BLOOMSBURY ACADEMIC
Bloomsbury Publishing Inc, 1359 Broadway, New York, NY 10018, USA
Bloomsbury Publishing Plc, 50 Bedford Square, London, WC1B 3DP, UK
Bloomsbury Publishing Ireland, 29 Earlsfort Terrace, Dublin 2, D02 AY28, Ireland

BLOOMSBURY, BLOOMSBURY ACADEMIC and the Diana logo are trademarks of Bloomsbury Publishing Plc

First published in the United States of America 2025

A catalog record for this book is available from the Library of Congress.

ISBN: HB: 978-1-6669-5084-7
ePDF: 979-8-2162-7702-6
eBook: 978-1-6669-5085-4

Typeset by Deanta Global Publishing Services, Chennai, India

Contents

Tables

Acknowledgments

This book grew out of an earlier research interest in psychological warfare and military neuroscience. When the media started to report the Havana Syndrome and suspicions of covert directed energy attacks that may be directed against US personnel, I was not surprised that this would happen, given the terrifying potential of neuroscience-enabled directed energy weapons (DEW) that are currently transforming warfare. This was already apparent to some analysts, concerned scientists, and visionaries many decades earlier. Along the way, I had the opportunity to talk to several people at the receiving end of DEW attacks, who have provided me generously with their stories and other relevant information and documentation. I am particularly thankful for the information I received from Cheryl Welsh, Richard Dowling, and Len Ber. I am thankful to several people with relevant insights and access, who have sent me information anonymously or confidentially. They have left little doubt in my mind that Havana Syndrome is real and that there are many people around the world who are subjected to DEW attacks that are destroying their health and their lives. The cases reported by the media seem to be merely the tip of the iceberg. I am very thankful to Professor Robert McCreight for reaching out to me and offering much information and encouragement. It was very generous of him to give a guest lecture at East Carolina University (ECU) on cognitive warfare. I want to thank my great colleagues at ECU, especially Alethia Cook and Hanna Kassab. I am also thankful to my wife, Svetlana, who has offered patience and encouragement in the process of research and writing.

Abbreviations

ADS	Active Denial System
AHI	Anomalous Health Incidents
BCI	brain-computer interface
CFT (DoD)	cross-functional team
CW	continuous wave
DARPA	Defense Advanced Research Projects Agency
DEW	directed energy weapons
DIA	Defense Intelligence Agency
DoD	Department of Defense
ELF	extremely low frequency
EMF	electromagnetic fields
EMP	electromagnetic pulse
ESP	extrasensory perception
ETC (DoD)	Emerging Threats Cell
HPM	high-powered microwaves
IC	intelligence community
MAE	microwave auditory effect
MUTS	Moscow Unidentified Technical Signal
NIH	National Institutes of Health
NLW	nonlethal weapons
PMC	private military company

PSC	private security company
RF	radiofrequency
SRI	Stanford Research Institute
TMS	transcranial magnetic stimulation
TUMS	Technically Unidentified Moscow Signal
UHI	Unexplained Health Incident

Introduction

Directed energy weapons (DEW) are silently transforming warfare as the technology is maturing and is put into the field with both defensive and offensive applications. They are being developed to clear minefields, shoot down artillery rounds and drone swarms, and obliterate ballistic missiles in flight. Offensively, DEWs can be used to disable electronics, attack vehicles and other ground targets from the air, and dazzle or otherwise incapacitate enemy personnel. According to Louis del Monte, "[a] new revolution in warfare is coming, and, if you will pardon the pun, it is coming at the speed of light. This revolution concerns the emergence of directed energy weapons, which promise to be even more potent than nuclear weapons."[1] Although DEWs are usually discussed in the context of anti-material weapons (weapons that target equipment rather than personnel), there has been extensive research into antipersonnel DEWs that goes back at least to the 1960s. The possibility of incapacitating humans or altering their behavior was first investigated in the United States in the context of the Moscow Signal that seemingly affected US diplomats by exposing them to low energy microwaves.[2] Although it remained inconclusive at the time as to whether US diplomats were harmed by way of electromagnetic exposure, research into potential electromagnetic antipersonnel weapons continued in the United States well into the 1980s, as speculations grew that the Soviets may have achieved a breakthrough in this area of weapons research.[3] Public information on anti-personnel DEWs, which includes acoustic weapons, millimeter wave weapons, and laser dazzlers, is scarce. That some of these weapon systems exist is undeniable, even though their characteristics and their effectiveness are hotly debated.

Speculation about a novel acoustic weapon with debilitating effects grew when it was reported by the international media in summer 2017 that American diplomats had been attacked in Havana with an unknown "sonic weapon."[4] For years, the media reported ever more cases of so-called "Havana Syndrome" in many different locations worldwide. Skeptics were quick to dismiss allegations of covert attacks as paranoia or as potentially politically motivated. One prominent theory has been that Havana Syndrome is nothing but a "mass psychogenic illness" caused by stress and social contagion.[5] Major media outlets such as the *New York Times* and *CBS* produced countless news stories and many documentaries that invariably presented the phenomenon as an unsolvable puzzle or a curiosity that satisfies their viewers' and readers' appetite for the inexplicable. The US government added to the uncertainty and mystery by conducting several investigations and producing numerous studies with contradictory findings.

However, the mystery may not be as big as the media made it out to be, and the "simple" explanation of mass psychogenic illness, paranoia, and delusion is not convincing either, given the following facts (as will be further demonstrated in this book):

1. Governments have been developing DEWs since at least the 1960s, which amounts to over sixty years in research and development. All major military powers are developing DEWs, including the United States, Russia, China, the United Kingdom, Israel, Iran, and many others.
2. Various types of DEWs are known to exist, including acoustic weapons, millimeter wave weapons, lasers, particle beams, and high-powered microwave weapons. They are currently presented to the public mainly as anti-material weapons, which obscures other potential applications.
3. The amount of public information on DEWs, especially their capabilities and any bioeffects that they may have, is very limited as governments prefer to keep the existence of certain weapons and capabilities secret, hence the mystery.
4. A weapon that can damage the brain or other organs or interfere with the central nervous system over a distance of tens or hundreds of meters through walls does not violate any laws of physics. Skeptics can only question the practicality of such weapons but cannot disprove their theoretical feasibility.
5. Intelligence services have a history of covertly harassing whom they see as foreign or domestic enemies, including dissidents, suspected foreign agents, foreign intelligence officers, and foreign diplomats, which makes harassment with novel DEWs no fundamental departure from past covert practices.
6. Many analysts and strategists believe that the brain or cognition is becoming a new battlespace or operational domain as advances in

neuroscience and technology make it increasingly possible to affect with some precision perception, emotion, mental capacity, thinking/reasoning, and behavior. A DEW that can degrade mental capacity is therefore just a stepping stone toward an entirely new vision of warfare that emphasizes non-kinetic approaches for subduing an enemy.

Military Neuroscience

Neuroscience is an interdisciplinary field that seeks to advance knowledge of the brain, which can lead to new therapies and drugs for treating brain diseases and mental disorders. Neuroscience can also be used for human enhancement in the form of boosting mental capacity, including by connecting brains directly to computers.[6] In 2013, the Obama administration announced the Brain Research through Advancing Innovative Neurotechnologies (BRAIN) Initiative, which provided $100 million in neuroscience research funding through the National Institutes of Health (NIH), to unlock the mysteries of the brain.[7] There is also a dark side to neuroscience as better knowledge of the brain and cognitive processes will allow militaries, authoritarians, and ruthless corporations to influence human perception and behavior and even exercise control over human minds at a societal level. According to neuroscientist James Giordano, "[a]dvancements in neuroscience could be used to create 'super soldiers,' link brains to weapon systems for command and control, or even manipulate groups or leaders into taking actions that they normally wouldn't do."[8] In other words, current military neuroscience programs could be pursuing mind control capabilities at a grand, perhaps global scale. This general vision and the associated research agenda came out of the 1950s MK ULTRA program and associated research projects that investigated the possibilities of interfering with the brain using drugs, sensual stimuli, subliminal messaging, and even electromagnetic radiation.[9]

A notable MK ULTRA researcher was Yale University scientist José Delgado, who suggested in 1970 that the electrical stimulation of the brain would help create a "happier, less destructive and better balanced man" and that "one day our computers will be sophisticated enough to be used to put thoughts into people's heads . . . [and] possibly exert some influence on gross emotional behavior."[10] In his book *The Physical Control of the Mind* Delgado promoted the idea that the technology for the broad control of humans through electric stimuli was available and that special agencies needed to be created for a "psychocivilized society" that could suppress all the problematic urges and behaviors of man. He wrote:

> These accomplishments should familiarize us with the idea that we may also control the biological functions of living organisms from a distance. Cats, monkeys, or human beings can be induced to flex a limb, to reject food, or to feel emotional excitement under the influence of electrical impulses reaching the depths of their brains through radio waves purposefully sent by an investigator.[11]

The sad reality is that we are not too far off from Delgado's radical vision of governments exercising direct control over their people's brains. Brain implants that could accomplish the remote control of mental states, the reading of minds, and the insertion of information (sensual perception, dreams, and memories) are under development.[12] The decoding of the brain could be the most consequential discovery in human history as it turns the brain into a biocomputer that can be connected to a network or "hive mind." Human brains could then be hacked remotely through a brain-computer interface (BCI).[13]

NATO's New Obsession with Cognitive Warfare

From 2020, NATO published a series of papers and commentaries on cognitive warfare that highlight the possibility of Russia or other foreign powers messing with the perceptions and mental states of populations.[14] These ideas grew out of NATO's think tank *Innovation Hub*, founded in 2012, which is part of NATO's Allied Command Transformation based in Norfolk, Virginia.[15] Its current manager and expert on cognitive warfare is the French officer Francois du Cluzel. NATO's *Innovation Hub* held its first scientific meeting on cognitive warfare in Bordeaux, France, in June 2021, and the anthology with the papers presented has been published online.[16] One of the NATO conference papers suggests that "Cognitive Warfare (CW) has emerged quickly in the past years and quite possibly presents one of the greatest threats to NATO countries."[17] Although the focus of this body of work seems to be largely on propaganda, disinformation, social media content manipulation, deep fakes, and other uses of AI for shaping human perceptions and predicting behavior, there is an acknowledgment of the potential for a more direct adversarial interference with brain function. Francois du Cluzel argued:

> The objectives for neuroweapons in warfare may be achieved by augmenting or degrading functions of the nervous system, so as to affect cognitive, emotional and/or motor activity and capability (e.g., perception, judgment, morale,

> pain tolerance, or physical abilities and stamina) necessary for combat. Many technologies can be used to produce these effects, and there is demonstrated utility for neuroweapons in both conventional and irregular warfare scenarios.[18]

However, one has difficulty finding any NATO discussion of Havana Syndrome. It is strangely absent from the cognitive warfare debate, despite the rather obvious potential of neuroweapons that can degrade mental capacity and damage the brain.[19] It is hard to believe that NATO and the respective governments would be so oblivious to a very real threat. This book argues that Havana Syndrome is caused by adversaries targeting US personnel with DEW and that it should be considered as an aspect of cognitive warfare, which is bound to become more prevalent. There is no reason to believe that Havana Syndrome or Anomalous Health Incidents (AHIs) would be going away.[20] It is time to go beyond the mystification of the incidents and the conditions and to have a serious debate about what needs to be done to mitigate, prevent, and deter these covert attacks.

Outline of the Book

The first chapter of the book discusses the argument made by skeptics that the most likely explanation for Havana Syndrome is mass psychogenic illness and that the idea of an adversary carrying out covert attacks on US diplomats for unknown reasons simply lacks any valid evidence. This line of reasoning has received some tailwinds in the form of the US intelligence community (IC) releasing the summary of an intelligence assessment that points at the absence of evidence for adversarial activity causing AHIs. It is therefore essential to point out the flaws in the reasoning of the skeptics. The second chapter argues that there is a relevant historical precedent, namely the Moscow Signal, which leaked to the public in the early 1970s when several US diplomats returned home from Moscow with severe illnesses. It is very plausible that the Moscow Signal should be seen as a primitive version of the weapons that may currently be used by adversaries to cause brain damage. The third chapter turns to the unconventional research conducted by the two superpowers in the areas of parapsychology and psychotronics, which coincided with the Moscow Signal and with MK ULTRA mind control research. Although the psychic warfare programs were eventually shut down for good after the Cold War, one must wonder as to whether they were at least partially a cover for the development of DEWs and mind control/brain research. In any case, Soviet "psychotronic weapons" were rumored to be able to debilitate and even kill people from a distance. The fourth chapter discusses the concept of nonlethal weapons (NLWs) and reviews some of the weapon technologies associated with them, with a particular focus on acoustic and electromagnetic weapons. NLWs remain controversial due to their inherent potential for causing permanent damage and even death when used against vulnerable people or when used inappropriately. The fifth chapter provides an overview of the publicized cases of Havana Syndrome and the US policy responses to the challenge. It will be shown that there is some variation in the cases that may indicate that different types of DEWs were used on different victims. The sixth chapter reviews the main studies and investigations related to Havana Syndrome, some of which support the idea that radiofrequency/microwave weapons could have produced the observed health effects while others remain skeptical. It will be shown that none of the studies could offer any definitive answer to the involvement of an adversarial actor in the AHIs. The seventh chapter speculates on who the responsible actors are and what their motivations are. The primary suspects are the governments of Cuba, Russia, and China, with the possible involvement of nonstate actors. It seems likely that many incidents are connected to Russia, with some incidents that could be connected to China. The final chapter puts the AHIs into the larger framework of NATO's cognitive warfare concept. It also proposes some options for defense, including the development of detection systems, shielding/jamming of signals, deterrence, and options for a response to AHIs.

Notes

1 Louis del Monte, *War at the Speed of Light: Directed-Energy Weapons and the Future of Twenty-First Century Warfare* (Lincoln: Potomac Books, 2022), 42.

2 Del Monte, *War at the Speed of Light*, 89–90.

3 Chuck De Caro, "Weapons of War: Is There an RF Gap?," *CNN Special Assignment*, November 1985, available at: https://rumble.com/v2fw85s-electromagnetic-frequency-weapons-1985-cnn-special-reports.html.

4 Matthew Lee and Michael Weissenstein, "Hearing Loss of U.S. Diplomats in Cuba Blamed on Covert Device," *Associated Press*, August 9, 2017, available at: https://apnews.com/article/51828908c6c84d78a29e833d0aae10aa.

5 Erin Anderssen, "Mad Gassers, Toxic Bussers, and the Havana Syndrome: What Society Still Gets Wrong About the Way Stress Can Make Us Sick," *The Globe and Mail*, May 22, 2019.

6 Ivan S. Kotchetkov, Brian Y. Hwang, Geoffrey Appelboom, Christopher P. Kellner, and Sander Connolly, "Brain-Computer Interfaces: Military, Neurosurgical, and Ethical Perspectives," *Neurosurgical Focus* 28, no. 5 (2010): 4.

7 Thomas R. Insel, Story C. Landis, and Francis S. Collins, "The NIH BRAIN Initiative," *Science* 340, no. 6133 (2013): 687.

8 James Giordano, "Weaponizing the Brain: Neuroscience Advancements Spark Debate," *National Defense*, May 11, 2017, available at: https://www.nationaldefensemagazine.org/articles/2017/5/11/weaponizing-the-brain-neuroscience-advancements-spark-debate.

9 Walter Bowart, *Operation Mind Control* (New York: Dell Publishing, 1978).

10 Maggie Scarf, "Brain Researcher José Delgado Asks—'What Kind of Humans Would You Like to Construct?'" *New York Times*, November 15, 1970.

11 José Delgado, *The Physical Control of the Mind: Towards a Psychocivilized Society* (New York: Harper & Row, 1969), 75.

12 Kyle Mizokami, "DARPA Wants Soldiers to Control Machines with Their Minds," *Popular Mechanics*, May 22, 2019, available at: https://www.popularmechanics.com/military/research/a27560088/darpa-soldier-machine/; Eric Bland, "Army Developing 'Synthetic Telepathy,'" *NBC News*, October 13, 2008, available at: https://www.nbcnews.com/id/wbna27162401; Dawn Lim, "Real-Life Inception: Army Looks to 'Counteract Nightmares' with Digital Dreams," *Wired*, October 21, 2011, available at: https://www.wired.com/2011/10/real-life-inception/.

13 Jonathan Pugh, Laurie Pycroft, Anders Sandberg, Tipu Aziz, and Julian Savulescu, "Brainjacking in Deep Brain Stimulation and Autonomy," *Ethics and Information Technology* 20, no. 3 (2018): 219–32.

14 Francois du Cluzel, "Cognitive Warfare," NATO Innovation Hub, June–November 2020, available at: https://innovationhub-act.org/wp-content/uploads/2023/12/20210113_CW-Final-v2-.pdf.

15 Yasmin Tadjdeh, "Innovation Hub Connects Industry, Academia and NATO," *National Defense* 102, no. 768 (2017): 28.

16 B. Claverie, B. Prébot, N. Buchler, and F. Du Cluzel, eds., *Cognitive Warfare: The Future of Cognitive Dominance* (Neuilly, France: NATO, 2022), available at: https://innovationhub-act.org/wp-content/uploads/2023/12/210601-Cognition-Workshop-Report-v3.pdf.

17 Robin Burda, "Detection Tools for Cognitive Warfare: Leveraging the Cyber Domain," NATO Science and Technology Organization, 2023, available at: https://www.sto.nato.int/publications/STO%20Meeting%20Proceedings/STO-MP-SAS-OCS-ORA-2023/MP-SAS-OCS-ORA-2023-28.pdf.

18 Du Cluzel, "Cognitive Warfare," 20.

19 James Giordano, "Nation Must Come Together to Tackle Havana Syndrome," *National Defense*, October 15, 2021, available at: https://www.nationaldefensemagazine.org/articles/2021/10/15/nation-must-come-together-to-tackle-havana-syndrome.

20 Eric Bazail-Eimil, "Havana Syndrome Won't Go Away," *Politico*, April 1, 2024, available at: https://www.politico.com/newsletters/national-security-daily/2024/04/01/havana-syndrome-wont-go-away-00149977.

1

Examining the Arguments of Havana Syndrome Skeptics

Havana Syndrome or the Anomalous Health Incidents as they were later called were from the very start viewed with some degree of skepticism by parts of the government, press, and the scientific community. The media kept reporting regularly on suspected Havana Syndrome cases from the middle of 2017 to 2020, but was generally more cautious as to the causes and the reality of the phenomenon. Havana Syndrome was frequently described as a "mystery" or even a potentially politically motivated fraud or deception to justify the demonization of the Cuban or Russian governments. Even some investigations from within the government, such as the first report of the JASONs and an FBI review of the known cases, seemed to suggest rather benign origins, such as crickets and/or a psychological origin. But how good are the arguments of the skeptics and how confident can one be in dismissing the possibility of a deliberate covert attack in *all* supposed Havana Syndrome incidents? This chapter evaluates the reasoning of the Havana Syndrome skeptics in light of the available evidence.

Debunking the Havana Syndrome Debunkers

The media debate on Havana Syndrome has included quite a few skeptical voices, which have tried to dismiss the phenomenon as a mix of hysteria, bad science, and politics. The most comprehensive effort to debunk Havana Syndrome was made by Robert Baloh and Robert Bartholomew in their 2020 book *Havana Syndrome: Mass Psychogenic Illness and the Real Story Behind the Embassy Mystery and Hysteria*. Baloh, a neurologist, and Bartholomew, a medical psychologist, have claimed that Havana Syndrome is merely a "mass psychogenic illness" or a form of mass hysteria, where people believe they have been exposed to something harmful and subsequently manifest symptoms that are only caused by their mind but have no material basis.[1] The authors make it clear that they believe the supposed attacks "*never happened*" and that Havana Syndrome is merely a "social construct."[2] They asserted that "[t]heir [the victims'] symptoms and suffering are real, but they are not from a mysterious energy force, they are due to physiological changes in the brain that are triggered by chronic stress."[3] They did not suggest that the affected individuals would be deliberately trying to deceive others or would be trying to make up health complaints that have no basis in reality. What they did suggest is that the underlying causes are psychosomatic and not physical in the way of some sort of harmful environmental exposure or a deliberate attack.

The book by Baloh and Bartholomew only devotes 55 out of its 190 pages to the discussion of Havana Syndrome itself, with the remainder of the book covering other historical cases of mass psychogenic illness to provide more context to the medical phenomenon and to make the overall Havana Syndrome debunking more plausible. To prove that *Havana Syndrome does not exist*, Baloh and Bartholomew needed to accomplish the following: (1) they must demonstrate that the covert attack hypothesis is implausible and lacks any evidence and (2) make the case that all the circumstances and characteristics observed in Havana Syndrome perfectly fit into the mass hysteria/mass psychogenic illness framework.

Ockham's Razor

One of Baloh's and Bartholomew's arguments presented in their book is Ockham's razor or the principle of parsimony, which suggests that the simplest explanation is most likely the correct one.[4] Ockham's razor is just a rule of thumb or an economy principle that advises scientists to first consider the simplest explanation before moving on to more fanciful and less likely explanations. Baloh and Bartholomew put it in the following way: "Instead of initially examining mundane explanations, State Department officials opted for the most exotic hypothesis early on. Instead of looking for horses, they began searching for zebras. Unicorns would be an even more accurate description because however unlikely, the existence of zebras is at least possible, whereas the use of sonic weapons would defy the laws of physics."[5]

Mass hysteria/mass psychogenic illness is, in their view, the most plausible explanation because it is the simplest explanation that does not require many contentious assumptions. The alternative explanation that some US personnel suffered covert attacks with an unknown weapon, device, or method would require a greater set of assumptions to be true, which would make it less likely to be true. One would have to assume: (1) a foreign adversary wanted to covertly hurt US personnel, (2) a foreign adversary possessed an unknown technology to do so, and (3) for some reason, for many years the US intelligence community has been unable to find any hard evidence for deliberate attacks taking place—all of which seems to indicate that there were no covert attacks causing Havana Syndrome to begin with.

Ockham's razor works well in the natural sciences, but it has not much applicability in the world of national security and strategy, where there are intelligent opponents who have an incentive to deceive and misdirect. A famous example of a military deception was the D-Day deception. The most trusted German agents reported that the location of the planned Allied invasion was Calais, open-source information indicated it was Calais, and reconnaissance flights indicated Allied forces preparing for an invasion at Calais. The simplest explanation for the observed phenomena would be that the Allied invasion was planned to take place at Calais, and the more fanciful explanation was that all German intelligence sources and methods had been manipulated and that the real location of the attack was somewhere else. The more fanciful explanation was the correct one. Similarly, it is a mistake to dismiss the hypothesis of Havana Syndrome having been caused by a deliberate attack from an unknown adversary with an unknown weapon from the outset as extremely unlikely. If an adversary had developed such a weapon and planned to use it covertly, they would take extreme care to hide the existence of the weapon and their tracks when using it.

It is important to note that mass hysteria or mass psychogenic illness as an explanation of Havana Syndrome would require some contentious assumptions too: (1) psychosomatic symptoms of US diplomats were incorrectly diagnosed early on by medical doctors, who should have known better; (2) there was a social contagion that caused more people with somewhat similar symptoms to believe that they were also under attack when this was not the case, which is unlikely to apply to the first Havana Syndrome cases of late 2016 and early 2017; and (3) many senior US officials, experts, and researchers bought into a theory that had hardly any plausibility or evidence behind it, which suggests these officials were either paranoid or engaged in a deliberate deception for political ends. It is therefore in the eye of the beholder as to which set of assumptions is more plausible or contentious.

Is It Implausible That a Foreign Power Would Harass Diplomats?

People less familiar with the intelligence world may find it somewhat implausible that any government would covertly harass foreign diplomats and intelligence officers. For example, Sharon Weinberger pointed out "the seeming absurdity of a hostile country randomly zapping diplomats and spies with their most advanced weaponry for no discernible reason other than harassment."[6] Assuming that a foreign government had an antipersonnel DEW suitable for covert attacks, would it be completely out of character for Russian or Chinese counterintelligence services to try to harm diplomatic personnel from an adversarial country? The historical record would suggest otherwise: US diplomats and intelligence officers have been subjected to all sorts of harassment when operating in adversarial states. Sometimes the harassment has been direct, and sometimes it has been covert.

Kyle Cunliffe has discussed some of the harassment techniques that US diplomats and intelligence officers have had to put up with in recent years. In countries like Russia, they not only face aggressive surveillance but also "burglaries, intimidation, harassment, defamation, physical assault, and even drink spiking."[7] He mentioned that a CIA officer in Russia was violently tackled and forced to the ground by a uniformed FSB guard on the way back to the US embassy. The CIA officer sustained injuries severe enough to require his evacuation from Russia. Keir Giles claimed that a US intelligence officer in Moscow was punched hard in the stomach by two people (likely FSB surveillance) in the metro a week after he arrived, while a NATO defense attaché had his own children briefly kidnapped as they were put deliberately on a wrong school bus and driven around Moscow for several hours.[8] According to a *Washington Post* story from June 2016, "diplomats reported that Russian intruders had broken into their homes late at night, only to rearrange the furniture or turn on all the lights and televisions, and then leave. One diplomat reported that an intruder had defecated on his living room carpet."[9] Others had their tires slashed or were harassed by traffic police or had their dogs killed during break-ins. According to US ambassador to the Czech Republic Norm Eisen, "[s]ince the return of Putin, Russia has been engaged in an increasingly aggressive gray war across Europe. Now it's in retaliation for Western sanctions because of Ukraine. The widely reported harassment is another front in the gray war."[10]

When US diplomats returned to Cuba after fifty-five years in 2015, they also experienced a lot of harassment by the Cuban security services. All US diplomats were under constant surveillance by the Cubans, both physical and electronic surveillance. The *Washington Post* reported that "[t]he American diplomats believed their homes and cars were all bugged, as well as restaurants they frequented."[11] There were break-ins into the residences of US diplomats where feces were left or where pictures of their children were deleted from their computers or where books were turned around on the book shelves to show them that there was no privacy.[12] Would it be extraordinary for an authoritarian regime to try to covertly injure the personnel of an adversarial state? Hardly. Authoritarian governments do not treat their perceived domestic enemies with any civility. In such countries, the domestic political opposition gets routinely intimidated, harassed, otherwise mistreated, and even assassinated. The East German Stasi (state security) covertly exposed dissidents to ionizing radiation (X-rays hidden behind walls) to induce cancer.[13] There is no surprise that foreign enemies would be treated any better than domestic ones.

No Brain Injury in Havana Syndrome Patients

Baloh and Bartholomew made a great effort to dismiss the evidence of brain injury sustained by some of the US and Canadian personnel since this contradicts their hypothesis of a psychosomatic origin of the experienced symptoms. In the absence of another diagnosed disease, brain injury simply must have an external cause, even if the cause cannot be readily identified. Edward Shorter, a psychiatrist, also suggested that "[i]nner ear damage is not psychogenic and means that the tissues of the inner ear itself have sustained some kind of assault."[14] Hence, Baloh and Bartholomew argued that the diagnosis of concussion or brain injury must have been wrong, possibly because of poor or inadequate medical testing methodology. They pointed in particular at inconsistencies between the study by a research team at the University of Miami and a different team at the University of Pennsylvania, with the former attributing the symptoms to vestibular damage and the latter attributing them to traumatic brain injury, and at disputes between the researchers, as well as at potential conflicts of interest.[15] Baloh and Bartholomew quoted R. Douglas Fields from the National Institutes of Health, who had stated that the brain imaging studies carried out did not support the claim of brain injury.[16] They commented on Shorter's support for the brain injury conclusion in the 2018 Journal of the American Medical Association (JAMA) article that "respected specialists, even on psychogenic illness, can be misled if they have either not read or understood the research."[17] The respective studies and the views of experts on it will be discussed at a later point in the book.

A recent NIH-funded study using brain imaging seems to strengthen the argument of Havana Syndrome skeptics. The researchers in this study stated that "there was no significant MRI-detectable evidence of brain injury among the group of participants who experienced AHIs compared with a group of matched control participants."[18] The findings were widely reported in the international press and taken as the final proof that Havana Syndrome is psychosomatic and not caused by a deliberate attack. Robert McCreight has criticized the media reporting of the NIH study since it misrepresented the actual findings to make "the uninformed public think there is nothing serious or harmful to worry about."[19]

When one reads the actual study, the authors have findings not in line with the mass psychogenic illness hypothesis, and they also acknowledge some important limitations of the study. In particular, they state that "increased connectivity in the salience network has been associated with posttraumatic stress disorder and anxiety; however, no such relationships were observed within the AHI cohort," which seems to suggest that brain imaging of thirty-one AHI patients has not indicated PTSD.[20] They mentioned the relatively small sample size, the time delay between the appearance of symptoms and the brain scans, and the use of Diffusion Magnetic Resonance Imaging (dMRI) instead of Functional Magnetic Resonance Imaging (fMRI) as the main limitations.

Neuroscientist James Giordano has pointed out in an interview after the publication of the NIH study that there is evidence of functional impairment in AHI patients, which may be like decompression sickness or a mini-stroke that does not show up in MRI scans as structural changes or brain damage.[21] David Relman, who led the National Academy of Sciences study on AHIs, commented that "NIH's methods were 'diluting important signals' by lumping alleged victims and real victims into the same pool."[22] The argument the critics of the NIH study seem to make is that it is hard to dispute the functional cognitive impairment in some AHI patients, even if this impairment does not show up as a structural change or lesions in brain scans.

No Weapon Exists That Could Cause Havana Syndrome

If the Havana Syndrome is caused by a type of weapon, most likely a DEW, it must be an unknown type of weapon since no government seems to have such a weapon officially in their arsenal. The "Updated IC Assessment on Anomalous Health Incidents" even stated that "there is no credible evidence that a foreign adversary has a weapon or collection device that is causing AHIs."[23] Baloh and Bartholomew quoted and referenced several highly reputed experts in the area of acoustics such as Professor Jürgen Altmann from the Technical University of Dortmund, Professor Emeritus Joseph Pompeii from MIT, and Professor Seth Horowitz from Brown University, who all stated that they did not believe sound or ultrasound could produce the Havana Syndrome symptoms.[24] Since high-energy microwaves could conceivably produce some of the Havana Syndrome symptoms, it must be still plausible that it could be done covertly or from a longer distance, which would be necessary for attacks in hotels or residencies, which Baloh and Bartholomew deemed to be unlikely.[25]

On the other side of the argument, there are also numerous highly reputed experts who have gone on the record stating that they consider it not only possible that there was a plausible physical mechanism for causing Havana Syndrome, but that they actually believe weapons that could cause Havana Syndrome symptoms already exist. Some experts have even accused the US government of a cover-up aimed at hiding the existence of such technology.[26] But is it completely implausible that governments could keep the development of highly advanced weapon systems secret?

Secret Weapons

One line of argument that is frequently stated by skeptics is the impossibility for governments to keep secrets in the information age. Secrets and secret technologies would always leak out to the public. However, it is widely known that the US government has a "black budget" (non-itemized government spending) that funds the intelligence community and a range of classified programs, including highly classified research and development of new weapons. The overall black budget request of the Trump administration for 2019 was over \$81 billion.[27] The most sensitive programs are called Special Access Programs (SAPs), which have special measures to prevent unauthorized disclosure. There are Unacknowledged SAPs that allow government officials and contractors to publicly deny their existence and even employ deception. Waived SAPs are only disclosed to eight ranking members of Congress, who receive oral briefings.[28] SAPs can also have subcompartments that are exempted from even those limited disclosure rules.[29] To complicate matters even more, secret weapons technology is developed by private defense contractors, who are not subject to the same degree of accountability and oversight as government agencies. There could be secret revolutionary technology tucked away in places like Area-51, which is a secret military base operated by private companies such as Lockheed Martin. For example, the US military likely developed a revolutionary hypersonic aircraft called "Aurora" (also referred to as TR3) in the 1980s and 1990s, which was never publicly acknowledged.[30] If the US government can manage to keep certain weapons technologies secret for years and even decades, it is a given that authoritarian states can do it as well and probably are much better at keeping such secrets.

Many weapons technologies have been developed in complete secrecy and have only been disclosed to the public after many years. A famous example is stealth technology, which was developed in the late 1970s and was only publicly disclosed over a decade later. The F-117A Stealth Fighter was operational for five years before the US government revealed its existence in 1988. It is not a stretch that a major government such as the United States, Russia, or China has a secret weapons program that develops revolutionary weapons technologies that remain hidden until they would be used openly in a major war. These weapons technologies could be secretly used on a smaller scale to see how well they would do in the field to make improvements or refine the tactics before they become operational.

Baloh and Bartholomew raise the issue that if Russia had a secret weapon, "why wasn't such a device used on the battlefield to save lives and avoid house-to-house combat in war zones, such as Iraq and Syria?"[31] First of all, it would be difficult to establish with any degree of certainty whether such a weapon was used in war since no medical personnel or international organizations such as the Red Cross would be familiar with the weapon and its effects, making it less likely that its existence or usage would be noticed, far less proven. Secondly, any government that was in possession of such a weapon would consider it prudent to keep its existence hidden as long as possible since it is perfect for deniable and covert attacks on key enemy personnel within and outside of war zones. If adversaries are not aware of it, they are less likely to develop similar weapons or develop any effective countermeasures. Wars of choice that do not pose an existential threat to a government possessing these weapons would not warrant the open or large-scale use of a secret weapon that could be used when the stakes are much higher. Besides, a weapon that could cause Havana Syndrome would violate international law, which would discourage overt usage to avoid war crime accusations.

Are Weapons That Could Cause Havana Syndrome Even Technologically Impossible?

Baloh and Bartholomew suggested that "any such device must adhere to the laws of physics, which are not conducive to the development of an effective device in the first place."[32] They quoted former CIA officer Fulton Armstrong, who stated: "No one has a device that can do that" and "no such device exists."[33] But expert opinions diverge greatly when it comes to the technical feasibility of antipersonnel DEWs, even though a couple of such weapons systems are known to exist, which include the Long-Range Acoustic Device (LRAD) and the Active Denial System (ADS). Skeptics are quick to point out that neither ultrasound nor microwaves are suitable for incapacitating enemy personnel and that the known antipersonnel DEWs use audible sound or millimeter waves, while proposed weapons systems such as Medusa have proven to be either impractical or unfeasible.

For example, Sharon Weinberger has claimed that the ADS' "massive size, energy consumption and technical complexity make it effectively unusable on the battlefield" and that after fifty years of R&D in electromagnetic weapons "progress is elusive."[34] Weinberger argued that the weapon was not working well in rainy conditions and that needed to be cooled for 16 hours before it could be fired. Her explanation as to why the US military (and other militaries) keeps funding DEWs is that the enormous secrecy of such weapons programs would encourage unrealistic expectations not in tune with the laws of physics.[35]

One of the experts quoted by Weinberger is bioengineering Professor emeritus Kenneth Foster, who claimed: "Since the intensity of the radiation falls off as a square of the distance, well, if I wanted to produce that sensation more than a few feet from the transmitter, I would have to have a much bigger transmitter," the size of a "shipping container" and "[a] small transmitter might look like a big refrigerator. This is not something that you can just pick up, put in the back of your car and drive away."[36] Foster commented in relation to the microwave weapon theory for Havana Syndrome: "It would require something like a major airport radar transmitter with the subject's head close to the antenna in its direct beam. . . . I guess it is possible, but not likely."[37] Similarly, chemist Cheryl Rofer has reasoned that "[a]side from the reported syndromes, there's no evidence that a microwave weapon exists—and all the available science suggests that any such weapon would be wildly impractical."[38]

On the other side of the argument, there is no shortage of experts with a national security background who believe that a weapon that can produce Havana Syndrome may exist. A study by the National Academy of Sciences from 2020, which will be discussed later, concluded that "the acute symptoms [of Havana Syndrome] were consistent with a directed radiofrequency (RF) attack."[39] Although Kenneth Foster disagreed with the pulsed microwave hypothesis, he did not completely dismiss the feasibility of a portable nonlethal DEW that could produce Havana Syndrome. He argued that IR lasers "can induce auditory/vestibular responses in humans via thermoelastic sound generation when directed against the head." He even suggested that "high-peak power pulsed lasers are commercially available" and that even though weapons of this kind would be hypothetical, they would be "of interest to governments around the world which have made already considerable investments in laser weapons."[40]

One of the most outspoken academic experts is neuroscientist James Giordano, who claimed in an interview with *The Guardian* that US adversaries had developed new weapons that used microwave frequencies and that could "disrupt brain function without any burning sensation."[41] Similarly, James Lin, a professor emeritus of electrical and computer engineering at the University of Illinois, has claimed that "a thermoelastic pressure wave" could penetrate the brain and cause damage. He opined that "[y]ou can certainly put together a system in a couple of big suitcases that will allow you to put it in a van or an SUV," and: "It's not something that you need to have enormous amounts of space or equipment to do it."[42] Electrical engineering professor Edl Schamiloglu has also argued that a DEW could be the best explanation for Havana Syndrome. He suggested that "high-power microwave weapons are generally designed to disable electronic equipment. But as the Havana Syndrome reports show, these pulses of energy can harm people as well."[43]

The statement of Lin is in line with the information provided by journalist Christo Grozev, who told the Homeland Security Committee: "I have seen a

1991 version of the [Havana Syndrome] weapon and it looks like a satellite dish with a unit this size [Grozev was pointing at a box in front of him about 15 inches wide] attached to it."[44] He claimed that it could be contained in the trunk of a car or even in a backpack. If the Havana Syndrome was caused by a small handheld device or a device that could be used from within a van or car while it was hidden, it would explain as to why the CIA or the FBI has been unable to catch the perpetrators of such attacks. The duration of an attack that causes some degree of brain damage and other symptoms may only be a couple of minutes, which would make it even harder to detect attacks at the time they were happening. In short, a DEW that could cause Havana Syndrome does not violate the laws of physics and does not have to be so large that it cannot be hidden inside a smaller vehicle.

Havana Syndrome as Mass Psychogenic Illness

Mass psychogenic illness was previously referred to in the medical literature as mass hysteria or mass panic that resulted from an imaginary rather than real threat. Mass hysteria has been observed throughout history in connection to superstitions and folklore such as witchcraft, demon possession, and public anxieties related to new technologies. The term mass psychogenic illness suggests that people who suffer from it have real symptoms, but the underlying causes are psychosomatic, which means that the illness is caused by the body's response to stress and faulty beliefs. Robert Bartholomew and Chandra Sekaran Muniratnam have defined mass psychogenic illness as

> the rapid spread of illness signs and symptoms within a cohesive social unit for which there is no plausible organic cause. Episodes are triggered by an anxiety-generating stimulus within the victims' immediate environment (either real or imagined), and symptoms appear within a close temporal proximity of exposure to the perceived harmful agent. Symptoms are transient and benign, have rapid onset and recovery, and victims are overwhelmingly female.[45]

Baloh and Bartholomew suggest that mass psychogenic illness is a "placebo effect in reverse": people imagine that they have been exposed to some specific harm and the stress and anxiety that result from this materialize in several typical psychosomatic symptoms. "Persons who believe they have been exposed to tainted food commonly experience abdominal pain, diarrhea, nausea, and vomiting, while persons who think they have been in contact with toxic gas typically exhibit dizziness, itchy eyes, and breathing problems."[46] They point out that "[p]sycongenic illness can affect anyone" and that "[m]ost victims are normal healthy people," meaning that they are not mentally ill or mentally unstable.[47] They argued that "[t]his condition is often prompted by stress," and that "[w]ith passage of time, these conditions tend to resolve on their own."[48] To what extent does this definition of mass psychogenic illness apply to Havana Syndrome?

Vague Symptoms

Baloh and Bartholomew pointed out that the symptoms for Havana Syndrome are so vague and generic that there could be numerous reasons as to why people could have these symptoms that have nothing to do with DEW or any exposure to a specific hazard. If one ignores the traumatic brain injury observed in some Havana Syndrome patients, one could end up with a range of symptoms that "are common in the general population." Baloh and Bartholomew mentioned that a female Canadian diplomat described her symptoms as "nausea, dizziness, ringing in the ears, pain behind the eyes, difficulty speaking, exhaustion, memory problems, and issues with her vision."[49] The symptoms varied also somewhat from individual to individual, which weakens the case for the existence of a "syndrome" or a distinctive pattern of symptoms associated with a particular disease or exposure. For example, symptoms experienced by other Canadian diplomats included

> neurological complaints resembling brain injuries, headaches and migraines, dizziness, balance problems, nausea, insomnia, fatigue, difficulty remembering and concentrating, emotional disturbances including depression, irritability, anger, anxiety, sadness, nervousness, worry, ear pain, tinnitus, sensitivity to light and sound, vision problems, nose bleeds, and even "loss of consciousness." Most of these symptoms are routinely encountered by a GP.[50]

In other words, Baloh and Bartholomew suggested that because symptoms experienced by people diagnosed with Havana Syndrome are also experienced by a large number of random people in the general population in different combinations and different contexts, it must be all psychosomatic, which is not entirely convincing. It still does not rule out the possibility that at least a subset of individuals who have reported Havana Syndrome could have suffered symptoms because of real physical conditions that caused them.

Baloh and Bartholomew point to the analysis of the recordings made by one of the individuals who experienced Havana Syndrome in Cuba that indicated that it "was virtually identical to the mating call of the Indies short-tailed cricket (*Anorogryllus celerinictus*)."[51] They alluded that US diplomats in Cuba with a high degree of anxiety heard some crickets and then suffered an episode of psychosomatic symptoms, which they misinterpreted as an attack with a sonic weapon. They concluded their book by stating: "The symptoms that begin in Cuba as a result of social paranoia and insect sounds, exemplify the power of belief. That same power holds the key to recovery."[52] The assumption is that symptoms would eventually disappear once anxiety and stress subside and an individual stops believing in having suffered an unspecified harm. This is simply not the case for the more severe AHI patients, who have been suffering from symptoms for many years, sometimes with little improvement in their condition.

High-Stress Environments

Baloh and Bartholomew claimed that the people who first reported Havana Syndrome were working demanding jobs in a high-stress environment. US diplomats only returned to Cuba in 2015, and they were aware of the harassment that American officials had been subjected by Cuban intelligence. They pointed out that "[t]he actions of Cuban agents against embassy personnel have been well-documented to the point where it has become part of American intelligence folklore. Diplomats were harassed in a myriad of ways. Cuban agents were known to enter homes, rearrange books and furniture, dump urine or feces onto the floor, deflate car tires, and find ways to disrupt their sleep."[53] This meant that US embassy personnel were likely suffering from some degree of anxiety even before they arrived and that they were perhaps overly perceptive of potential threats. When psychosomatic symptoms materialized, they were interpreted as possible attacks, and their superiors, who were aware of a history of Cubans harassing US diplomats, were quite willing to accept this interpretation.

The counterargument here is that a subset of the people afflicted with Havana Syndrome are not ordinary civilians, but people who are accustomed to stress and who are not easily scared or fooled. What is known now is that many of the early supposed Havana Syndrome victims were CIA operations officers or case officers. The first four individuals to report an AHI in Cuba were all CIA officers working under diplomatic cover, as were two additional individuals who suffered Havana Syndrome in Cuba some time later.[54] It is a normal part of the job of a case officer to go to adversarial countries and to take risks without cracking under pressure. Marc Polymeropoulos, who suffered an AHI in Moscow in 2017, stated: "Back-alley high-risk operational meetings with agents in Afghanistan, or being second in the door on a Naval Special Warfare raid in Iraq, or hunting High Value Targets in places I'd better not mention, were walks in the park compared to the sheer terror I faced that night in the chic center of the Russian capital."[55] The idea that CIA operations officers could get spooked by rumors, hearing some crickets, and having some headaches seems highly implausible. One would need to then assume that they had a personal motive to lie (perhaps to get benefits and early retirement), or that their agency told them to lie about the covert attacks they supposedly suffered (perhaps to advance a political agenda), both of which seem implausible. The victims faced major disadvantages in their careers for going public, and their former employers failed to support them in the aftermath, which they would have if it had been an agency-sanctioned hoax.

Havana Syndrome in Children and Pets

It is notable that the close family members of US personnel have also been also affected by Havana Syndrome, which includes not only spouses but even infant children and pets. US Department of Commerce official Robyn Garfield was afflicted with Havana Syndrome and so were his wife and his two children.[56] He stated: "I can tell you I've personally seen balance issues in children that have never had that. Trouble with finding their words, stuttering. And then continuing challenges around vision. One of the things that we have heard from some parents is that these are manifesting in the classroom in real, tangible ways." Garfield also mentioned that he knows of eight other children who had been similarly impacted.[57]

Another *CBS News* report puts the number of impacted children at altogether twenty, stating that "a mother and her infant were affected while the baby was breastfeeding. Both have been diagnosed with a traumatic brain injury."[58] It does not make sense to assume that an infant child would psychosomatically materialize "concussion-like" symptoms in response to any anxiety about its environment that may have been imprinted on it by the infant's parents. Nevertheless, Bartholomew claims that "[a] more mundane explanation is sleep or night terrors, which affect up to half of all children and are triggered by an array of factors including stress."[59] In response to the assertion that an infant suffered from traumatic brain injury, he merely points out that it has "never been demonstrated in published patient studies of the U.S. diplomats in Cuba" and without that one would end up with "the classic symptoms of mass psychogenic illness."[60]

US diplomat in China, Catherine Werner, who was posted to Guangzhou, China, in 2017, reported that not only were she and her family affected but also their dog began acting strangely. The dog shivered, vomited blood, and did not want to go back into the apartment after long walks.[61] A Canadian diplomat using the pseudonym "Allen," who was in Havana in 2017, also reported strange behaviors of his three Shih Tzu dogs. According to a story in the *Ottawa Citizen*, "[a]lmost every night, the dogs would run to the corner of their yard backing onto a house where American diplomatic staff lived and bark frantically, for no apparent reason. 'There was nothing there.'" Other strange behaviors included "suddenly biting at non-existent flies, arching its back and lying on its back and putting its feet in the air. A veterinarian diagnosed seizures and told the family there was something wrong with the dog's brain."[62] Baloh and Bartholomew commented that "[o]ne of the diplomats in China dismissed the mass hysteria hypothesis by noting that her dog had vomited and could not have been influenced by media coverage about the symptoms, yet vomiting was not one of the complaints listed in Cuba."[63] However, nausea has been publicly stated as a major symptom by several of the individuals afflicted with Havana Syndrome. Nausea is listed in the CDC report on Havana Syndrome as one of the common symptoms.[64] Besides, the physiology of a dog is different from humans, and vomiting blood was not the only observed change in the behavior of the dog.

Political Motivations for Creating a Fake Scandal

Proponents of the mass psychogenic illness hypothesis must come to terms with the fact that many national security officials, some senior government officials, and some members of Congress not personally affected by Havana Syndrome not only considered the theory that US diplomats and intelligence officers were targets of deliberate attacks a possibility but also believed that this was actually happening. Former acting secretary of defense Chris Miller called the suspected directed energy attacks on US personnel "an act of war" if that could be confirmed.[65] Former National Security Advisor John Bolton expressed in an interview that he thought "there's very likely some hostile adversary behavior here, whether it's Russia, China, maybe somebody else, more than likely Russia."[66] The Trump administration was taking various steps to punish governments they believed were responsible or complicit. The Havana Syndrome has endured for over eight years and spanned two very different US administrations, which makes it far less plausible that it was just mass hysteria and a false belief by a couple of US government employees that they were covertly attacked. Why would so many senior people in the US government go along with giving credence to the idea of covert attacks for so long when there was absolutely no evidence for it? Why did leading US media outlets such as the *New York Times*, the *Washington Post*, and *CNN* produce hundreds of news stories and reports that were uncritically advancing the idea that US diplomats were under attack around the world when supposedly the most likely explanation for it all was, from early on, some kind of mass hysteria? Bartholomew's response to the strange persistence of the Havana Syndrome story was that it had to be "a grand case of mass deception. Human beings have deceived themselves," and that it was "one of the craziest stories" he had ever encountered.[67] The only logical way of reconciling the persistence of the story with the mass psychogenic illness hypothesis is to assume some kind of political conspiracy aimed at promoting Havana Syndrome in the media in the pursuit of a particular political agenda. While the assumption of a political conspiracy is not entirely without some plausibility, it still fails to convince when it gets scrutinized.

Trump Administration's Stance of Reversing the Obama-Era Policies toward Cuba

US–Cuba diplomatic relations were severed in 1961, following the Bay of Pigs invasion. Cuba was under heavy US sanctions once it had established close economic and military ties with the Soviet Union. The Fidel Castro regime considered the United States their enemies and this enmity endured even after the end of the Cold War. The Obama administration decided to reopen diplomatic relations with Cuba in late 2014, and the United States established an embassy in July 2015. The United States and Cuba started in 2015 to cooperate in intelligence gathering, drug interdiction, and maritime security while US companies explored business opportunities in Cuba, especially in the tourism industry.[68] President Obama visited Cuba in March 2016 to normalize US–Cuba relations. According to John Kirk, "there is no doubt that on many levels the new arrangement was generally beneficial to both countries."[69] It seemed in 2015 to 2016 that much friendlier relations between the United States and Cuba were on the horizon. Then something happened that threatened the diplomatic progress made—Donald Trump was elected as president.

The timing of the start of the Havana Syndrome is curious to say the least—the first incident happened in late 2016, which was shortly after one of the most contentious political elections in American history. Donald Trump's election signaled that a major shift in US foreign policy was imminent. Baloh and Bartholomew themselves make this connection by stating that "in early November 2016, shortly after the election of President Trump, a small number of workers at the US Embassy in Havana began to experience symptoms that were accompanied by the presence of mysterious high-pitched sounds."[70] They allude that the Trump administration was trying to deliberately sabotage improvements in US–Cuba relations that had occurred late in the Obama administration, using the Havana Syndrome as a pretext for this major US foreign policy reversal. They pointed out that "[t]he episode threatened to derail a 2-year initiative that began under the Obama administration to renew diplomatic ties and normalize relations with the government in Havana."[71] They also stressed that the Cuban government "were keen to cooperate with the United States over the claims" of their responsibility for the Havana Syndrome because they genuinely wanted better relations.[72]

Branko Marcetic, a journalist for the *Jacobin*, claimed that the Trump administration was keen to overthrow the Cuban government when they came into office and that the Havana Syndrome "played a role in a concerted campaign begun by the Donald Trump administration to lay the groundwork for regime change in Cuba."[73] This was supposedly part of the administration's plan to put "maximum pressure" on Cuba, which began two months before the Havana Syndrome story was reported in the news. Marcetic suggested that Havana Syndrome was "only one instance of the media lending authority to unsubstantiated and ultimately debunked claims made by those in power that are meant to ratchet up hostilities with another country, even potentially lay the groundwork for war."[74] In other words, Havana Syndrome may have been either invented by US intelligence or may have been opportunistically exploited by a reckless administration to bully other countries.

While it is true that the Trump administration from the very beginning demanded a "better deal" from the Cuban government for improved relations, it does not mean that Havana Syndrome was invented or even opportunistically exploited by those who wanted to see an end to socialism in Cuba. If Havana Syndrome was a political deception to return to the pre-2014 US–Cuba policy, why were there other incidents around the world announced by the Trump administration that had nothing to do with Cuba? Was there a more ambitious political agenda at work to upset the international order?

A Deliberate Effort by the US Government to Restart the Cold War

It has been speculated that Havana Syndrome was part of an overall effort by neoconservative political forces in the United States to restart the Cold War, which had been put on pause between 1991 and 2014. The surprise election win of Donald Trump in November 2016 almost immediately resulted in accusations by the IC that the election had been manipulated by Russia. On December 10, 2016, former CIA case officer Robert Baer stated his opinion on CNN that he believed the Russians interfered in the elections, that the election result was illegitimate, and that new elections should be held as this was common practice in other countries.[75] A subsequent Intelligence Community Assessment produced by the outgoing Obama administration asserted that "Putin and the Russian Government aspired to help President-elect Trump's election chances when possible by discrediting Secretary Clinton and publicly contrasting her unfavorably to him."[76] This led to the Special Counsel investigation by Robert Mueller and several years of Russia hysteria in which Russia was framed as the major threat to US national security. The American foreign policy establishment as represented in the Council on Foreign Relations declared in February 2018 that "Cold War II" had already begun.[77]

Havana Syndrome undoubtedly represented a great opportunity for the Russia hawks in American politics to go back to a Cold War footing with Russia, which promised to boost defense spending at a time when the War on Terror was winding down and not many other threats were on the horizon. It was also an opportunity for President Trump's political enemies to accuse him of being soft on Russia, possibly because he had been compromised by Russian intelligence.[78] A report on *Epoch Times* went so far as to suggest that many of the supposed Havana Syndrome victims (Marc Polymeropoulos, Mark Lenzi,

Olivia Troye, and Miles Taylor) and some of their advocates (Greg Edgreen and Mark Zaid) were rabid anti-Trumpers and may be in on a hoax aimed at undermining Donald Trump's presidency (and later his reelection campaign), while also seeking personal financial benefits from this hoax.[79] National Security Advisor John Bolton even admitted that he did not brief the president on Havana Syndrome incidents because "we didn't feel we would get support from President Trump if we said, 'We think the Russians are coming after American personnel,'" which implies that Trump was unwilling to confront Russia over it, a view in line with the then popular argument of Trump being a Russian agent.[80]

In short, the barrage of media stories about potential Russian DEW attacks on US personnel constantly highlighted the Russia threat and undermined President Trump's legitimacy since he was not doing enough about Russia. It is not far-fetched that the US intelligence community would be conducting a psyop on the American people, which was aimed at promoting a nonexistent threat in the mainstream media.[81] When Donald Trump lost the 2020 election, the intelligence services increasingly acknowledged that the original hypothesis of Russian DEW attacks on US personnel may have been wrong, as the psyop had already fulfilled its purpose. Havana Syndrome also suspiciously reemerged in spring 2024 when the odds greatly increased that Trump might return to the presidency in 2024, which could prepare the American public for another round of Russia hysteria.

This interpretation of the Havana Syndrome as a primarily political phenomenon linked to geopolitical maneuvering and domestic politics seems plausible, but is not really convincing, as attempts to discredit and "cancel" the Havana Syndrome by the incoming Biden administration were not successful: new cases continued to happen early into the Biden administration, and several parts of the government still take the Havana Syndrome and its potential connection to DEW very seriously, especially the Pentagon. Somebody seems to be targeting US personnel and other individuals around the world with a new kind of weapon since—the incidents have not ended, and the evidence increasingly points toward a foreign power being responsible. The stance of the Biden administration that involvement of a foreign power was highly unlikely has not changed as of summer 2024, making it far less plausible that it was all a political hoax to discredit Trump and push for Cold War 2.0.

Conclusion

Baloh and Bartholomew have made the argument that Havana Syndrome should be considered nothing but a mass psychogenic illness that was originally triggered by anxious and stressed-out US and Canadian diplomats hearing crickets in Cuba. Of course, it is very reasonable to assume that perhaps the majority of the 1,500 cases reported so far could be completely psychosomatic with no unique external cause. However, this does not rule out the possibility that a subsection of Havana Syndrome sufferers acquired their condition from a particular external cause such as an attack with DEW. Baloh and Bartholomew are generally too quick in their book in attributing many mysterious health conditions to mass psychogenic illness, even in cases when the evidence goes against this explanation.

A good example is Gulf War Syndrome (GWS), which the two authors attribute to "war neurosis" after claiming that "[n]umerous studies . . . have failed to find evidence of a unique Gulf War Syndrome or toxic or infectious cause for the symptoms."[82] This conclusion seems to misrepresent the overall research in this field, as it does not discuss or acknowledge some of the newer studies that rejected the PTSD hypothesis and have looked more closely at potential exposure to biological or chemical agents. A 465-page report issued by the Research Advisory Committee on Gulf War Veterans' Illness from 2008 concluded that "Gulf War illness is not the result of combat or other deployment stressors, and that rates of posttraumatic stress disorder (PTSD) and other psychiatric conditions are relatively low in Gulf War veterans."[83] A 2016 study by Roberta White et al. concluded that "exposure to pesticides and/or to PB are causally associated with GWI and the neurological dysfunction in GW veterans. . . . The health consequences of chemical exposures in the GW and other conflicts have been called 'toxic wounds' by veterans."[84] More recently, a study led by Robert Haley argued that over 95,000 US personnel who suffered from GWS were within the hypothetical plume caused by the demolition of the Khamisiyah munition depot and were likely exposed to nerve agents.[85]

The point is that the US government was keen on attributing GWS to PTSD or psychological factors as they were not willing to pay for the necessary healthcare of veterans who had been injured by chemical exposure, which explains the low rate of approval for GWS Veterans Affairs claims.[86] Over thirty years later, the US government has accepted that GWS was not just caused by PTSD and that there was an identified external cause for about 40 percent of all reported GWS cases.

Similarly, Havana Syndrome could be partially psychological and partially caused by yet-to-be-determined environmental conditions. Is it that surprising that the US government has been reluctant to officially acknowledge the existence of Havana Syndrome, even though it has provided some compensation to victims for hardship or injury in the line of duty, considering how GWS was handled? Havana Syndrome cannot be universally dismissed as mass psychogenic illness, and it is also not plausible that it was just some kind of political deception. Havana Syndrome is not an entirely new phenomenon. It likely has happened before and was then called the "Moscow Signal."

Notes

1 Robert W. Baloh and Robert E. Bartholomew, *Havana Syndrome: Mass Psychogenic Illness and the Real Story Behind the Embassy Mystery and Hysteria* (Cham, Switzerland: Springer, 2020).
2 Baloh and Bartholomew, *Havana Syndrome*, 2, 4.
3 Baloh and Bartholomew, *Havana Syndrome*, 5.
4 William Safire, "Ockham's Razor's Close Shave," *New York Times*, January 31, 1999.
5 Baloh and Bartholomew, *Havana Syndrome*, 23.
6 Sharon Weinberger, "Microwave Weapons Are Real, But They Can't Explain 'Havana Syndrome,'" *Wall Street Journal*, April 6, 2024.
7 Kyle S. Cunliffe, "Hard Target Espionage in the Information Era: New Challenges for the Second-Oldest Profession," *Intelligence and National Security* 36, no. 7 (2021): 1020.
8 Keir Giles, *Russia's War on Everybody and What It Means for You* (London: Bloomsbury Academic, 2022), 148.
9 Josh Rogin, "Russia Is Harassing U.S. Diplomats All Over Europe," *Washington Post*, June 27, 2016.
10 Rogin, "Russia Is Harassing U.S. Diplomats All Over Europe."
11 Joshua Partlow, "In Cuba, Harassment of U.S. Diplomats Even Extends to Their Pets. Will That Now Change?," *Washington Post Online*, January 1, 2015.
12 Frances Robles and Kirk Semple, "'Health Attacks' on U.S. Diplomats in Cuba Baffle Experts," *New York Times*, August 11, 2017.
13 BBC Staff, "World: Europe Dissidents Say Stasi Gave Them Cancer," *BBC*, May 25, 1999, available at: http://news.bbc.co.uk/2/hi/europe/352461.stm.

14 Edward Shorter, "'Havana Syndrome' Symptoms of Diplomats in Cuba Are Not Mass Hysteria," *The Conversation*, July 3, 2019, https://theconversation.com/havana-syndrome-symptoms-of-diplomats-in-cuba-are-not-mass-hysteria-118678.

15 Baloh and Bartholomew, *Havana Syndrome*, 35.

16 Baloh and Bartholomew, *Havana Syndrome*, 49.

17 Baloh and Bartholomew, *Havana Syndrome*, 50.

18 Carlo Pierpaoli, Amritha Nayak, Rabikul Hafiz et al., "Neuroimaging Findings in US Government Personnel and Their Family Members Involved in Anomalous Health Incidents," *JAMA* 331, no. 13 (2024): 1122–34.

19 Robert McCreight, "Analyzing & Refuting Various JAMA/NIH Claims on Havana Syndrome," Statement from March 19, 2024.

20 Pierpaoli, Nayak, Hafiz et al., "Neuroimaging Findings in US Government Personnel and Their Family Members Involved in Anomalous Health Incidents," 1132.

21 Matthew Phelan, "New NIH Study Sheds Light on 'Mysterious Havana Syndrome': Victims' Symptoms Are 'Real' and 'Quite Profound'—But Injuries Don't Show Up on MRI Much Like a 'Mini-Stroke', One Pentagon Medical Consultant Tells Daily Mail," *Daily Mail*, March 18, 2024, available at: https://www.dailymail.co.uk/sciencetech/article-13210727/NIH-study-Havana-Syndrome-Victims-symptoms-energy-weapons-microwave-acoustic-mystery.html.

22 Phelan, "New NIH Study Sheds Light on 'Mysterious Havana Syndrome.'"

23 US Office of the Director of National Intelligence, "Updated Assessment of Anomalous Health Incidents," *Intelligence Community Assessment*, March 1, 2023, 1.

24 Baloh and Bartholomew, *Havana Syndrome*, 12.

25 Baloh and Bartholomew, *Havana Syndrome*, 39.

26 The question of a potential government cover-up of the existence of a DEW that could produce Havana Syndrome was raised at the Homeland Security Committee on Foreign Anomalous Health Incidents conducted on May 8, 2024, where key witnesses Christo Grozev and Mark Zaid alluded to a government cover-up. Zaid told the committee that "I will say that the public statements that the executive branch is making is inconsistent with the classified record." US Congress, "House Homeland Security Committee Holds Hearing on Foreign Anomalous Health Incidents," *Forbes Breaking News*, May 8, 2024, available at: https://www.youtube.com/watch?v=bwlCmtLCM2U.

27 Yuval Rosenberg, "Trump Administration Asks for $81.1 Billion 'Black Budget', the Largest Ever," *Fiscal Times*, February 28, 2018, available at: https://www.thefiscaltimes.com/2018/02/28/Trump-Administration-Asks-811-Billion-Black-Budget-Largest-Ever.

28 Tim McMillan and Tyler Rogoway, "Special Access Programs and the Pentagon's Ecosystem of Secrecy," *The Warzone*, December 1, 2019, available at: https://www.twz.com/29092/special-access-programs-and-the-pentagons-ecosystem-of-secrecy.
29 Marc Ambinder and D. B. Grady, *Deep State: Inside Government Secrecy* (Hoboken: Wiley & Sons, 2013), 166.
30 Alex Hollings, "SR-91 Aurora: The U.S. Military's Secret Mach 5 Plane?," *The National Interest*, October 29, 2023, available at: https://nationalinterest.org/blog/buzz/sr-91-aurora-us-militarys-secret-mach-5-plane-207093.
31 Baloh and Bartholomew, *Havana Syndrome*, 12.
32 Baloh and Bartholomew, *Havana Syndrome*, 13.
33 Baloh and Bartholomew, *Havana Syndrome*, 13.
34 Sharon Weinberger, "Wasted Energy: Despite 50 Years of Research on High-Power Microwaves, the US Military Has Yet to Produce a Usable Weapon," *Nature* 489, no. 7415 (2012): 198–9.
35 Weinberger, "Wasted Energy," 200.
36 Weinberger, "Microwave Weapons Are Real, But They Can't Explain 'Havana Syndrome.'"
37 Dominique Mosbergen, "Microwave Weapons Could Be the Culprit Behind the Mysterious U.S. Embassy Attacks," *Huffington Post*, September 2, 2018, available at: https://www.huffpost.com/entry/microwave-weapons-embassy-attack-cuba-china_n_5b8bdaf4e4b0cf7b00370cc8.
38 Cheryl Rofer, "Claims of Microwave Attacks Are Scientifically Implausible," *Foreign Policy*, May 10, 2021, available at: https://foreignpolicy.com/2021/05/10/microwave-attacks-havana-syndrome-scientifically-implausible/.
39 David A. Relman and Julie A. Pavlin, eds., *An Assessment of Illness in U.S. Government Employees and Their Families in Overseas Embassies* (Washington, DC: National Academies Press, 2020), 17.
40 K. R. Foster, D. C. Garrett, and M. C. Ziskin, "A Commentary on Can Microwave Auditory Effect Be 'Weaponized?,'" *Frontiers in Public Health* 9 (2021): 1–3.
41 Julian Borger, "Microwave Weapons That Could Cause Havana Syndrome Exist," *The Guardian*, June 2, 2021, available at: https://www.theguardian.com/science/2021/jun/02/microwave-weapons-havana-syndrome-experts.
42 Borger, "Microwave Weapons That Could Cause Havana Syndrome Exist."
43 Edl Schamiloglu, "Microwave Weapon Behind Havana Syndrome: Report," *Asia Times*, February 7, 2022, available at: https://asiatimes.com/2022/02/microwave-weapon-behind-havana-syndrome-report/.
44 US Congress, "House Homeland Security Committee Holds Hearing on Foreign Anomalous Health Incidents."

45 Robert E. Bartholomew and Chandra Sekaran Muniratnam, "How Should Mental Health Professionals Respond to Outbreaks of Mass Psychogenic Illness?," *Journal of Cognitive Psychotherapy* 25, no. 4 (2011): 235.
46 Baloh and Bartholomew, *Havana Syndrome*, 3.
47 Baloh and Bartholomew, *Havana Syndrome*, 4.
48 Baloh and Bartholomew, *Havana Syndrome*, 3.
49 Baloh and Bartholomew, *Havana Syndrome*, 45.
50 Baloh and Bartholomew, *Havana Syndrome*, 45.
51 Baloh and Bartholomew, *Havana Syndrome*, 14.
52 Baloh and Bartholomew, *Havana Syndrome*, 188.
53 Baloh and Bartholomew, *Havana Syndrome*, 38.
54 Peter Kornbluh, "What the U.S. Government Is Not Telling You About Those 'Sonic Attacks' in Cuba," *The Nation*, March 7, 2018, available at: https://www.thenation.com/article/archive/what-the-us-government-is-not-telling-you-about-those-sonic-attacks-in-cuba/.
55 Marc Polymeropoulos, "'All I Wanted Was to See a Doctor': Ex-CIA Officer Tells All About His Battle with Havana Syndrome—and His Former Agency," *The Insider*, March 31, 2024, available at: https://theins.ru/en/opinion/marc-polymeropoulos/270427.
56 Scott Pelley, "Havana Syndrome: High-Level National Security Officials Stricken with Unexplained Illness on White House Grounds," *CBS News*, February 20, 2022, available at: https://www.cbsnews.com/news/havana-syndrome-white-house-cabinet-60-minutes-2022-02-20/?ftag=CNM-00-10aab7d&linkId=153082702.
57 Pelley, "Havana Syndrome."
58 Brit McCandless Farmer, Michael Rey, and Oriana Zill de Granados, "The Youngest Victims of 'Havana Syndrome,'" *CBS News*, February 20, 2022, available at: https://www.cbsnews.com/news/havana-syndrome-children-60-minutes-2022-02-20/.
59 Robert E. Bartholomew, "60 Minutes Whips Up 'Havana Syndrome' Hysteria, Airs Sensational Segment on White House 'Attacks,'" *The Skeptic*, March 4, 2022, available at: https://www.skeptic.com/reading_room/60-minutes-whips-up-havana-syndrome-hysteria-airs-sensational-segment-on-white-house-attacks/ - note03.
60 Bartholomew, "60 Minutes Whips Up 'Havana Syndrome' Hysteria, Airs Sensational Segment on White House 'Attacks.'"
61 USA Today, "Victim of Suspected Health Attacks Speaks Out," *USA Today*, November 20, 2018, available at: https://www.youtube.com/watch?v=pOdXVye-4X0.
62 Elizabeth Payne, "Havana Syndrome Part 2: How a Dog's Brain May Help Solve the Mystery of Canadian Diplomats' Cuban Nightmare," *Ottawa Citizen*, February 27, 2019, available at: https://ottawacitizen.com/news/local-news/havana-syndrome

-part-2-how-a-dogs-brain-may-help-solve-the-mystery-of-canadian-diplomats-cuban-nightmare.

63 Baloh and Bartholomew, *Havana Syndrome*, 46.

64 US Centers for Disease Control, "Cuba Unexplained Events Investigation—Final Report," December 3, 2019, 5.

65 Lara Seligman and Andrew Desiderio, "'It Is an Act of War': Trump Acting Pentagon Chief Urges Biden to Tackle Directed Energy Attacks," *Politico*, March 5, 2021, available at: https://www.politico.com/news/2021/05/03/acting-pentagon-chief-miller-attacks-485236.

66 Germania Rodriguez Poleo, "Ex-National Security Advisor John Bolton Warns Russia 'Very Likely' Behind Havana Syndrome Amid Fears It's Being Used as Energy Weapon—as He Claims 'It Isn't Being Taken Seriously,'" *Daily Mail*, April 1, 2024, available at: https://www.dailymail.co.uk/news/article-13260299/john-bolton-russia-havana-syndrome.html.

67 CBS Staff, "Havana Syndrome Symptoms Suggest Who May Be Responsible for Mysterious Brain Injuries," *60 Minutes*, March 31, 2024, available at: https://www.youtube.com/watch?v=JdPSD1SUYCY.

68 John M. Kirk, "The Strange Case of the Havana 'Sonic Attacks,'" *International Journal of Cuban Studies* 11, no. 1 (2019): 26.

69 Kirk, "The Strange Case of the Havana 'Sonic Attacks,'" 26–7.

70 Baloh and Bartholomew, *Havana Syndrome*, 9.

71 Baloh and Bartholomew, *Havana Syndrome*, 7.

72 Baloh and Bartholomew, *Havana Syndrome*, 7.

73 Branko Marcetic, "Havana Syndrome Is Fake. But Mainstream Media Couldn't Get Enough of It for Years," *The Jacobin*, March 4, 2023, available at: https://jacobin.com/2023/03/havana-syndrome-government-report-debunking-intelligence-establishment-media.

74 Marcetic, "Havana Syndrome Is Fake."

75 CNN, "Ex-CIA Operative Calls for New Election," *CNN*, December 10, 2016, available at: https://www.youtube.com/watch?v=erRf6CONfco.

76 US Office of the Director of National Intelligence, "Assessing Russian Activities and Intentions in Recent US Elections," *Intelligence Community Assessment*, January 6, 2017.

77 Richard Haas, "Cold War II," *Council on Foreign Relations*, February 23, 2018, available at: https://www.cfr.org/article/cold-war-ii.

78 Tim Weiner, "The Unanswered Question of Our Time: Is Trump an Agent of Russia?," *Washington Post*, September 21, 2020, available at: https://www.washingtonpost.com/outlook/2020/09/21/russian-agent-trump-counterintelligence/.

79 Hans Mahncke, "New Russia Hoax: Report Blames Kremlin for 'Havana Syndrome', But Evidence Suggests Otherwise," *Epoch Times Truth Over News*, April 5, 2024, available at: https://www.theepochtimes.com/epochtv/new-russia-hoax-report-blames-kremlin-for-havana-syndrome-but-evidence-suggests-otherwise-truth-over-news-5622714.

80 Martin Pengelly, "John Bolton Chose Not to Brief Trump on Russia Havana Syndrome Suspicion," *The Guardian*, March 13, 2023, available at: https://www.theguardian.com/us-news/2023/mar/13/john-bolton-donald-trump-russia-havana-syndrome.

81 Russiagate was in itself a hoax perpetrated by senior intelligence officials, which is pretty well-documented in books such as Dick Morris and Eileen McGann, *Rogue Spooks: The Intelligence War on Donald Trump* (New York: St. Martin's Press, 2017), Dave Erickson, *Framing Flynn: The Scandalous Takedown of an American General* (New York: Post Hill Press, 2021), and Oliver Boyd-Barrett and Stephen Marmura, *Russiagate Revisited: The Aftermath of a Hoax* (Cham, Switzerland: Palgrave Macmillan, 2023).

82 Baloh and Bartholomew, *Havana Syndrome*, 67.

83 Research Advisory Committee on Gulf War Veterans' Illness, *Gulf War Illness and the Health of Gulf War Veterans: Scientific Findings and Recommendations* (Washington, DC: US Government Printing Office, 2008), 4–5.

84 Roberta F. White, Lea Steele, James P. O. Callaghan, Kimberly Sullivan, James H. Binns, Beatrice A. Golomb, Floyd E. Bloom, James A. Bunker, Fiona Crawford, Joel C. Graves, Anthony Hardie, Nancy Klimas, Marguerite Knox, William J. Meggs, Jack Melling, Martina A. Philbert, and Rachel Grashow, "Recent Research on Gulf War Illness and Other Health Problems in Veterans of 1991 Gulf War: Effects of Toxicant Exposures During Deployment," *Cortex* 74 (2016): 449–75.

85 Robert W. Haley, Gerald Kramer, Junhui Xiao, Jill A. Dever, and John F. Teiber, "Evaluation of a Gene-Environment Interaction of P0N1 and Low-Level Nerve Agent Exposure with Gulf War Illness: A Prevalence Case-Control Study Drawn from the U.S. National Health Survey's National Population Sample," *Environmental Health Perspectives* 130, no. 5 (2022): 1–16.

86 Baloh and Bartholomew, *Havana Syndrome*, 67.

2

The Moscow Signal

Between 1953 and 1976, the Soviets radiated sections of the US embassy with microwaves, which became known as the "Moscow Signal." The Moscow Signal is frequently mentioned in discussions of Havana Syndrome as a potential early incident of Russia using DEW against US diplomats during the Cold War.[1] Since some analysts have suggested that pulsed microwaves could be responsible for the Havana Syndrome, a close examination of the Moscow Signal may offer important insights into the Havana Syndrome.[2] The Moscow Signal is well documented, but it remains controversial as to the Soviet intent and the health effects that it may have caused to US personnel at the time. Since the 1960s, there was speculation based on scientific research into the bioeffects of microwaves that the signal was designed to harm or "brainwash" US personnel, with much public speculation once the microwave "attacks" were leaked to the public in 1972.[3]

The Moscow Signal started also a public debate about Soviet "psychotronic weapons" that used RF or microwaves to attack the central nervous system and the brains of people. While the Moscow Signal was in itself a seemingly insignificant episode in the Cold War, it became also part of a much broader scientific debate regarding the potentially harmful bioeffects of electromagnetic fields (EMF) at low-energy density levels (below the threshold of thermal effects). Some scientists have argued that the Moscow Signal proved the dangers of low-energy nonionizing radiation and others have claimed that there was no evidence of harm. For example, Robert O. Becker, who had researched the bioeffects of microwaves for the US government at the time, became convinced that the Moscow Signal "could affect the central nervous system, put people to sleep, interfere with decision-making capacity and induce chronic stress."[4] Other research discussed below, such as Project Pandora, seemed to contradict Becker's claims. The question of harmful bioeffects of microwaves below thermal levels remains unresolved in the academic debate.

This chapter argues that the Moscow Signal did produce adverse health effects and that a covert attack (or deliberate harmful exposure) on US personnel did very likely occur. Soviet intentions could have been to test a new DEW or to punish the United States for intelligence gathering or other covert activities directed against the Soviet Union from the Moscow embassy. If true, the Moscow Signal may also indicate the feasibility of DEWs that attack the central nervous system at low energy levels. It also lends much greater credibility to the idea that US diplomats affected by the Havana Syndrome since at least 2016 were victims of DEW attacks.

The Moscow Signal

The Cold War was a protracted conflict between the two superpowers over world domination, fought primarily by indirect and non-military means such as diplomacy, economic influence, propaganda, covert action, and intelligence. Embassies became both major bases and targets for intelligence collection, as intelligence services often operated out of embassies, and as secret diplomatic information could be obtained by penetrating these embassies. Since the Soviet Union was a "denied territory" that was difficult to access for Western spies, most intelligence gathering in the Soviet Union had to be carried out from the US embassy in Moscow. This included both human intelligence operations and technical collection through antennas that picked up Soviet radio communications.[5] The Soviets were very successful in penetrating the US embassy with various kinds of sophisticated listening devices (colloquially referred to as "bugs") and occasionally with human agents who had physical access to the embassy. In 1963, a Soviet defector revealed that the KGB had placed numerous bugs inside the embassy.[6] A thorough bug sweep conducted in 1964 discovered forty hidden microphones, some deeply embedded in the building's structure.[7] Project Gunman revealed in 1985 that the Soviets had managed to bug US typewriters and hence could read some of the classified documents produced in the embassy.[8] The situation was so bad in the 1980s that CIA officers inside the embassy even turned to "silently passing notes to each other at the water fountain" to prevent Soviet eavesdropping.[9] Because of the intensive bugging of the old embassy building, the US government decided to construct a new one. But despite strong security measures at the construction site, the KGB managed to "put permanent eavesdropping systems into the actual structure of the building . . . so sophisticated that it could not be removed from the steel and concrete columns."[10] This is the larger context of the so-called Moscow Signal that was first discovered in the early 1950s and continued into the 1980s.

The Thing

The origins of the Moscow Signal are said to go back to a novel listening device or bug (called "The Thing") that was contained in a carved wood Great Seal presented to US ambassador to the Soviet Union Averell Harriman in 1945. The Great Seal was placed on the wall of the library of the ambassador's official residence, Spaso House in the Moscow mission, where it allowed the Soviets to listen to confidential conversations of at least four US ambassadors from 1945 to 1951.[11] Unlike conventional listening devices, *The Thing* did not have any battery since it could be remotely powered and activated with radio waves. The technique was called "RF imposition," which, according to Eric Haseltine, "captured voice signals from vibrations of different kinds of electrical conductors that reflected radiofrequency (RF) energy."[12] *The Thing* was powered by a continuous 800 MHz signal directed at the Great Seal and it picked up voices through privations and reflected them back as a radio signal.[13]

This radio signal was only discovered by chance in 1951 by a British radio operator in the Moscow embassy trying to monitor Russian military aircraft traffic, where he could hear the voice of the British Air Attaché.[14] No bugs were found in the British embassy, but a bug sweep in the American ambassador's residence in preparation for a visit of the secretary of state in 1952 uncovered a strange signal, which led to the discovery of *The Thing* inside the Great Seal. US intelligence called the discovered Soviet RF signal the "Technically Unidentified Moscow Signal" (TUMS), which had been active since the 1940s and was related to *The Thing*.[15] Robert Wallace and Keith Melton suggested that "[t]he concept behind *The Thing* represented a remarkable leap forward in eavesdropping technology."[16] Because of the discovery of *The Thing*, US intelligence started, from 1952, to routinely monitor any strange RF or microwave signals detected in US embassies around the world.[17]

Microwaving the US Embassy

In 1952, the decision was made to move the US chancery in Moscow from Mokhovaya Street near the Kremlin to a new location several miles away on Chekhovsky Street. Soon after the completion of the move, US intelligence detected a constant microwave beam that targeted one side of the US embassy in Moscow in May 1953.[18] However, the signal varied from 2 GHz to 7 GHz and there was no apparent pattern.[19] Since it occurred irregularly, it did not cause much concern.[20] Meanwhile in the United States, the CIA sponsored highly classified research under the MK ULTRA program, which interestingly also included research into the behavioral effects of radio frequency energy. NIH neuroscientist Maitland Baldwin was, in 1957, contracted to study "the effects of radio-frequency energy on primate cerebral activity." In a status report, Baldwin claimed that "certain kinds of radio frequency energy have been found to effect reversible neurological changes in chimpanzees."[21] The CIA was hence aware in the late 1950s of the potential for behavioral and health effects of microwave exposure.

When Vice President Richard Nixon was scheduled to travel to Moscow in 1959, a security sweep was conducted of the ambassador's apartment where Nixon was supposed to sleep. They discovered dangerously high levels of ionizing radiation.[22] Secret Service agents who had detected the radiation with dosimeters in Nixon's quarters in Spaso House loudly denounced the dirty trick to the benefit of Soviet eavesdroppers, which resulted in the Soviets turning down the levels.[23] It was also discovered at this time that the signal pointing at the US embassy had become constant. By the early 1960s, a decision was made to place equipment in all areas of the chancery to monitor and record any signals that could be detected.[24] According to Kenneth Pollack, who had investigated the microwave signal on behalf of the State Department, "there was a single source beam illuminating the west facade of the chancery building starting at about the sixth floor, peaking at around the tenth floor and the roof. The north, south, and east had no evidence of any beaming whatsoever."[25] The US government was fully aware of the microwave exposure of parts of the US embassy, mostly the upper floors on the west side of the building, but kept the information from the diplomats and staff.

From TUMS to MUTS

By 1962, two new signals were detected that were coming from inside a ten-story building about a hundred meters away from the US embassy, called Moscow Unidentified Technical Signal, or MUTS-1 and MUTS-2.[26] There was little doubt that the signal was "a carefully manufactured beam of radiation aimed at the embassy and its personnel."[27] The frequencies and strength of the signal fluctuated over the years, and it was in the range from 0.5 GHz to 10 GHz and had an average intensity of 0.005 mW/cm^2 over 9 hours per day.[28] It was decided to monitor the signal and not to inform the affected US embassy personnel.

It seems obvious that the US government became increasingly concerned about the nature of the Moscow Signal, which they suspected to be deliberately harmful to US personnel. Secretary of State Dean Rusk raised the issue of an electromagnetic signal targeting the US embassy in Moscow during a meeting with Soviet ambassador Andrei Gromyko in Glassboro, New Jersey, in 1967. According to the meeting memo, Rusk said that "we were very much concerned at an electro-magnetic signal directed against our Chancery building in Moscow. The radiation from this signal was of a higher level than Soviet experts consider safe."[29] Rusk formally requested the signal to be stopped, and Gromyko said that he would look into the matter.

In 1969, the Soviet Foreign Ministry provided its official response to the American request, and it was a simple denial that there was any intentional radiation pointed toward the US embassy. The US reply by Ambassador Jacob Beam was that there could not be any doubt about a low energy, high-frequency signal coming from a nearby Soviet apartment building. Beam stated that US animal research had indicated physiological changes and that there were concerns about long-term health effects. He also stressed that the matter could not be kept secret for much longer, as US personnel had gotten ill, with one former employee whose wife had died of cancer suing the State Department on the basis that the Soviet signal may have caused the cancer.[30] A State Department telegram from June 1969 stated that many employees had become aware of the Moscow Signal and the possible connection to medical problems.[31]

The Press Leak of MUTS

All Americans eventually learned about the Moscow Signal from a newspaper article by Jack Anderson from May 1972.[32] Anderson pointed out that the Soviet scientific literature suggested that "microwaves can cause nervous tension, irritability, even disorders," which led to US speculations that "the Russians were trying to drive American diplomats stir crazy with the waves."[33] The article mentioned Project Pandora and that one of the Pandora scientists believed that microwaves could cause behavioral changes in monkeys. Two months after Anderson's revealing of the Moscow Signal, the world chess championship took place in Reykjavik where Bobby Fischer was playing against Boris Spassky, which was one of the most iconic moments in sports during the Cold War. When Fischer surprisingly defeated the world champion Spassky, the Soviets claimed that Fischer (or his supporters) had used unspecified "electronic devices and chemical substances" to degrade Spassky's mental abilities. In light of the Moscow Signal, the Soviet complaint seemed to suggest that the Soviets did believe that microwaves could have disrupted the brain of Spassky.[34]

In late May 1975, the US embassy was hit with two microwave beams from different directions. The microwave bombardment had also increased substantially in duration and intensity. According to Pollack, "one from the east on the other side of Chekovsky Street and one from the south from a high rise Soviet building."[35] Lin claimed that the energy density increased from 0.005 mW/cm^2 to up to 0.015 mW/cm^2 and that the signal could be detected for up to 18 hours a day (an increase from a previous average of 9 hours per day).[36] However, many people working in the embassy had little or no exposure to the microwaves since only the upper floors were targeted and not all sides of the building were covered. They were primarily hitting the upper floors and the ambassador's office.

Secretary of State Henry Kissinger called Soviet ambassador Anatoli Dobrynin in December 1975 to discuss the recent changes in the Moscow Signal, pointing out that there were now three signals, that the operation time of the signals had doubled, and that they would have recall Ambassador Stoessel because of his illness.[37] Stoessel suffered serious symptoms, including bleeding eyes, but decided to keep the matter quiet after Kissinger had asked him to.[38]

In February 1976, the *New York Times* reported that Ambassador Stoessel had developed leukemia and that his condition was potentially caused by microwave exposure in Moscow.[39] A month later, *Time Magazine* published a story claiming that, in addition to Stoessel's leukemia, two other former US ambassadors to the Soviet Union had died from cancer (Charles Bohlen and Llewellyn Thompson), another diplomat had died from cancer, five women had undergone cancer-related mastectomies, and other former US embassy personnel and family members had recalled strange ailments when they were in Moscow.[40] According to *Time Magazine*, the US government made a deal with the Soviets to reduce the intensity of the microwaves to the level before May 1975.[41] The State Department also launched a full-scale medical investigation to determine as to whether diplomats were harmed. To address some of the health concerns of embassy personnel, some of the embassy windows were equipped with aluminum screens that further reduced the microwave exposure.[42] After this shielding measure, the microwave exposure inside the embassy dropped to below 0.001 mW/cm^2, which was below the Soviet safety standard.[43]

The Mystery of the Purpose of the Moscow Signal

There was a lot of speculation about the purpose of the microwave bombardment, especially since published Soviet research on the bioeffects of microwaves seemed to suggest a potential for affecting the behavior and health of US diplomats.[44] There were at least four different theories regarding the purpose of the microwave signals targeting the embassy: (1) the Soviets were trying to eavesdrop on the embassy in a manner that was not understood by the CIA technical experts; (2) the Soviets tried to interfere with the electronic equipment in the US embassy to prevent or reduce the ability of US intelligence to collect signals; (3) the Soviets tried to harm US embassy personnel to punish them for intelligence collection from the US embassy; and (4) the Soviets were testing new DEWs to mind control or "brainwash" US diplomats. All these theories had some degree of plausibility, especially in light of the times.

According to Eric Haseltine, the purpose of MUTS was to spy on the embassy using a technique they called "RF imposition," where voice signals could be captured and reflected back as an RF signal.[45] The Soviet government denied the existence of an intentional microwave signal beamed at the embassy until 1976 when they suggested that its purpose was actually to jam American eavesdropping equipment inside the embassy.[46] The fact that the Moscow Signal exceeded Soviet safety standards for microwave exposure, combined with the reported cancer cases, seemed to suggest that the Soviets either did not care about the health consequences for US embassy personnel or were deliberately trying to harm US personnel.[47] Even the least likely explanation of potential Soviet behavioral manipulation through microwaves was seriously considered by scientists of Project Pandora, some of whom believed that this was indeed the real intention behind MUTS.[48]

The Pandora Project

Luigi Galvani discovered in the late eighteenth century that animals generate electricity, which was the beginning of a new discipline called biophysics. The human body is electric in the sense that the brain and central nervous system use weak currents and generate weak EMFs. Small electric charges transmitted through the central nervous system allow the brain to control the body and to receive sensory input. In 1924, Hans Berger, a German psychiatrist, discovered that there were measurable fluctuations in voltage on the scalp later called brain waves.[49] These fluctuations are translated by an electroencephalogram (EEG) into frequencies in the range between 0 Hz and 100 Hz used for coordinating brain functions. Certain frequency ranges are associated with particular mental states.[50] This frequency range of the brain waves is called extremely low frequency (ELF) waves. There have been long-standing concerns that radio waves in the ELF range or microwaves pulsed in the ELF range could interfere with the brain and affect human well-being.[51] It is therefore quite plausible, if not logical, that exposure to EMF would somewhat affect biological functions and human health.[52] There were numerous studies carried out in the 1950s and 1960s to determine whether there were any bioeffects of radiofrequency or microwaves and at what levels, types, or intensity human exposure could result in harm. One of these early research projects was Project Pandora.

The Start of Project Pandora

The CIA also consulted a New York ophthalmologist Dr. Milton Zaret in connection to the Moscow Signal in early 1965, who had conducted research for the US military on the health effects of microwaves. He was told about the still highly classified Moscow Signal that "[i]t was being generated at multiple frequencies and wildly fluctuating patterns and at power densities that never exceeded four milliwatts per square centimeter."[53] It should be noted here that other studies put the maximum energy density of the Moscow Signal much lower at about 0.005 mW/cm^2.[54] Zaret advised the CIA that they should urge the Soviets to stop the signal at once, that they should conduct thorough medical examinations of US embassy personnel, and that they should conduct experiments on monkeys using the exact same signal to determine the behavioral and biological effects of the signal.[55]

These suggestions led to the start of a secret research effort by the Pentagon's Advanced Research Projects Agency (now known as DARPA) called Project Pandora that was active from 1965 to 1970. The project manager was Richard Cesaro, who was assisted by Dr. Herbert Pollack, a professor of clinical medicine at George Washington University, Dr. Joseph Sharp, a medical doctor at Walter Reed Military Hospital, and Mark Grove, an engineer and microwave expert.[56] Other prominent contributors to the study were Milton Zaret of the Zaret Foundation, Ross Adey of UCLA, and Maitland Baldwin, a scientist for the NIH and a witting MK ULTRA researcher.[57] Some of the Pandora scientists have claimed that they had found evidence for behavioral and harmful effects of microwaves while the official conclusion was that the Project Pandora findings were inconclusive.

Health Survey

From March 1965, a secret study was conducted to monitor the health of US Moscow embassy personnel, which included a review of their files, mandatory health checkups before they came to Moscow and after they left Moscow, and blood tests and eye examinations. The embassy personnel were told that there was a concern about possible viral contamination, which was a cover story.[58] The health records for 139 US embassy personnel (out of a total of 229) and those of their family members were reviewed, which was a total of 409 records in this study. According to a US Department of State document quoted by Steneck, "no recognizable patterns of disease or evidence of recurring problems" was discovered.[59]

Primates Experiments

Richard Cesaro described the purpose of this part of Project Pandora in the following way: "A program has been outlined to irradiate a group of primates under carefully controlled conditions simulating the dosages and complex modulation of the threat. . . . The trained primates will be carefully observed under varying and controlled irradiated conditions to determine if any changes in their behavior or physiological condition can be detected."[60] The primate research was codenamed “Project Bizarre.” The primate experiments were carried out in a special laboratory at Walter Reed Army Institute for Research.

A 1966 memo by Richard Cesaro described the experiment and commented on the results. Monkeys were radiated with microwaves at an energy density of 5 mW/cm^2 for twenty-eight days with stoppages in between. When the microwave exposure stopped, the monkeys fell into deep sleep. The memo noted that

> [t]here is no question that penetration of the central nervous system has been achieved, either directly or indirectly into that portion of the brain concerned with the changes in the work functions and the effects observed. . . . On the 12th day of radiation (10 hours/day), a definite slowdown was recorded in the monkey’s ability to time his work functions. On the 13th day of radiation, the monkey further degraded and finally stopped working.[61]

In the memo, Cesaro claimed that there were definitive behavioral effects of microwaves on at least one monkey and that there was a potential for human behavior to be affected by low-level microwave exposure. However, the experiment was seemingly conducted with a much higher energy level than the Moscow Signal. When another experiment used energy densities below 0.1 mW/cm^2 or signals modulated in the “S” band, there was no observed change in the behavior or capacity of the monkey.[62] Since this experiment did not examine the monkey’s biological functions such as EEG, EKG, genetic effects, blood chemistry, and so on, it is unclear whether there were such bioeffects. The memo further suggests that human experiments would be necessary for understanding behavioral and other bioeffects.

Human Experiments

Herbert Pollack was tasked with collecting data from crew members of the aircraft carrier U.S.S. *Saratoga* in late December 1968, which was codenamed “Project Big Boy.” The idea was to study the physiological and psychological effects of radar by taking blood samples of twenty-one crew members, whose work put them at a higher exposure to microwaves, which were measured to be up to one milliwatt per square centimeter.[63] The exposure of the crew never exceeded 1 mW/cm^2. A cover story was used to deceive the crew members about the purpose of the research. The conclusion of the research was that some abnormalities were found in the blood samples, but they were still within the normal range.[64]

Further research tried to determine whether performance was impacted by microwave exposure by dividing crew members into those with exposure (crew members on the flight deck) and those with no exposure (crew members in the hangar), using a set of tests given immediately after the end of their work time. These tests included psychomotor, sensory-perceptual, and cognitive tests. Some of the tests were simple questionnaires. The results indicated that "[t]here are no meaningfully significant differences between the test performances of the Flight Deck and the Hangar Deck crews," leading to the conclusion that "[n]o exposure effect was demonstrated."[65] A later discussion of the Pandora committee suggested that the levels of microwave radiation and the exposure time were too low to have much of an effect.[66] The question was also raised as to whether the specific modulation of the Moscow Signal may have been responsible for adverse health effects and that the experiment had not accurately replicated the Moscow Signal, thus causing the negative results.

Inconclusive Results

ARPA ended Project Pandora after five years, which resulted in the transfer of the research to the US Army on July 1, 1970. The Army continued the funding of similar research at Walter Reed Army Institute of Research. A research report from 1969 that described the primate experiments and summarized its findings suggested that

> I am forced to conclude that the data do not present any evidence of a behavioral change due to the presence of the special signal within the limits of any reasonable scientific criteria. There is evidence of behavioral change in some cases but this change could be attributed to a variety of causes or systematic measurement errors all well within the limits of experimental methodology. Evidence of other effects such as EEG, histology, and chromosomal analyses have not accumulated with either adequate detail or control to tell whether effects due to radiation are present.[67]

Incidentally, project manager Cesaro disagreed with these findings. Cesaro claimed: "In our experiments we did some remarkable things. And there was no question in my mind that you can get into the brain with microwaves."[68] According to Paul Brodeur, Cesaro claimed at a meeting of the science advisory committee that "there was evidence that low-level radiation could penetrate the central nervous system of monkeys and that it was now necessary to determine how such penetration occurred and what microwave characteristics and biomedical engineering principles were involved." Furthermore, he claimed that the effects of the Moscow Signal "could be physiological, behavioral, and genetic."[69] Cesaro urged DARPA to pursue further studies to investigate weapons applications.[70]

Nicholas Steneck argued that the Moscow Signal had created a dilemma for policymakers as there were two prevailing viewpoints on the matter of the dangers of nonionizing radiation: the orthodox viewpoint that disregarded nonthermal effects of the kind of low-energy density Moscow Signal and the viewpoint embraced by senior intelligence professionals, who claimed that there was some probability for adverse bioeffects.[71] Two Directors of Central Intelligence, William Colby and George H. W. Bush, believed that the microwave bombardment was a matter of serious concern.[72] Pandora project leader Cesaro was convinced that the primates exposed to microwaves experienced adverse health effects.[73]

The Continuing Question of Bioeffects of Microwaves

What came up in several of the Project Pandora meetings was the need to review US safety standards for RF and microwave exposure, which were possibly inadequate. The US safety standard of 10 mW/cm^2 was 2,000 times higher than the average exposure of US personnel in the US embassy in Moscow of about 0.005 mW/cm^2 before June 1975, although it somewhat exceeded the Soviet safety standard of 0.001 mW/cm^2.[74] US safety standards are based entirely on the thermal effects of microwaves on cell tissue, which means that they do not consider possible nonthermal bioeffects. During the 1970s, there was a public debate on the dangers of microwaves as the science did not seem to be settled. One of the journalists warning of the dangers of microwaves was Paul Brodeur, who wrote numerous articles and a popular book on the subject. He pointed out how high the stakes were for the US government and the telecommunications and entertainment industries because of their high dependence on microwave technology: for the US government it was a national security issue, and for the industry it was a matter of enormous profit that could be derived from this technology. He stated: "[G]iven the mass addiction to television, and the widespread use of microwaves in all manner of communication, it seems questionable whether today's society would even want to do much about it."[75] Some forty-five years later, microwave technology is ubiquitous since it is used for mobile phones, Wi-Fi, and all kinds of smart devices. Although the great majority of the population does not seem to experience identifiable negative health effects, the general concerns about constant human exposure to low-energy microwaves and EMF have endured.

The Frey Effect

Allan Frey was a biophysicist who is mostly known for the discovery of the microwave auditory effect (MAE). In 1961, Frey was a research scientist at Cornell University working on an Office of Naval Research grant to investigate "the effects of radio-frequency on the nervous system and on behavior."[76] A technician at the General Electric radar test facility in Syracuse told him that he could hear the radar, which went against the established scientific paradigm that only acoustical energy was audible. Frey decided to test this claim himself and found out that

> depending upon the width of the pulse and its rate of repetition, radio-frequency sound was perceived as buzzing, ticking, hissing, or knocking; that it could be induced several hundred feet from an antenna the instant an antenna's transmitter was turned on; that it could occur at average power densities far below the ten-milliwatt level; that it could be perceived by people who were blindfolded and people who were deaf; and that it always seemed to come from within or short distance behind the head.[77]

Frey published his findings in a scientific article in 1962, where he tried to explain why people can hear inaudible microwave energy. He speculated that "it is reasonable to suspect that possibly the electromagnetic field could interact with neuron fields."[78] In other words, the microwaves could penetrate the skull and directly stimulate the auditory cortex to generate the perception of sounds, bypassing the ear and cochlea.

Don R. Justesen, a neuropsychologist and expert on the behavioral effects of microwaves, confirmed the Frey effect. He suggested that humans can hear microwaves that are modulated in the form of a series of high-amplitude pulses and that the MAE occurs "at least an order of magnitude below the current permissible limit in the United States for continuous exposure to microwaves, which is 10 mW/cm^2."[79] The Frey effect hence is possible well below the threshold for thermal effects of microwaves. Justesen pointed at a 1975 experiment that demonstrated that information could be transmitted with the help of the Frey effect using Morse Code. He also claimed that "Sharp and Grove found that appropriate modulation of microwave energy can result in direct 'wireless' and 'receiverless' communication of speech. . . . By radiating themselves with these 'voice modulated' microwaves, Sharp and Grove were readily able to hear, identify, and distinguish among the 9 words."[80] This phenomenon was also confirmed by Soviet research. A 1976 report by the Defense Intelligence Agency (DIA) on Soviet research on the bioeffects of electromagnetic radiation stated that "[t]he potential for the development of a number of antipersonnel applications is suggested by the research published in the USSR, East Europe, and the West. Sounds and possibly even words which appear to be originating intracranially can be induced by signal modulation at very low average power densities."[81] The Frey effect is a possible explanation for the sounds heard by people suffering from Havana Syndrome.[82]

Thermal Effects of Microwaves

At the same time, it is uncontroversial that microwaves at energy density levels above the threshold for thermal effects are harmful to humans and may cause severe damage to the brain and other internal organs, and even death. Numerous animal studies were conducted in the 1950s and 1960s to identify potential health hazards related to microwave exposure. In 1956, the Department of Defense started a major study called the "Tri-Service Research Program" to determine the bioeffects of microwaves.[83] This study proposed the current 10 mW/cm^2 US safety standard.[84] The study suggested that injury was observed in experimental animals because of the absorption of microwave energy that was associated with a rise in body and tissue temperature.[85] The study used healthy dogs, rabbits, rats, and mice, which were irradiated with microwaves up to an energy density of 165 mW/cm^2.

One experiment with dogs managed to raise the body temperature of the animals by two or three degrees Fahrenheit within forty to sixty minutes, resulting in distress, collapse, and sometimes death thirty minutes after exposure.[86] Burns on the body were also observed, with the rib cage being particularly susceptible to this injury.[87] There were also hematological, EKG, and central nervous system changes observed at high exposure levels, including altered brain function, loss of equilibrium, and vomiting.[88] Effects on the eyes, such as a darkening of the lens and shrinking of eyeballs, were observed in rabbits. The authors of the study concluded:

> When tissues are exposed to microwaves, the radiant energy absorbed is transformed into increased kinetic energy of the absorbing molecules, thereby producing a general heating of the entire medium. This effect on biologic systems is modified by mechanisms of heat loss primarily neurocirculatory in type. When the thermoregulatory capability of the animal is exceeded, death can result.[89]

They also suggest that "[t]he biologic effects of microwaves are related to microwave frequency, field intensity, and duration of exposure. Other important factors are environmental temperature, the influence of any medication on the subject, and mode of exposure (pulsed or CW [continuous wave])."[90]

A Department of Defense review of research on the bioeffects of microwaves declassified in 2006 discusses the effects on humans. The document suggests that "microwave hyperthermia (even with only a 1°C increase in brain temperature) may disrupt working memory, thus resulting in disorientation."[91] Prolonged hyperthermia can lead to severe brain damage and death. "Periods of hyperthermia are accompanied by cerebral edema that damage neurons, and the victim exhibits disorientation, delirium, and convulsions." The document mentions the Frey effect and the possibility to disrupt "the function of the spinal motor neurons which control muscle contractions and body movements. Persons suffering from this condition lose voluntary control of their body."[92] It is not hard to see the potential for weaponizing the thermal effects of microwaves as all humans and animals would be equally and predictably affected by microwave heating and by the Frey effect.

The Johns Hopkins University Study

The State Department contracted Dr. Abraham Lilienfeld of Johns Hopkins University in June 1976 to conduct a two-year epidemiological study on the approximately 3,500 US diplomats and dependents who had served in the Moscow embassy from 1953 to 1976, to compare their health with other US government personnel who had been posted to Eastern European embassies and consulates during the same time.[93] The comparison group consisted of about 8,000 individuals who had served in embassies and consulates in locations with a similar "climate, diet, geographic location, disease problems, and general social milieu," namely Budapest, Leningrad, Prague, Warsaw, Belgrade, Bucharest, Zagreb, and Sofia.[94] The study was an epidemiological survey of the mortality and morbidity of US government personnel and dependents in those locations, utilizing the medical records of the State Department Office of Medical Services, a health questionnaire, and phone interviews. The study reviewed death certificates for the Moscow embassy group and the comparison group for deceased individuals, as far as they were available. In addition, the study attempted to determine whether health conditions associated with microwave exposure, such as infertility, high blood pressure, audio or visual impairment, higher white blood cell count, and several other conditions, could be determined from the medical records.

Foreign Service personnel are required to undergo physical examinations before employment, prior to transfer from a foreign post, when they return to the United States, and when they separate or retire, which amounted to an average of six or seven examinations for each of the reviewed medical records. The Lilienfeld study found no significant difference in mortality between the Moscow embassy group and the comparison group, with the overall mortality for both groups lower than the average for the US population.[95] There were also no significant differences between the Moscow embassy group and the comparison group concerning health conditions associated with microwave exposure. The report stated that there was a "very close similarity between the study groups both in terms of the lifetime history and in the reporting of diseases and conditions after arrival at the index post."[96] The health survey indicated that the Moscow group reported more frequently than the comparison group the following conditions: "depression, irritability, more difficulty concentrating and more memory loss."[97] The authors of the study concluded: "No convincing evidence was discovered that would directly implicate the exposure to microwave radiation experienced by the employees at the Moscow embassy in the causation of any adverse health effects as of the time of this analysis."[98] The Lilienfeld study is even today sometimes invoked as proof that low-energy microwave exposure is safe, but these findings have been questioned by many other researchers.

The Johns Hopkins Study Revisited

John Goldsmith reviewed the statistical data produced by the Lilienfeld study almost twenty years later and argued that some of the findings were incorrect since there was a higher cancer incidence rate in both the Moscow and the comparison group relative to the general US population. Goldsmith alleged that there was "some evidence that the other embassies also may have been irradiated."[99] Goldsmith claimed that the investigators had called the finding of a higher cancer incidence rate "disturbing," but that this word was removed upon request from the State Department contracting officer.[100] Goldsmith also pointed out that the group that was impacted most by the microwaves was the cohort that served from June 1975 to February 1976 when the microwave energy density and the daily duration of the signal were highest. Since the Lilienfeld study was completed in July 1978, there was not enough time for adverse health effects of this more intense exposure to appear.[101] Follow-up research was not conducted, which possibly distorts the findings. It is conceivable that the Johns Hopkins University research team was biased toward dismissing the hypothesis that microwave exposure of the Moscow group was responsible for worse health outcomes, as this was the finding that the State Department preferred at the time. Needless to say, this finding also saved the government some money by not compensating State Department employees for health damage suffered in the line of duty.

A more recent review of the data related to the Moscow Signal by Jose Martinez found that the statistical data is inconclusive as to the harmful effects of microwave exposures at the Moscow embassy that were somewhat higher than typical exposures today. According to Soviet scientific literature on microwaves published at that time, "Soviet scientists were absolutely convinced of the biological effects of microwaves at low intensities, that radiation could be used as a weapon to disorient and affect the behavior of military and diplomatic personnel, and that it could also be used in interrogations."[102] Martinez pointed out that two US ambassadors died of cancer and one of leukemia at the ages sixty-nine, sixty-seven, and sixty-six, and that their offices in the US embassy received the highest microwave exposure.[103] Many other US embassy employees received much lower levels of exposure and hence were less likely to die from cancer. The cancer incidence rate was unusually high for both the Moscow and comparison groups and reportedly, the first cohort to serve in the new US embassy in Moscow from 1953 had the highest cancer incidence rate of all.[104]

Martinez pointed out the following flaws in the Lilienfeld study that make the findings questionable: (1) it includes family members of US Moscow embassy personnel when they had far less microwave exposure, (2) the medical records for both groups were incomplete as some records could not be found, (3) some US embassy personnel could not recall their workplace in the embassy, in which case it was assumed that they were not or little exposed, (4) cancer cases of individuals whose medical records were not found or who could not be tracked down were not included, which could have affected the findings due to the altogether low numbers of cancer deaths, (5) the study excluded deaths where causes could not be determined, (6) the health survey had a generally low response rate, (7) causes of death were not obtained from death certificates in 36 percent, (8) there is a contradiction between observed lower mortality for Moscow embassy personnel while there was higher morbidity for certain health problems, (9) all-cause mortality was much lower compared to the general population but cancer mortality was much closer to the general population, and (10) no control variables were used to account for health differences between the two groups.[105]

Martinez also cautioned that newer research suggests a safety limit for electromagnetic radiation (EMR) exposure that is three orders of magnitude lower than the safety standards of most countries.[106] Furthermore, it is important to understand that the intensity of EMR exposure is only one aspect to consider, and that microwaves that are modulated in a certain way could produce more harmful effects than exposure intensity alone would suggest. In other words, energy density is just one aspect of the potential harm caused by microwaves: duration of exposure, frequency, and modulation of the wave also matter.

Current Research on EMF Dangers

The issue as to whether EMF is harmful to human health at lower energy density and exposure levels remains highly controversial and is seemingly unresolved, even though the average EMF exposure of people around the world has gone up dramatically since the 1970s when the first health concerns were voiced. People are now constantly exposed to EMFs generated by the electricity grid, power outlets, electric and electronic devices, Wi-Fi, cell phones, radars, and radio and microwave broadcasting. More recent research into the dangers of "electrosmog" or the constant human exposure to low-energy EMF has indicated the following potential hazards: "cancers, neurodegenerative diseases, genotoxicity, DNA damage, alteration of the blood-brain barrier, oxidative stress, inflammatory factors, autism," and many other problems.[107]

An article by Dominique Belpomme et al. suggests: "We have definitive evidence that use of a mobile phone results in changes in brain metabolism. We know that low-intensity ELF and RF-EMFs generate reactive oxygen species (ROS), alter calcium metabolism and change gene expression through epigenetic mechanisms, any of which may result in development of cancer and/or diseases or physiological changes."[108] The International Agency for Research on Cancer, which is a World Health Organization suborganization, classified ELF-EMFs as "possibly carcinogenic to humans."[109] A major challenge in determining the extent to which cell phones or other low-intensity EMF exposures are carcinogenic is that cancer might only appear with substantial delay, which can be decades. The dramatic increase in daily EMF exposure has been accompanied by a dramatic increase in cancer rates for people under fifty years, which is up worldwide 79 percent from 1990 to 2019.[110]

There are specific concerns with respect to the negative health effects of EMF exposure on children because their bodies are much weaker and more vulnerable. It has been suggested that different EMF safety standards would be required for children compared to adults.[111] A Korean study conducted in the 1990s on the harms of EMF on children found that children living within 2 kilometers of an AM radio transmitter had a 2.5 times higher risk for leukemia and brain tumors compared to a control group.[112] Another study found that mobile phone microwave radiation more easily penetrates the skulls of children as it is thinner, which could affect cognitive functions, although the findings were inconclusive. As there are few studies on the bioeffects of EMF on children, the WHO has recommended reducing personal exposure and minimizing EMF exposures in kindergartens and schools.[113] Since governments have not taken action, some schools have introduced their own increased safety measures in response to cancer and leukemia cases observed in children, possibly associated with nearby cell phone towers and classroom Wi-Fi.[114]

Conclusion

The consensus view that emerged in the late 1970s was that the Soviets did not target US diplomats with microwaves to harm them but to eavesdrop on what was going on inside the embassy.[115] The explanation offered by the Soviet government in 1976 was that they tried to jam electronic equipment inside the US embassy. Both explanations are dubious, considering the amount of deception that characterized both the way the US government and the Soviet government handled the affair.[116] The US government faced the dilemma that they had to be concerned about the health of their embassy personnel in light of several cases of cancer and other negative health conditions among embassy workers and that the US government's own safety standards seemed to indicate that the Moscow Signal could not possibly have been harmful. Anecdotal evidence from some of the diplomats who served in the embassy seemed to suggest that they did face a higher health risk. James Schumaker, who was a Foreign Service Officer serving in the Moscow embassy from 1977 to 1979, recounted that he was completely unconcerned about the microwave exposure when he arrived, but that his cavalier attitude toward the threat soon changed. At the end of his tour, the routine medical examination found that he had a much higher than normal white blood cell count, which led to a later diagnosis of lymphocytic leukemia.[117] The Moscow Signal also followed a familiar pattern where the US government initially tried to keep it secret, then denied it had any major health effects, and eventually paid out money for "hardship" to some of their personnel affected by it to keep them quiet.[118] The Moscow Signal would be an important test case for the reality of Havana Syndrome: if US personnel were deliberately or inadvertently harmed by way of directed energy exposure back then, it becomes a lot more plausible that such covert attacks could have occurred after the Cold War and may still be occurring.

Notes

1 Casey Michel, "The Time Russians Really Did Target Americans with Microwaves," *Politico*, March 10, 2023, available at: https://www.politico.com/news/magazine/2023/03/10/russians-americans-microwaves-00086482.

2 Jose Martinez, "The 'Moscow Signal' Epidemiological Study, 40 Years On," *Reviews on Environmental Health* 34, no. 1 (2019): 14.

3 Jack Anderson, "'Brainwash' Attempt by Russians?," *Washington Post*, May 10, 1972.

4 Annie Jacobsen, *Phenomena: The Secret History of the U.S. Government's Investigations Into Extrasensory Perception and Psychokinesis* (New York: Little, Brown and Co., 2017), 193.

5 Jeffrey Richelson, *The Wizards of Langley: Inside the CIA's Directorate of Science and Technology* (Boulder: Westview Press, 2001), 209–10.

6 Antonio Mendez and Joanna Mendez, *Moscow Rules: The Secret CIA Tactics that Helped America Win the Cold War* (New York: Public Affairs, 2019), 13.

7 Richard Reston, "Soviet 'Bugs' Find in U.S. Embassy Walls," *Los Angeles Times*, May 20, 1964.

8 Eric Haseltine, *The Spy in Moscow Station: A Counterspy's Hunt for a Deadly Cold War Threat* (New York: St. Martin's Griffin, 2019), 182.

9 Mendez and Mendez, *Moscow Rules*, 13.

10 Elaine Sciolino, "The Bugged Embassy Case: What Went Wrong," *New York Times*, November 15, 1988.

11 Robert Wallace and H. Keith Melton, *Spycraft: Inside the CIA's Top Secret Spy Lab* (London: Bantam Press, 2008), 164.

12 Haseltine, *The Spy in Moscow Station*, 22.

13 Wallace and Melton, *Spycraft*, 165.

14 Peter Wright, *Spycatcher! The Candid Biography of a Senior Intelligence Officer* (New York: Viking, 1987), 24.

15 Haseltine, *The Spy in Moscow Station*, 42.

16 Wallace and Melton, *Spycraft*, 165.

17 Anderson, "'Brainwash' Attempt by Russians?"

18 Herbert Pollack, "Epidemiologic Data on American Personnel in the Moscow Embassy," *Bulletin of the New York Academy of Medicine*, April 9–10, 1979.

19 Pollack, "Epidemiologic Data on American Personnel in the Moscow Embassy," 1183.

20 Nicholas H. Steneck, *The Microwave Debate* (Boston: MIT Press, 1984), 93.

21 Colin A. Ross, *The C.I.A. Doctors* (Richardson: Manitou Communications Inc, 2006), 103.

22 Steneck, *The Microwave Debate*, 93.

23 William Burr and Peter Kornbluh, eds., "The Moscow Signals Declassified: Irradiating Richard Nixon," *National Security Archive*, September 22, 2022, available at: https://nsarchive.gwu.edu/briefing-book/intelligence-nuclear-vault-russia-programs/2022-09-22/moscow-signals-declassified.

24 Pollack, "Epidemiologic Data on American Personnel in the Moscow Embassy," 1183.

25 Pollack, "Epidemiologic Data on American Personnel in the Moscow Embassy," 1183.

26 Jacobsen, *Phenomena*, 75.

27 Steneck, *The Microwave Debate*, 93.

28 James C. Lin, "Microwave Signal at the US Embassy in Moscow," *IEEE Microwave Magazine* 3 (2018): 20.

29 US Department of State, "Memorandum of Conversation," June 25, 1967, available at: https://nsarchive.gwu.edu/document/28809-document-1-memorandum-conversation-25-june-1967-attached-letter-ambassador-llewellyn.

30 US Department of State, "U.S. Embassy Telegram to State Department," August 19, 1969, available at: https://nsarchive.gwu.edu/document/28811-document-3-us-embassy-moscow-telegram-4343-state-department-tums-19-august-1969.

31 US Department of State, "For Ambassador from Under Secretary Richardson," June 7, 1969.

32 Anderson, "'Brainwash' Attempt by Russians?"
33 Anderson, "'Brainwash' Attempt by Russians?"
34 Nicholas Wade, "Fischer-Spassky Charges: What Did the Russians Have in Mind?," *Science* 177, no. 4051 (1972): 778.
35 Pollack, "Epidemiologic Data on American Personnel in the Moscow Embassy," 1184.
36 Lin, "Microwave Signal at the US Embassy in Moscow," 20.
37 US Department of State, "Kissinger Telephone Conversation with Ambassador Dobrynin," December 23, 1975, available at: https://nsarchive.gwu.edu/document/28818-document-10-kissinger-telephone-conversation-ambassador-dobrynin-23-december-1975.
38 Gordon Corera, "'Havana Syndrome' and the Mystery of the Microwaves," *BBC*, September 8, 2021, available at: https://www.bbc.com/news/world-58396698.
39 New York Times Staff, "U.S. Moscow Envoy Reported to Be Ill: Embassy Denies," *New York Times*, February 17, 1976.
40 Time, "The Microwave Furor," *Time Magazine* 107, no. 12 (1976): 15.
41 Time, "The Microwave Furor," 15.
42 Bernard Gwertzman, "U.S. Radio Spying in Soviet Suffers," *New York Times*, May 2, 1976.
43 Martinez, "The 'Moscow Signal' Epidemiological Study, 40 Years On," 15.
44 Steneck, *The Microwave Debate*, 93.
45 Haseltine, *The Spy in Moscow Station*, 22.
46 Gwertzman, "U.S. Radio Spying in Soviet Suffers."
47 Bernard Gwertzman, "Soviet Dim Beams at U.S. Embassy," *New York Times*, July 8, 1976.
48 Paul Brodeur, *The Zapping of America: Microwaves, the Deadly Risk, and the Cover-Up* (New York: W.W. Norton & Co., 1977), 61.
49 Robert O. Becker and Gary Selden, *The Body Electric: Electromagnetism and the Foundation of Life* (New York: William Morrow, 1985), 88.
50 Becker and Selden, *The Body Electric*, 88.
51 Robert O. Becker, *Cross Currents: The Perils of Electropollution, the Promise of Electromedicine* (New York: Penguin, 1990), 202.
52 Becker, *Cross Currents*, 187.
53 Brodeur, *The Zapping of America*, 61.
54 Martinez, "The 'Moscow Signal' Epidemiological Study, 40 Years On," 14.
55 Brodeur, *The Zapping of America*, 61.
56 Anderson, "'Brainwash' Attempt by Russians?"
57 Richard Cesaro, "Memorandum for the Director, Advanced Projects Agency," October 15, 1965.

58 Steneck, *The Microwave Debate*, 98.
59 Steneck, *The Microwave Debate*, 99.
60 US Advanced Research Projects Agency, "Justification Memorandum for Project Pandora," October 15, 1965, available at: https://nsarchive.gwu.edu/document/28787-document-3-arpa-richard-s-cesaro-memorandum-justification-memorandum-project-pandora.
61 US Advanced Research Projects Agency, "PANDORA-BIZARRE Test Results," Memorandum, December 15, 1966.
62 US Advanced Research Projects Agency, "Memorandum for Director, Defense Research & Engineering," Memorandum, September 27, 1967.
63 Brodeur, *The Zapping of America*, 119.
64 Brodeur, *The Zapping of America*, 119.
65 Joseph F. Kubis, "Saratoga Report," Institute for Defense Analysis, May 8, 1969.
66 US Advanced Research Projects Agency, "Minutes of Pandora Meetings," August 12 and 13, 1969.
67 Stephen Lukasik, "Review of Project Pandora Experiments," *RAND Corporation*, October 4, 1969.
68 Quoted from Jacobsen, *Phenomena*, 75.
69 Brodeur, *The Zapping of America*, 120.
70 David Guyatt, "Anti-Personnel 'Soft Kill' Weaponry," *World Affairs* 9, no. 2 (2005): 45.
71 Steneck, *The Microwave Debate*, 97.
72 Barton Reppert, "Zapping an Embassy: 35 Years Later the Mystery Lingers," *Times Daily* (1988): 6d."
73 Jacobsen, *Phenomena*, 75.
74 Martinez, "The 'Moscow Signal' Epidemiological Study, 40 Years On," 14.
75 Brodeur, *The Zapping of America*, 317.
76 Brodeur, *The Zapping of America*, 50.
77 Brodeur, *The Zapping of America*, 51.
78 Allan H. Frey, "Human Auditory System Response to Modulated Electromagnetic Energy," *Journal of Applied Physiology* 17, no. 4 (1962): 692.
79 Don R. Justesen, "Microwaves and Behavior," *American Psychologist* (March 1975): 395.
80 Justesen, "Microwaves and Behavior," 396.
81 Ronald M. Adams and R. A. Williams, "Biological Effects of Electromagnetic Radiation (Radiowaves and Microwaves)—Eurasian Communist Countries," Defense Intelligence Agency, March 1976, VIII.
82 James Lin, "Weaponizing the Microwave Auditory Effect and the Havana Syndrome," *The Radio Science Bulletin* 376 (2021): 36–8.
83 Steneck, *The Microwave Debate*, 38.

84 Sol M. Michaelson, Roderick A. E. Thomson, and Joe W. Howland, "Biologic Effects of Microwave Exposure," University of Rochester, September 1967.
85 Michaelson, Thomson, and Howland, "Biologic Effects of Microwave Exposure," 1.
86 Michaelson, Thomson, and Howland, "Biologic Effects of Microwave Exposure," 4.
87 Michaelson, Thomson, and Howland, "Biologic Effects of Microwave Exposure," 15.
88 Michaelson, Thomson, and Howland, "Biologic Effects of Microwave Exposure," 44.
89 Michaelson, Thomson, and Howland, "Biologic Effects of Microwave Exposure," 66.
90 Michaelson, Thomson, and Howland, "Biologic Effects of Microwave Exposure," 87–8.
91 US Department of Defense, "Bioeffects of Selected Nonlethal Weapons," Declassified December 6, 2006, 2.
92 US Department of Defense, "Bioeffects of Selected Nonlethal Weapons," 8.
93 Abraham M. Lilienfeld, "Evaluation of Health Status of Foreign Service and Other Employees from Selected Eastern European Posts," Department of Epidemiology, School of Hygiene and Public Health, Johns Hopkins University, July 31, 1978, 1.
94 Lilienfeld, "Evaluation of Health Status of Foreign Service and Other Employees from Selected Eastern European Posts," 1.
95 Lilienfeld, "Evaluation of Health Status of Foreign Service and Other Employees from Selected Eastern European Posts," 88.
96 Lilienfeld, "Evaluation of Health Status of Foreign Service and Other Employees from Selected Eastern European Posts," 125.
97 Lilienfeld, "Evaluation of Health Status of Foreign Service and Other Employees from Selected Eastern European Posts," 245.
98 Lilienfeld, "Evaluation of Health Status of Foreign Service and Other Employees from Selected Eastern European Posts," 246.
99 John R. Goldsmith, "Balancing the Interests of Patients, Science and Employees: Case Study of RF (Microwave) Exposure of US Embassy Staff in Eastern European Posts," *The Science of the Total Environment* 184 (1996): 84.
100 Goldsmith, "Balancing the Interests of Patients, Science and Employees," 85.
101 Goldsmith, "Balancing the Interests of Patients, Science and Employees," 86.
102 Martinez, "The 'Moscow Signal' Epidemiological Study, 40 Years On," 15.
103 Martinez, "The 'Moscow Signal' Epidemiological Study, 40 Years On," 19.
104 Martinez, "The 'Moscow Signal' Epidemiological Study, 40 Years On," 19.
105 Martinez, "The 'Moscow Signal' Epidemiological Study, 40 Years On," 19–20.
106 Martinez, "The 'Moscow Signal' Epidemiological Study, 40 Years On," 23.

107 Fabien Deruelle, "The Different Sources of Electromagnetic Fields: Dangers Are Not Limited to Physical Health," *Electromagnetic Biology and Medicine* 29, no. 2 (2020): 166.

108 Dominique Belpomme, Lennart Hardell, Igor Belyaev, Ernesto Burgio, and David O. Carpenter, "Thermal and Non-Thermal Health Effects of Low-Intensity Non-Ionizing Radiation: An International Perspective," *Environmental Pollution* 242 (2018): 644.

109 Belpomme, Hardell, Belyaev, Burgio, and Carpenter, "Thermal and Non-Thermal Health Effects of Low-Intensity Non-Ionizing Radiation," 644.

110 Janet Shamlian, "New Study Finds Alarming Rise in Cancer Rates Among People Under 60," *CBS Evening News*, September 6, 2023, available at: https://www.cbsnews.com/news/study-alarming-rise-cancer-people-under-50/.

111 Jin-Hwa Moon, "Health Effects of Electromagnetic Fields on Children," *Clinical and Experimental Pediatrics* 63, no. 11 (2020): 422.

112 Moon, "Health Effects of Electromagnetic Fields on Children," 425.

113 Moon, "Health Effects of Electromagnetic Fields on Children," 425.

114 CBS Staff, "After Several Childhood Cancer Cases at One School, Parents Question Radiation from Cell Tower," *CBS News*, April 4, 2019, available at: https://www.cbsnews.com/news/cell-tower-shut-down-some-california-parents-link-to-several-cases-of-childhood-cancer/.

115 Haseltine, *The Spy in Moscow Station*, 42.

116 Martinez, "The 'Moscow Signal' Epidemiological Study, 40 Years On," 17.

117 James Schumaker, "Before Havana Syndrome, There Was Moscow Signal," *The Foreign Service Journal*, January/February 2022, available at: https://afsa.org/havana-syndrome-there-was-moscow-signal.

118 Becker and Selden, *The Body Electric*, 317.

3

ESP Research and Psychotronic Weapons

The reason why parts of the US government, especially the State Department, CIA, and DIA, believed that the Moscow Signal was possibly a Soviet plot to harm and/or mind control US personnel in the embassy was the existence of a large amount of Soviet literature that clearly suggested bioeffects of low-energy RF and microwave exposure. Some of this literature discussed these bioeffects in relation to extrasensory perception (ESP) and so-called "psychotronic weapons," which were believed to affect the human mind or consciousness from a distance, exploiting paranormal phenomena. Soviet parapsychology research suggested that all paranormal phenomena are based on the principles of physics and hence can be objectively researched. A central idea of Soviet research was that paranormal phenomena are related to bioelectromagnetics and can be enhanced by technical means. In other words, in the 1960s and 1970s, there was a strange overlap between paranormal research (parapsychology) and what could be called nonlethal DEWs (to be explored in the next chapter). In any case, the Soviet concept of psychotronic weapons and the many references in Soviet and Russian military literature make it worthwhile to have a closer look, since a Havana Syndrome weapon may be based on much older Soviet psychotronic weapons research and technology. The chapter will trace the origins of Soviet and US parapsychology research, will discuss the reality of paranormal phenomena, and will establish the connection to psychotronic weapons.

The Beginning of Parapsychology

Parapsychology is the scientific investigation of paranormal abilities and phenomena, which includes diverse areas such as ghosts, spirits, dowsing, telepathy, hypnosis, telekinesis, clairvoyance, near-death experiences, synchronicity, and precognition. These are sometimes called "psi phenomena," which is a catchall term for the paranormal element in observed empirical phenomena. Extrasensory perception (ESP) is an umbrella term that includes telepathy, out-of-body experiences, and clairvoyance (the ability to see future events). Related to parapsychology, but not officially included, is research into UFOs, occultism, and other inexplicable phenomena such as cryptozoology. Although such phenomena have existed (or at least have generated human interest) for millennia, the idea that they can be subjected to serious and rigorous scientific investigation is relatively new (as is modern science).

Interest in the paranormal was quite popular in Europe in the late nineteenth and early twentieth centuries when it was fashionable among the upper class to have an interest in the occult, such as holding seances to consult with the spirits of the dead. It was this kind of upper-class pursuit that led to the attempted inclusion of parapsychology as a new discipline in the academy. In 1911, a generous gift by Thomas Welton Stanford to Stanford University established a permanent fellowship for psychical research, which sponsored a research program into ESP.[1] In 1930, a Parapsychology Laboratory was created at Duke University by John Banks Rhine, who was the leading parapsychology researcher of this era.

Not surprisingly, parapsychology was not welcomed by the academy and has been considered from the start as a pseudoscience that has been relegated to the fringes of scientific exploration. Even some of its early practitioners, such as John Edgar Coover, who occupied the Stanford Fellow in Psychical Research for twenty-five years, joined the camp of the skeptics as so little progress was made in the documentation, let alone the explanation, of ESP.[2] Parapsychologists have mainly relied on laboratory experiments to generate data for statistical analysis to determine whether an individual has displayed paranormal abilities such as ESP or psychokinesis. Rhine developed the so-called Zener cards, which are a deck of twenty-five cards with different symbols that a test subject must guess. If there are enough correct guesses to be statistically significant, it can be hypothesized that psi, or specifically ESP, enabled the higher number of correct guesses. Zener cards have also been used in telepathy experiments where a sender looks at a set of Zener cards and a receiver in a distant location must guess which cards were viewed by the sender.

Parapsychologists have also used hypnosis as it is connected to the subconscious, which is considered to be more capable of accessing paranormal abilities. A major interest of parapsychologists has been how the mind or consciousness relates to matter and whether particular mental states can be associated with psi phenomena such as ESP. There are hence notable connections between parapsychology research, the exploration of consciousness, and mind control research, which may also explain some of the long-lasting military and intelligence interest in parapsychology. There are significant differences in paranormal research in the West and in the East/Russia. Western parapsychology research seems to have largely refrained from postulating a hypothetical energy source or mechanism for psi phenomena, while Russian parapsychology research, from early on, tried to connect paranormal phenomena and hypnosis to physical principles.

Russian/Soviet Parapsychology Research

Russian researchers suggested that paranormal phenomena could be based on electromagnetism, which was assumed to play a role in ESP or the transmission of information from and between biological organisms. In the late nineteenth century, the psychiatrist V. L. Ohotrovich hypothesized that all living organisms produce a magnetic field and that there is a transmission of low-level energy that is physical and can be measured.[3] This kind of bioenergy was later supposedly captured with the help of Kirlian photography, developed by Semyon Davidovich in 1939, which uses high frequency electrical fields and a photographic plate.[4] Kirlian photography is said to show an energy field that surrounds a living being, or the "aura." A key idea of bioenergetics is that people could be healed (or made sick) by manipulating their biological energy.

Parapsychology was included in the academy in the early twentieth century. Tsar Nicholas II established the St. Petersburg Research Institute of Neuropsychiatrics in 1907, which later conducted unconventional research into paranormal phenomena.[5] According to Serge Kernbach, in the 1920s, the Moscow biophysics laboratory carried out a research project "to investigate the physical nature of telepathy."[6] When test subjects were placed inside Faraday cages it did not affect their psychic abilities, which effectively meant that there was no apparent connection to electromagnetism. It was hence assumed that there was a telepathic radiation that transmits information among biological organisms, which was "high-penetrating" and "non-electromagnetic."[7] According to research by Serge Kernbach on the early Soviet parapsychology research,

> the works with EM emission have shown that mechanisms of higher nervous activity can be affected by technical means, in particular by microwave radiation.

> In this context, the effects discovered by B.G. Michaylovski can be mentioned. It is about impact of medium/short EM waves modulated by low frequency signals on separate areas of the brain, which are responsible for emotional state and functionality of different organs.[8]

In short, the Soviet researchers believed that microwaves can be used to stimulate the brain and the central nervous system by using low-energy electromagnetic waves modulated to be in the frequency range of the brain, which is called ELF. This means that although telepathy cannot be entirely explained in terms of an electromagnetic phenomenon, electromagnetics may still play a role in telepathic information transfer as the non-electromagnetic telepathic radiation must interact with the body in some way. Later hypotheses for the mechanisms of psi phenomena were the metaethereal hypothesis that proclaims the existence of metaethereal energy, the psychic energy hypothesis that assumes brain processes can produce psychic energy, and the gravitational hypothesis that suggests gravitational fields may interact with the brain and enable telepathic communication.[9]

Soviet state security (OGPU/NKVD) was conducting their own research into behavioral modification or mind control, which also intersected with parapsychology research. A special department of the OGPU (a predecessor organization of the KGB) may have established a "neuro-energetic" laboratory in the 1920s to explore various paranormal phenomena related to "healers shamans, psychics, and hypnotists."[10] However, little is known about what was discovered in this research. Because of the Stalinist show trials in the 1930s, there was the suspicion in the West that the communists may have achieved a breakthrough in the development of mind control techniques that enabled them to "brainwash" people into believing the most absurd lies and acting as if they were remotely controlled. These assumptions motivated the CIA's own mind control research that began in 1950 (under the codenames Bluebird, Artichoke, MK ULTRA, and MK SEARCH).[11]

The Nazi elites, in particular Heinrich Himmler and the SS, also had a strong interest in the occult. The SS organization Ahnenerbe ("ancestral heritage") conducted expeditions around the world to discover ancient artifacts and ancient knowledge. According to Annie Jacobsen, "Ahnenerbe was vast and well funded" and included Occult Sciences or research into "extrasensory perception, astrology, map dowsing, spirit channeling, and other forms of anomalous mental phenomena and divination."[12] After the Second World War, American and Soviet intelligence captured some of the Ahnenerbe documents and researchers, which sparked renewed interest in paranormal phenomena and the occult in the West and the East and may have been the start of a new type of Cold War arms race in the paranormal arena.[13]

Parapsychology Research for National Security Purposes

The interest of the US national security state in the paranormal precedes the Cold War. The Canadian psychiatrist George Estabrooks, a specialist in hypnosis, worked as a contractor for the US Department of War during the Second World War, and he later claimed that he had used hypnosis to create spies with multiple personalities that could be triggered by cues such as codewords, who could resist enemy interrogation.[14] This may have been the beginning of American mind control research under MK ULTRA, which also explored the use of hypnosis and the possibility to induce hypnotic states with drugs or electromagnetic waves.[15]

After the Second World War, a medical doctor and US Army officer by the name of Andrija Puharich, with a keen private interest in parapsychology, promoted the study of paranormal phenomena within the US military and later the CIA. In the mid-1950s, Puharich worked as a medical officer at Edgewood Arsenal, Maryland, where the Army's Special Operations Division, together with the CIA, conducted drug experiments on US service members in the context of MK ULTRA mind control research.[16] Puharich developed a theory that there was a body energy force that radiated electromagnetic energy, which could not yet be detected or measured.[17] One of the ideas he pursued was that ELF waves could be responsible for ESP. ELF are waves in the frequency range between 3 and 30 Hz, which is the frequency range of the human brain. They are also extremely long with wavelengths between 100,000 and 10,000 kilometers. Puharich conducted experiments with psychic individuals who were tested inside and outside of a Faraday cage, and it was discovered that electromagnetic shielding seemed to enhance rather than stop paranormal abilities.[18]

The US military funded parapsychology research at Duke University in relation to ESP abilities of dogs to detect landmines, the ability of homing pigeons to find their way, and whether man could telepathically communicate with a cat.[19] The CIA investigated in their MK ULTRA subproject 58 whether altering states of mind with hallucinogenic drugs would enhance ESP abilities. The CIA sent Gordon Wasson, a pediatrician, to Indian tribes in Mexico in search of hallucinogenic mushrooms that could enable people to access or enhance ESP.[20] Since few of the MK ULTRA documents have survived after DCI Helms ordered their destruction in late 1972 to prevent public disclosure, it is largely unknown as to what the CIA may have discovered in their paranormal research of the 1950s and 1960s.

The Fear of a "Psychic Gap"

Scientific research in the Soviet Union was heavily affected by communist ideology, which sometimes led to pseudoscientific theories such as Lysenkoism and limited what could be researched at Soviet universities. The problem with parapsychology research in the Soviet Union was that it seemed to contradict materialism, which is the philosophical foundation of Marxism. Hence, during the Stalin era, there was no government support for parapsychology research. After the death of Stalin in 1953, there was some more open-mindedness in the Soviet Union that allowed for some parapsychology-related research to take place. Even so, Soviet researchers were still afraid to venture into a field as controversial as parapsychology.[21] What seemingly propelled the psychic arms race was a supposed successful American telepathy experiment of 1958.

The Nautilus Story

In 1959, the French magazine *Constellation* published a sensational report about an American military telepathy experiment involving the nuclear submarine U.S.S. *Nautilus*, which sparked Soviet fears that the West may have had some kind of breakthrough in paranormal research.[22] A more detailed version of the story appeared in the French science magazine *Science et Vie* in February 1960, written by one of the editors, Gérald Messadié.[23] According to the article, President Eisenhower had received a study from the RAND Corporation that suggested communication with dived submarines may be possible via telepathy. The US submarine *Nautilus* was dispatched to the North Pole to receive telepathic messages from Westinghouse's Friendship Laboratory. An assistant (Smith) was looking at randomly selected Zener cards and then transmitting the information telepathically to a *Nautilus* crew member (Jones), who drew the received Zener card symbols and put them into an envelope that was sealed. When the *Nautilus* returned to port, the sealed envelope was taken to the Westinghouse laboratory in Baltimore, and the symbols recorded in the envelope were compared with the selected Zener cards: Jones had a 70 percent accuracy rate.[24] This seemingly defied the odds for random guessing.

Professor Leonid L. Vasiliev from the Department of Physiology at the University of Leningrad believed that the United States had demonstrated the reality of telepathy, which confirmed older Soviet experiments and proved that a revival of psychic studies was needed to investigate the physical foundations of telepathy. Vasiliev claimed: "The discovery of the energy underlying ESP will be equivalent to the discovery of atomic energy."[25] Vasiliev was successful in his lobbying for Soviet ESP research as he was put in charge of a special laboratory to study biocommunications or telepathy at the University of Leningrad in 1962.[26]

According to Ostrander and Schroeder, the Kremlin made it a top priority in 1963 to include parapsychology in the biological sciences.[27] Soviet scientists were seemingly convinced that the *Nautilus* experiment was real and that it indicated the existence of a potentially larger and secret US military parapsychology research effort that they felt the Soviet Union needed to counter with their own groundbreaking research. The official denial of the US Navy that no such telepathy experiment had taken place only strengthened the Soviet view that parapsychology research had become a new arena for superpower competition.[28]

Strangely, there seems to be no evidence that the *Nautilus* experiment had actually happened. The main source for the story was Jacques Bergier, a French physicist of Ukrainian origin and former spy, who possibly made it up. Martin Ebon, who tried to track down key individuals in the story and any confirmatory documentation many years later, discovered that the captain of the *Nautilus* denied that any such experiment took place and that there was no documentary evidence.[29]

Vaughan Purvis suggested that the *Nautilus* story was a CIA disinformation operation that was aimed to distract Soviet intelligence from some other research, secret, or operation: it could have been a cover for the hydrophones the United States was placing in the ocean to track Soviet submarines, to conceal a new technology of using very low frequency (VLF) waves for communicating with submerged submarines, a ruse to fuel Soviet paranoia and superstitions, or an effort to make the Soviets waste resources on useless research.[30] Ebon also suggested that the *Nautilus* story may have been a cover for testing ELF underwater transmission.[31] ELF waves are known to be used by submarines to communicate when submerged. Purvis pointed out the irony that the likely US *Nautilus* disinformation did lead to a massive Soviet parapsychology effort, which was seen as threatening enough to inspire similar US research, including a real telepathy experiment involving a US submarine in 1977, which could mean that this was the first time the United States had carried out this particular experiment.[32]

Pentagon Reports on Soviet ESP Research

Throughout the 1970s, the US military and the CIA produced several intelligence reports assessing Soviet parapsychology research in terms of applications for mind control, intelligence collection, and remote influencing and assassination. In July 1972, John LaMothe produced for the DIA a classified report on Soviet mind control research titled "Controlled Offensive Behavior" (declassified in 1976), which alleged that the Soviets were leading in key areas such as ESP, mind control, and electromagnetic weaponry.[33] The report suggested an "ever increasing link between the psychology and psychiatry fields with the pharmacology, human engineering, bioelectronics, physics, and parapsychology disciplines."[34] It provided a very comprehensive overview of the research that was known to have been carried out in these areas in the Soviet Union. The report claimed that "[t]he major impetus behind the Soviet drive to harness the possible capabilities of telepathic communication, telekinetics, and bionics are said to come from the Soviet military and KGB," which funded this research to the tune of $21 million annually to support twenty or more research centers.[35]

The Soviets did not use the term parapsychology but preferred biocommunication, psycho-physiology, psychotronics, psychoenergetics, or biophysical effects.[36] The Soviet research suggested that electromagnetic waves in the super-high frequency spectrum can be used to alter human behavior and that, according to Soviet studies, "[l]ethal and non-lethal aspects [of electromagnetic waves] have been shown to exist."[37] The DIA report speculated that

> before the end of the 1970s, Soviet diplomats will be able to sit in their foreign embassies and use ESP . . . to steal the secrets of their enemies . . . a spy would be hypnotized, then his invisible "spirit" would be ordered to leave his body, travel across barriers of space and time to a foreign government's security facility, and there read their top-secret documents and relay back their information.[38]

A follow-up report by Louis Maire and John LaMothe on "Soviet and Czechoslovakian Parapsychology Research" from 1975 cautioned that "official hostility towards parapsychology increased in the Soviet Union" and that "Soviet scientists are just as divided among themselves as scientists elsewhere."[39] It was pointed out that Edward Naumov, a leader in Soviet parapsychology, had been arrested and sentenced to years of hard labor for what looked like a bogus corruption charge. It was clear that the scientific opposition to parapsychology had grown in the Soviet Union and that the Soviet government wanted to distance itself from what was called a pseudoscience.

Despite this increased opposition by the Soviet scientific establishment, there were important advances made in the field in the 1970s, especially by Czech parapsychologists. The Czech researcher M. Cernousek developed a theory that telepathy was a regressive phenomenon in the sense of accessing an older or primitive state of the mind. Telepathy would be enabled by empathy between individuals that allows them to transfer information by simultaneously accessing similar information stored in the minds of sender and receiver.[40] The model of the brain used is cybernetics, or the assumption that the brain is a biological computer. The brain would have a large reserve capacity in the form of the subconscious that allows the brain to process a lot more information than the conscious mind. Parapsychology research could therefore help with the development of creative computers and enable man-machine interfaces. The report suggested: "The Soviet-Czech team approach to parapsychology research . . . will advance them into direct man-machine communication, creative computers, and eventually into cyborgs, i.e., human inductors coupled with physical psychotronic instrumentation."[41] According to this theory, there is a still unknown source of psychic energy produced by the brain that is responsible for psi phenomena and that can in principle be detected and manipulated with technical equipment. The report concludes:

> The bulk of recent telepathy research in the USSR has been concerned with the transmission of emotional or behavioral impulses and the study of physiological responses to PK exercises, etc. In their exploration of telepathy, they are seeking the eventual capability to reproduce and to amplify the phenomena so that control is feasible. Control and manipulation of the human consciousness must be considered a primary goal.[42]

The journal *Military Review* published an article by Colonel John B. Alexander in 1980, which suggested that "[i]t is generally believed that the Soviets and their allies are well in the lead in parapsychological research."[43] Alexander referenced the two aforementioned studies and alleged that "[t]he Soviets have further developed techniques to control and actively employ their knowledge of parapsychology," which seems to indicate that there was some kind of operational capacity for using psi phenomena, including the ability to heal or induce disease over distance, telepathic behavior modification, and psychokinesis.[44] Alexander claimed that "psychotronic weapons already exist; only their capabilities are in doubt."[45] He advised that there should be more coordinated parapsychology research in the United States.

Project Stargate

In 1946, Stanford University created the Stanford Research Institute (SRI) as a nonprofit organization focused on innovation and economic development. SRI, in 1977 renamed SRI International, received 75 percent of its funding from the US government and about 40 percent came from the Department of Defense.[46] SRI became the center of American parapsychology research during the 1970s because of the initiative of physicist and specialist in laser technology Harold "Hal" Puthoff, who pitched the idea to the CIA in a letter from March 1972.[47] Puthoff was, according to Jim Schnabel, a former NSA employee who had completed his military service at Fort Meade in the 1960s and later stayed with the NSA as a civilian employee before joining SRI.[48] He was also an active member of the Church of Scientology, which may explain his interest in fringe sciences and mind control.[49] He teamed up with Russell Targ as his assistant, who was also a physicist specialized in lasers with a keen interest in paranormal phenomena, and whose sister was coincidentally married to world chess champion Bobby Fischer. In April 1972, Targ met with members of the CIA Office of Scientific Intelligence (OSI) to discuss Soviet parapsychology research, which eventually led to CIA funding of ESP research at SRI.[50]

The Stanford Research Institute Experiments

Russell Targ and Hal Puthoff decided to start their exploration of the paranormal by contacting famous New York psychic and artist Ingo Swann to test his abilities under laboratory conditions. Swann arrived at SRI in June 1972, where he was asked to alter the output of a highly sensitive magnetometer, known as the Varian Hall experiment.[51] Swann was successful in doing so using his psychic ability. A CIA report on paranormal research from 1977 suggested that "these variations [to the magnetometer induced by Swann] were never seen before or after the visit."[52] The experiment convinced the CIA's Office of Technical Services to provide $2,500 in funding for parapsychology research at SRI in August 1972, with additional $50,000 approved in October 1972.[53] The money was used to involve more psychics, most notably the Israeli medium Uri Geller, who was invited to SRI in fall 1972.[54]

Geller's visit was arranged by Andrija Puharich on recommendation of Apollo astronaut Edgar Mitchell and on behalf of the CIA.[55] Geller had worked with the Israeli Mossad and Shin Bet before, and the CIA wanted to know whether Geller's psychic abilities were real or whether he was a fraud, as many suspected.[56] Puthoff and Targ conducted a series of experiments with Geller over five weeks leading up to Christmas in 1972 and another one in March 1974, testing him for clairvoyance, metal bending, psychokinesis, and remote viewing.[57] These tests were conducted under laboratory conditions to eliminate the possibility of cheating, which included Geller and other psychics being placed inside an electromagnetically and acoustically shielded room. SRI was also working with another exceptional psychic by the name Pat Price. Price was a retired Burbank police commissioner who claimed to have successfully used psychic abilities in police investigations.[58] In particular, Price demonstrated an ability to psychically view locations when given coordinates on a map, which later came to define the practice of "remote viewing."

Targ and Puthoff eventually published the results of their experiments with Swann, Geller, Price, and others in the October edition of the prestigious journal *Nature* in 1974.[59] In the article, they described the experiments in detail, including the remote viewing experiments with Price, where he had to accurately describe verbally randomly selected locations visited by experimenters. After an analysis of the results, it was concluded that "Price's ability to describe correctly buildings, docks, roads, gardens and so on, including structural materials, colour, ambience, sometimes in great detail, indicated the functioning of a remote perceptional ability."[60] Price described six out of nine locations correctly.

Opinions diverged greatly as to the validity of the SRI experiments of 1972 to 1974. Critics have suggested that the experiments may have been flawed because of three major factors that make the results unreliable: "1) loose laboratory controls; 2) skewing of data; and 3) the premise that the attitude of the scientists conducting the experiment . . . could negatively influence the subject or psychic."[61] Geller's psychic abilities were called into question by the magician James Randi, who demonstrated that Geller may have relied on magic stage tricks and sleight of hand to perform his paranormal feats, which convinced many parapsychologists that he likely was a fraud.[62] More difficult to dismiss as fraud were the remote viewing experiments, which seemed to suggest that psychic espionage was a viable addition to US national security.

The Pentagon's Psychic Spies

Puthoff and Targ developed a new method for testing ESP, which consisted of providing a psychic with map coordinates of locations and then having them draw or describe what they saw in their minds, called Project Scanate. In May 1973, Swann and Price were given each separately the coordinates of a secret NSA facility called Sugar Grove in West Virginia, and their job was to provide as many details as possible about this location. Both the experimenter providing the coordinates and the two psychics were unfamiliar with the location, making it impossible for the experimenter to provide subconscious cues to the remote viewers.[63] Price described a military underground facility in great detail and even documents with codewords contained in a file cabinet in that location, including the codeword for the facility itself: "Sugar Grove." Apparently, Price's description of Sugar Grove was so accurate that the CIA launched an internal investigation into a potential security breach.[64]

In another experiment, the CIA selected for the remote viewers a number of targets in the Soviet Union and China that were scheduled for satellite surveillance in two or three months.[65] The descriptions of the remote viewers were mostly, but not always, correct, which resulted in the recommendation by a consultant to the CIA that the results were good enough to explore practical applications.[66] However, the CIA's star remote viewer Pat Price died in July 1975 from a heart attack or possible assassination.[67] In 1977, the new DCI of the Carter administration, Stansfield Turner, had no interest in parapsychology research and therefore cancelled the funding with the dry comment that although the CIA "had an individual who from time to time was able to draw very elementary sketches of street scenes of foreign countries where he had not been . . . [but] [h]e died and we haven't heard from him since."[68]

SRI got new funding from the US Navy worth $50,000 to determine whether the psychics could detect electromagnetic emanations of submarines, which are extremely difficult to find in the oceans using conventional methods. The contract was completed in 1978 and seemed to have yielded few exploitable results.[69] Another Navy research contract with SRI was "to study the influence of extremely low frequency (ELF) electromagnetic radiation on the human mind," to disprove that there were negative effects on health, which were alleged by environmentalists.[70] From 1976 to 1979, the US Air Force also funded research into remote viewing, which, according to a DIA report, demonstrated: (1) "[r]emote viewing can be used to monitor real-time activities," (2) "[a]ccuracy and resolution are not a function of distance," (3) "[s]patial resolution is accurate down to millimeters," and "4) "[e]lectrical shielding does not block remote viewing."[71]

In 1977, the US Missile Intelligence Agency awarded a contract to SRI to study remote viewing, and in the same year, the US Army Intelligence and Security Command (INSCOM) launched a program called Gondola Wish "to integrate the Soviet and Eastern psychoenergetic Intelligence collection into the all-source operations (OPSEC) support scenario."[72] Gondola Wish was replaced in 1978 with Project Grill Flame, which attempted to turn remote viewing into an operational intelligence collection capability. This included the development of procedures for the selection and training of psychics.[73] Grill Flame was curiously located at Fort Meade, which happens to be also the location of the NSA headquarters. The NSA's specialization is the collection of signals intelligence and electronic warfare, not psychic spying, raising the question as to how those two may have been connected.

Grill Flame shifted from a pure research project to operational usage in 1979. In their first operational mission, the remote viewers were tasked in September 1979 to locate a Soviet electronic intelligence aircraft that had crashed in Zaire so that it could be recovered. According to Joe McMoneagle, a warrant officer at the time and one of the Pentagon's most talented psychics, the remote viewer's information was very accurate: "Search teams were sent into the area and the plane was located within a kilometer of the location provided by the SRI remote viewer."[74] In November 1979, American diplomats were taken hostage in Tehran, which started a 444-day hostage crisis. McMoneagle was given pictures of the American hostages and asked to provide every bit of information he could obtain via ESP on the location, condition, and circumstances of the hostages.[75] Inadvertently, the remote viewers discovered also information about the secret plan to rescue the hostages, which resulted in some of the remote viewers getting captured and interrogated by Army counterintelligence over fears of deficient operational security.[76]

SRI International's involvement with Grill Flame/remote viewing started in 1980 and continued until 1989. In 1990, the research contract was awarded to the defense company SAIC, which is when the program was renamed Project Stargate. The SAIC research was led by Edwin May, who is a nuclear physicist and who had previously taken over SRI International's parapsychology research after the departure of both Hal Puthoff and Russell Targ in 1985.[77]

Shutdown of Project Stargate

The CIA decided to contract out a scientific review of its Stargate remote viewer program to the American Institutes for Research, a Virginia-based nonprofit organization, which produced a final report in September 1995. The study consisted of a review of about eighty publications and reports related to the Stargate experiments, interviews with end users, remote viewers and program managers, and an assessment of the value of remote viewing reports based on feedback from end users.[78] The report suggested that there was very limited evidence that remote viewing worked, far less that it had any operational utility. The report suggested that "[t]he conditions under which remote viewing is observed under laboratory settings do not apply to intelligence gathering situations," that "the remote viewing reports failed to produce the concrete, specific information valued in intelligence gathering," that "[t]he information provided was inconsistent, inaccurate with regard to specifics, and required substantial subjective interpretation," and that "[i]n no case had the information provided ever been used in intelligence operations."[79]

The criticism of the lacking successes and/or utility of psychic spying seems overly harsh in light of various earlier reviews that indicated remote viewers sometimes could provide quite accurate information and may have been influenced by a general scientific skepticism toward parapsychology. In any case, the US Department of Defense decided to follow the report's recommendation to shut down the remote viewing unit. The overall cost of the over twenty-year program to the taxpayer was very modest, with only $20 million spent.[80] It has been speculated that psychic spying may have been merely privatized to avoid public scrutiny. There is also a bigger question of whether Pentagon research was also looking into weapons applications related to parapsychology research since such Soviet parapsychology-related efforts were occasionally described in intelligence reports and military journal articles.

Soviet Psychotronic Weapons

The term "psychotronics" was officially adopted at a Soviet bloc parapsychology conference in Prague in 1973 to name this particular field of scientific research. Psychotronics is a combination of the words psyche and electronics and it refers to devices meant to amplify psychic energy.[81] The term psychotronics was hence more acceptable to the Soviet government, as it implied a close connection between psychic phenomena and technology and as it did not sound like it was connected to superstition or inexplicable phenomena, which is implied by the Western term "paranormal."[82] It also indicates an assumed connection of parapsychology or psychic abilities to cybernetics, electronics, and electromagnetic waves. In the 1970s and 1980s, there was a lot of speculation in the West about Soviet psychotronic weapons that used psychic energy to manipulate or harm people from a distance. One can find occasional references to them in the Soviet/Russian and Western military literature to psychotronic weapons. For example, military analyst Timothy Thomas published an influential article on Russian psychotronics in 1998 titled "The Mind Has No Firewall." Thomas claimed there was

> [a]n entirely new arsenal of weapons, based on devices designed to introduce subliminal messages or to alter the body's psychological and data-processing capabilities, might be used to incapacitate individuals. These weapons aim to control or alter the psyche, or to attack the various sensory and data-processing systems of the human organism. In both cases, the goal is to confuse or destroy the signals that normally keep the body in equilibrium.[83]

In this article, Thomas reviewed Russian military literature and Russian research in the area of psychotronics and mind control, suggesting that "these weapons are used against the mind to induce hallucinations, sickness, mutations in human cells, 'zombification,' or even death."[84] However, it is difficult to conclusively prove that psychotronic weapons exist since their usage is difficult to detect and their existence is not officially acknowledged by any government.

Psychotronic Generators

The Czech parapsychologist Robert Pavlita developed psychotronic generators that supposedly can draw biological energy from humans and store it for future use. These machines are described in some detail in the 1975 DIA report on

Czech and Soviet parapsychology research. The report suggests: "[T]he devices are fabricated from various metals (steel, bronze, iron, gold) and their effects are result of their form. Pavlita's generators can be charged by direct contact (e.g., rubbing or touching to the temporal region of the head) or by visually directing mental concentration on them from distance."[85] It is suggested that the generators could have a variety of applications not directly related to parapsychology, such as enhancing plant growth or purifying water. There is speculation by the author that the Czechs were working on weaponizing the psychotronic generators: "biological energy might be an effective antipersonnel weapon. It would be difficult to defend against, since it apparently penetrates most common forms of insulation and its reported effects (changes in brain wave characteristics, disturbance of equilibrium, dizziness) could result in personality changes or physical discomfort which might alter combat effectiveness."[86]

The psychotronic generators are also described in a book by Sheila Ostrander and Lynn Schroeder, who claimed to have seen them in Moscow at a parapsychology conference.[87] Pavlita demonstrated his machine by way of a psychokinesis experiment. He managed to stop and even reverse the movement of a small copper strip rotating with the power of an electric motor in a sealed metal box that also contained a psychotronic generator from a six-foot distance by simply staring at it. According to Pavlita's theory, it was his psychic energy that charged the psychotronic generator and that was used to achieve the psychokinetic effect.[88]

Thomas Bearden, who was an army intelligence analyst, technical consultant for the US Army, and a psychotronics enthusiast, defined a psychotronic generator as

> a device which produces observable effects by collecting, condensing, amplifying, and/or processing subtle anenergies or scalar waves. Classic examples are the psychotronic generators of the Czech engineer, Robert Pavlita. Psychotronic devices are virtual state engineering devices that process and utilize scalar EM waves of massless charge flux. Most of Pavlita's devices are "charged" by the natural scalar electromagnetic emissions of the human brain and nervous systems.[89]

Scalar waves theory seems to be based on ideas of inventor Nikola Tesla going back to the 1920s. Scalar waves are hypothetical non-electromagnetic waves that function differently from normal physics. A DIA document that discusses scalar waves in reference to Bearden and that seems to be from the 1980s suggests that scalar waves "appear to have some properties of soliton waves: they may not attenuate like EM waves do, but if they exist their energy source is not clear. They have quantum mechanical flavor about them."[90] Bearden claimed that the Soviets had started a "psychotronic Manhattan Project" in the 1950s.[91] In particular, Bearden alleged that

> the radiation of the U.S. Embassy (and the U.S. ambassador to the Soviet Union) in Moscow with weak radiofrequency microwaves containing psychotronic modulations began about 1959–60 . . . this radiation was in fact another very clever Soviet intelligence probe: By observing how the U.S. reacted, they could determine whether the U.S. had any knowledge of psychotronics and thus whether or not the U.S. had developed secret psychotronic weapons and counters of its own.[92]

Although Bearden's work seems to lack scientific validation, it was apparently taken seriously by parts of the US military during the 1980s. Electromagnetic scalar waves, as hypothesized by Bearden, seem to be fundamental to Soviet psychotronic weaponry, which Bearden believed could be used for all sorts of effects, including death rays, disease induction, telepathy, brain links, brain probes, and for causing earthquakes.[93]

Robert McCreight has more recently argued that scalar waves could be a relevant mechanism for what he calls "NeuroStrike technology" (the technology that may cause Havana Syndrome). He wrote:

> [W]e must confront the reality that fundamental aspects of Tesla wave [or scalar wave] technology include certain discernible effects on human biology. Scalar waves are three dimensional self-contained waves that spin on one fixed axis. These non-linear waves disseminate throughout the bodies through crystalline lattices of elaborate collagen networks as they help in increasing every hydrogen atom's energy covalent level in the body.[94]

The scalar waves would be using a frequency close to the Schumann resonance of 7.83 Hz, which is in the ELF and brain wave range. According to McCreight, "[e]vidence from research shows a degree of cellular, neuronic, and immune suppressive factors influenced by elements of scalar waves."[95]

Psychotronic Weapons

One of the believers in psychotronic weaponry is Col. John B. Alexander, who wrote an influential article on the military applications of parapsychology in

1980. He defined psychotronics as "the interaction of mind and matter." In this article, he suggested that a weaponization of this interaction had been explored and that "there are weapons that operate on the power of the mind and whose lethal capacity has already been demonstrated."[96] Hence, a psychotronic weapon is a hypothetical weapon that can manipulate the minds and bodies of people from a distance using psychic abilities and electromagnetic energy. Alexander suggested that psychotronic weapons "would be able to induce illness or death with little or no risk to the operator. . . . The psychotronic weapon would be silent, difficult to detect and would require only a human operator as a power source."[97] Ostrander and Schroeder quoted in their book the Russian parapsychologist Edward Naumov, who claimed that "[a] psychotronic generator can influence an individual or a whole crowd of people. It can alter a person's psyche mentally and emotionally. It can affect memory and attention span. A psychotronic device can cause physical fatigue, disorientation, and alter a person's behavior."[98]

Former KGB major general Oleg Kalugin, who was part of the political opposition in the Soviet Union and emigrated to the United States in the early 1990s, claimed that it was chairman of the KGB Yuri Andropov (and later general secretary of the CPSU) who decided to go ahead with psychic warfare.[99] Parapsychology research was officially shut down in the Soviet academy in the mid-1970s and was subsequently transferred under the control of the KGB, according to a Soviet émigré, August Stern. Stern said in an interview with the *New York Times* that he had worked in a secret laboratory in Novosibirsk, deceptively named the Institute of Automation and Electrometry, to determine the physical source of psychic energy and that the research was moved to an even more secretive lab under KGB control near Moscow.[100] Naumov claimed in a 2007 interview on *ABC News* that "the Ministry of Defense, the KGB, and other organizations did build psychotronic generators. I know that over half a billion rubles were spent to develop psychotronic equipment, which brings up the question: where are all those devices?"[101] This statement implied that Russian intelligence may have retained control over them in order to use them covertly.

Parapsychologist Edwin May interviewed several former high-ranking officers of the KGB for his book *ESP Wars*, which offers incredible insights into Soviet parapsychology research and psychotronic weaponry.[102] One of his Russian sources told him that a psychotronic weapon is essentially a NLW that "ostensibly utilizes psychic energy (or other mental or life energies) stored in batteries often referred to as psychotronic generators. They were hardware devices—often with nothing inside the shell . . . to affect, influence, or control the minds of targets, potentially affect a target's health . . . or even to drive them to suicide or accidental death."[103] The same source claimed that "a program of integrated ESP research and psychotronic weapons creation did not exist in the USSR, nor could it exist. Such a program would have required the authorization from the top ideologues of the Central Committee of the Communist Party, which was absolutely impossible because parapsychology was considered inconsistent with ideological dogma."[104] This remark seems to suggest that the psychotronic weapons may have been just props to sell the Soviet state security apparatus the idea of psychic abilities and their offensive utility. However, there was also clearly a directed energy connection to KGB psychotronic research, discussed in May's book.

According to KGB Major General Nikolei Alekseevich Sham, the KGB developed "a combined psychophysical technique of collecting information from remote objects by using operational radio-commands as a physical base of remote viewing. . . . Experiments were conducted on Dickson island in the Russian Arctic."[105] He further stated in relation to psychotronic weapons that "complex programs for the covert manipulation of an enemy life force using technologies of mental and psychophysical influence were develop on the basis of a great deal of research at our scientific research institutes."[106] The KGB had even an electronic sleep installation that could induce sleep over several kilometers distance and was working on "space platforms that could influence entire cities and areas and cause laughter, tears, dreams, diarrhea, etc. at certain frequencies."[107] These weapons would be actually "radio-biological weapons" that fall in-between the definition for a psychotronic weapon and a purely physical weapon.[108]

Have Psychotronic Weapons Been Used?

Psychotronic and radio-biological weapons seem to have been used, according to Bearden, Kalugin, and a few other sources. Bearden claimed in his *Excalibur Briefing* that the Soviets had developed in the 1960s an incredibly powerful weapons technology called "time reversed waves" (TR waves), which are produced by radars and phase-conjugate mirrors that receive an ordinary wave. The TR waves can be amplified and returned to the radar object that produced the radar reflection to destroy the object.[109] "Thus a TR wave radar weapon can deliver a powerful TR pulse against a distant vehicle carrying a nuclear warhead, and the resultant EG pulse penetrating the nuclear material of the warhead will electrogravitationally explode it in a full-order nuclear detonation."[110] He claimed that this technology was also used against the US Moscow embassy in the 1960s and that it was used to destroy the US submarine U.S.S. *Thresher* in the North Atlantic in April 1963.[111]

The Soviets built the Duga over-the-horizon radar in Northern Ukraine in 1976, which sent an electromagnetic signal to the United States, which became known as the "Woodpecker signal" since ham operators could hear a constant knocking sound in their transmissions. In Bearden's view, the Woodpecker signal was capable of producing "similar conditions [as those suffered by the Moscow embassy personnel] in distant target populations. . . . They also are probably capable of killing large numbers of the targeted population."[112] Bearden claimed that Woodpecker was used to alter the weather in the United States and that it could be used for destroying missiles and aircraft.[113]

In August 1991, a group of communist hardliners made a coup attempt against Gorbachev, which may have involved a psychotronic attack on the leading opposition politician Boris Yeltsin. Kalugin said on *ABC News* that during the coup against Gorbachev in 1991, a person in charge of a Ukrainian military lab told him that there would be an attempt on Yeltsin's life with a psychotronic generator.[114] Yeltsin did suffer a heart attack shortly after the coup, which caused Yeltsin to seek help from a psychic healer, who was to shield him from further psychic attacks.[115]

In 1993, the FBI reached out to a Russian psychotronics expert by the name of Dr. Igor Smirnov of the Moscow Medical Academy to provide some help with the siege of the Branch Davidian ranch at Waco. Smirnov was the inventor of a new technology that he called "psycho-correction," which he had used to treat post-traumatic stress, alcoholism, and drug addiction of Soviet soldiers who had fought in Afghanistan.[116] Smirnov travelled to the United States with psychotronic devices and attended a meeting with US intelligence community officials to discuss the usage of the technology. The idea was to change the thoughts and behavior of cult leader David Koresh.[117] However, Smirnov only brought entry-level devices and could not promise zero-risk as requested by the US officials. Hence, the psychotronic devices were not used, and the siege ended tragically. In 2007, DHS decided to test Smirnov's psychotronic technology by awarding a contract to his company Psychotechnology Research Institute, later run by his wife after the inventor's death in 2004.[118]

Psychotronic Weapons in Russian Military Thought

In the 1990s, Russian military analysts embraced the concept of information warfare, which originated from the West and was part of the so-called Revolution in Military Affairs (RMA) debate. The RMA school suggested that warfare was undergoing a revolutionary change because of IT, which had become central to conducting military operations. Russian theorists had a much broader understanding of information warfare that spans both peacetime and wartime. According to Timothy Thomas, "[i]n its peacetime use, the term refers to a broader category, the information security of society and the government in the psychological, scientific, cultural, and production aspects, with special emphasis on protecting state information resources and attempting to influence enemy information resources."[119] Thomas wrote that "subcommittees of the State Duma commissioned studies on both information warfare and 'psychotronic' warfare, and Kremlin advisors and the security community are studying how information security issues may affect the country's political, technical, economic, and military policies."[120] In Thomas' view, several books by military experts published in Russia in the 1990s demonstrated a "fixation on behavior and on the mind itself."[121]

In March 2012, the Russian defense minister, Anatoli Serdjukov announced: "The development of weaponry based on new physics principles; direct-energy weapons, geophysical weapons, wave-energy weapons, genetic weapons, psychotronic weapons, etc., is part of the state arms procurement program for 2011–2020."[122] According to a report by the *Daily Mail* in response to the announcement, Russia wanted to develop weapons that attack the central nervous system of victims and turn them into zombies. Putin said that these electromagnetic weapons would be "entirely new instruments for achieving political and strategic goals" and that "[s]uch high-tech weapons systems will be more acceptable in terms of political and military ideology."[123]

Conclusion

It is difficult to make sense of the interest of the military and intelligence establishments of the United States and the Soviet Union in parapsychology research. The conventional explanation is that this psychic warfare arms race was merely motivated by the Cold War paranoia that the other side could achieve a breakthrough in this area and hence that it was necessary to stay abreast of any hypothetical advances. When the Cold War ended, both sides supposedly realized that psychic warfare was a dead end (or worse, a scam perpetrated by fraudsters) and thus ended all government-sponsored research. This explanation is not convincing, given the fact that psi phenomena seemed to have been demonstrated under laboratory and operational conditions, which was the justification for continuing funding for such research in the United States for over twenty years (and for even longer in Russia). Strangely, no documentation could be found that the US military reproduced any of the Soviet psychotronic weapons, even though they were discussed in US intelligence reports that identified them as potential threats to US national security. This alone suggests that the public account of US government interest in this area is at best partial and that there are more secrets to be discovered. Former high-ranking Soviet KGB and military officers have also confirmed after the Cold War that psychotronic devices and weapons were developed in the Soviet Union and that they supposedly had the ability to enhance/enable psi phenomena, such as telepathy and psychokinesis, and that they could be used to affect the minds and health of people from a distance. The Soviet research was seemingly very different from the US research in the sense that the Soviets were trying to use electromagnetic energy to enhance or produce bioenergetic effects. It seems difficult to draw a clear line in the Soviet context between a psychotronic weapon powered by psychic energy and an electromagnetic weapon. The fact that apparently none of the Soviet psychotronic weapons have been publicly shown or demonstrated makes the matter even more mysterious. In Western terminology, a psychotronic weapon would be considered a NLW, which is the subject of the next chapter.

Notes

1 Frederick C. Dommeyer, "Psychical Research at Stanford University," *The Journal of Parapsychology* 39, no. 3 (1975): 173.

2 Dommeyer, "Psychical Research at Stanford University," 180.

3 Serge Kernbach, "Unconventional Research in USSR and Russia: Short Overview," Cybertronica Research, Research Center of Advanced Robotics and Environmental Science, Stuttgart, 2013, 3.

4 Sheila Ostrander and Lynn Schroeder, *Psychic Discoveries* (New York: Marlow & Co., 1997), 164–5.

5 Kernbach, "Unconventional Research in USSR and Russia," 3.
6 Kernbach, "Unconventional Research in USSR and Russia," 4.
7 Kernbach, "Unconventional Research in USSR and Russia," 4.
8 Kernbach, "Unconventional Research in USSR and Russia," 4.
9 Louis F. Maire and John D. LaMothe, "Soviet and Czechoslovakian Parapsychology Research," Defense Intelligence Agency, September 1975, 16.
10 Kernbach, "Unconventional Research in USSR and Russia," 5.
11 John Marks, *The Search for the "Manchurian Candidate": The CIA and Mind Control* (New York: W.W. Norton & Co., 1979), 30–1.
12 Annie Jacobsen, *Phenomena: The Secret History of the U.S. Government's Investigation into Extrasensory Perception* (New York: Little, Brown and Co., 2017), 18.
13 Jacobsen, *Phenomena*, 18.
14 Colin A. Ross, *The C.I.A. Doctors* (Richardson: Manitou Communications, Inc., 2000), 155, 160.
15 Walter Bowart, *Operation Mind Control* (New York: Dell Publishing, 1978), 75, 262–3.
16 H. P. Albarelli, *A Terrible Mistake: The Murder of Frank Olson and the CIA's Cold War Experiments* (Walterville: TrineDay, 2009), 53.
17 Jacobsen, *Phenomena*, 25.
18 Jacobsen, *Phenomena*, 34.
19 Jacobsen, *Phenomena*, 43–4.
20 Jacobsen, *Phenomena*, 62.
21 Ron McRae, *Mind Wars: The True Story of Government Research into the Military Potential of Psychic Weapons* (New York: St. Martin's Press, 1984), 92.
22 Ostrander and Schroeder, *Psychic Discoveries*, 6–7.
23 Martin Ebon, *Psychic Warfare: Threat or Illusion* (New York: McGraw-Hill, 1983), 22–3.
24 Ebon, *Psychic Warfare*, 24.
25 Ostrander and Schroeder, *Psychic Discoveries*, 7.
26 John LaMothe, "Controlled Offensive Behavior—USSR," Defense Intelligence Agency, January 31, 1972, 25.
27 Ostrander and Schroeder, *Psychic Discoveries*, 7.
28 Jim Schnabel, *Remote Viewers: The Secret History of America's Psychic Spies* (New York: Dell Publishing/Kindle, 1997), 101.
29 Ebon, *Psychic Warfare*, 25.
30 Vaughan Purvis, "The Nautilus Affair," 1997, available at: https://www.transformation.dk/www.raven1.net/mcf/hambone/nauti.html.
31 Ebon, *Psychic Warfare*, 127.

32 Purvis, "The Nautilus Affair."
33 LaMothe, "Controlled Offensive Behavior—USSR."
34 LaMothe, "Controlled Offensive Behavior—USSR," 13.
35 LaMothe, "Controlled Offensive Behavior—USSR," XI.
36 LaMothe, "Controlled Offensive Behavior—USSR," 21.
37 LaMothe, "Controlled Offensive Behavior—USSR," 18.
38 LaMothe, "Controlled Offensive Behavior—USSR," 30.
39 Maire and LaMothe, "Soviet and Czechoslovakian Parapsychology Research," 5.
40 Maire and LaMothe, "Soviet and Czechoslovakian Parapsychology Research," 24.
41 Maire and LaMothe, "Soviet and Czechoslovakian Parapsychology Research," 25.
42 Maire and LaMothe, "Soviet and Czechoslovakian Parapsychology Research," 31.
43 John B. Alexander, "The New Mental Battlefield—Beam Me Up, Spock," *Military Review* 60, no. 12 (1980): 48.
44 Alexander, "The New Mental Battlefield—Beam Me Up, Spock," 48–9.
45 Alexander, "The New Mental Battlefield—Beam Me Up, Spock," 53.
46 McRae, *Mind Wars*, 93.
47 Jacobsen, *Phenomena*, 118.
48 Schnabel, *Remote Viewers*, 1455.
49 Jeffrey Richelson, *The Wizards of Langley: Inside the Directorate of Science and Technology* (Boulder: Westview Press, 2001), 177.
50 Richelson, *The Wizards of Langley*, 177.
51 Schnabel, *Remote Viewers*, 1338.
52 Kenneth A. Kress, "Parapsychology in Intelligence: A Personal View and Conclusions," *Studies in Intelligence* 24, no. 4 (1977): 8.
53 Kress, "Parapsychology in Intelligence," 8.
54 Schnabel, *Remote Viewers*, 1954.
55 Jonathan Margolis, *CIA Masterspy? The Secret Life of Uri Geller* (New York: Osprey Publishing, 2013), 3.
56 Schnabel, *Remote Viewers*, 2027.
57 Margolis, *CIA Masterspy?*, 34.
58 McRae, *Mind Wars*, 100.
59 Russell Targ and Harold Puthoff, "Information Transmission Under Conditions of Electromagnetic Shielding," *Nature* 251, no. 5476 (1974): 602–7.
60 Targ and Puthoff, "Information Transmission Under Conditions of Electromagnetic Shielding," 605.
61 Jacobsen, *Phenomena*, 145.
62 McRae, *Mind Wars*, 83–4.
63 Jacobsen, *Phenomena*, 155.
64 Jacobsen, *Phenomena*, 161.

65 McRae, *Mind Wars*, 99.
66 McRae, *Mind Wars*, 102.
67 Jacobsen, *Phenomena*, 182.
68 McRae, *Mind Wars*, 115.
69 McRae, *Mind Wars*, 105.
70 McRae, *Mind Wars*, 106.
71 US Defense Intelligence Agency, "Psychoenergetics Research," Defense Intelligence Agency Directorate of Scientific and Technical Intelligence, August 7, 1984, 17.
72 US Defense Intelligence Agency, "Project Sun Streak," Directorate of Science and Technology, undated, available at: https://nsarchive2.gwu.edu/NSAEBB/NSAEBB534-DIA-Declassified-Sourcebook/documents/DIA-21.pdf.
73 Defense Intelligence Agency, "Psychoenergetics Research," 3.
74 Edwin C. May, Victor Rubel, Joseph W. McMoneagle, and Loyd Auerbach, *ESP Wars East and West: An Account of the Military Use of Psychic Espionage as Narrated by Key Russian and American Players* (Crossroad Press Kindle, 2015), 122.
75 May, Rubel, McMoneagle, and Auerbach, *ESP Wars East and West*, 120–1.
76 May, Rubel, McMoneagle, and Auerbach, *ESP Wars East and West*, 121–2.
77 May, Rubel, McMoneagle, and Auerbach, *ESP Wars East and West*, 74.
78 Michael D. Mumford, Andrew M. Rose, and David A. Goslin, "An Evaluation of Remote Viewing: Research and Applications," The American Institutes for Research, September 29, 1995, E-2.
79 Mumford, Rose, and Goslin, "An Evaluation of Remote Viewing," E-4.
80 Mark Pilkington, "The Remote Viewers," *The Guardian*, June 4, 2005, available at: https://www.theguardian.com/science/2003/jun/05/research.science1.
81 McRae, *Mind Wars*, 125.
82 Ebon, *Psychic Warfare*, 99.
83 Timothy Thomas, "The Mind Has No Firewall," *Parameters* 28, no. 1 (1998): 85.
84 Thomas, "The Mind Has No Firewall," 89.
85 Maire and LaMothe, "Soviet and Czechoslovakian Parapsychology Research," 33.
86 Maire and LaMothe, "Soviet and Czechoslovakian Parapsychology Research," 34.
87 Ostrander and Schroeder, *Psychic Discoveries*, 285.
88 Ostrander and Schroeder, *Psychic Discoveries*, 288.
89 Thomas Bearden, *Excalibur Briefing: Explaining Paranormal Phenomena* (San Francisco: Strawberry Hill Press, 1988), 316, note 163.
90 US Defense Intelligence Agency, "Scalar Waves," Memo, undated, available at: https://www.cia.gov/readingroom/docs/CIA-RDP96-00792R000500240001-6.pdf.
91 Bearden, *Excalibur Briefing*, XXXII.

92 Bearden, *Excalibur Briefing*, 100, 103.
93 Dolan M. McKelvy, "Psychic Warfare: Exploring the Mind Frontier," Montgomery, Air War College, Research Report, 1988, 28.
94 Robert McCreight, "The War Inside Your Mind: Unprotected Brain Battlefields and Neuro-Vulnerability," *Academia Biology*, February 6, 2024, 4, https://doi.org/10.20935/AcadBiol6156.
95 McCreight, "The War Inside Your Mind," 4.
96 Alexander, "The New Mental Battlefield—Beam Me Up, Spock," 47.
97 Alexander, "The New Mental Battlefield—Beam Me Up, Spock," 52.
98 Ostrander and Schroeder, *Psychic Discoveries*, 330.
99 Ostrander and Schroeder, *Psychic Discoveries*, 329.
100 Flora Lewis, "Émigré Tells of Research in Soviet Parapsychology for Military Use," *New York Times*, June 19, 1977.
101 Paranormal TV, "KGB Psychic Weapons Research," November 15, 2007, available at: https://www.youtube.com/watch?v=jexw2TAliRc&t=126s.
102 May, Rubel, McMoneagle, and Auerbach, *ESP Wars East and West.*
103 May, Rubel, McMoneagle, and Auerbach, *ESP Wars East and West*, 155.
104 May, Rubel, McMoneagle, and Auerbach, *ESP Wars East and West*, 155.
105 May, Rubel, McMoneagle, and Auerbach, *ESP Wars East and West*, 174.
106 May, Rubel, McMoneagle, and Auerbach, *ESP Wars East and West*, 174.
107 May, Rubel, McMoneagle, and Auerbach, *ESP Wars East and West*, 174.
108 May, Rubel, McMoneagle, and Auerbach, *ESP Wars East and West*, 174–5.
109 Bearden, *Excalibur Briefing*, 286.
110 Bearden, *Excalibur Briefing*, 287.
111 Bearden, *Excalibur Briefing*, 287, 289.
112 Bearden, *Excalibur Briefing*, 290.
113 Bearden, *Excalibur Briefing*, 292.
114 Paranormal TV, "KGB Psychic Weapons Research."
115 Ostrander and Schroeder, *Psychic Discoveries*, 331–2.
116 Mark Tapscott, "DOD, Intel Agencies Look at Russian Mind Control Technology, Claims," *Defense Electronics,* July 1993, 17.
117 Ostrander and Schroeder, *Psychic Discoveries*, 333–4.
118 Sharon Weinberger, "The Weird Russian Mind-Control Research Behind a DHS Contract," *Wired*, September 28, 2007, available at: https://www.wired.com/2007/09/mind-reading/.
119 Timothy Thomas, "The Russian View of Information War," in *The Russian Armed Forces at the Dawn of the Millenium*, ed. Michael C. Crutcher (Carlisle: US Army War College, December 2000), 340.
120 Thomas, "The Russian View of Information War," 337.

121 Thomas, "The Russian View of Information War," 346.
122 Sputnik International Staff, "Russia Eyes Development of Futuristic Weaponry," *Sputnik International*, March 23, 2012, available at: https://sputnikglobe.com/20120322/172332421.html.
123 Christopher Leake and Will Stewart, "Putin Targets Foes with 'Zombie' Gun Which Attack Victims' Central Nervous System," *Daily Mail*, March 31, 2012, available at: https://www.dailymail.co.uk/news/article-2123415/Putin-targets-foes-zombie-gun-attack-victims-central-nervous-system.html.

4

Nonlethal Weapons and Directed Energy

A weapon that can induce Havana Syndrome would be considered a NLW since it does not kill people targeted with it outright. Although there is no public documentation of the US military having successfully developed "psychotronic weapons," there is some literature on the research into and development of many kinds of NLWs that are designed to disorient and otherwise incapacitate people using directed energy. NLW is a very broad category of weapons that includes electromagnetic weapons, chemical options, physical restraints, low kinetic impact munitions, acoustic weapons, information warfare, and biological agents.[1] The focus of the chapter will be on nonlethal DEWs since this is the most likely type of weapon that could be responsible for Havana Syndrome. Some of the US NLW research of the 1980s and beyond seems to be based on Soviet psychotronic weapons research, as far as it concerns the connections to electromagnetic and acoustic devices and subliminal/hypnosis-based devices. Not surprisingly, these aspects of NLW research and development seem to be highly classified as there is relatively little information on them in the public domain.[2] It is therefore quite difficult to find good information on nonlethal DEWs, despite general discussions of these types of weapons that indicate that they are feasible and may exist.

The Concept of Nonlethal Weapons

NLW are weapons that are specifically designed to incapacitate rather than kill people, which does not mean that NLW would be always nonlethal. The Department of Defense (DoD) defines NLW as "Weapons, devices and munitions that are explicitly designed and primarily employed to incapacitate targeted personnel or materiel immediately, while minimizing fatalities, permanent injury to personnel, and undesired damage to property in the targeted area or environment. NLW are intended to have reversible effects on personnel or materiel."[3] Furthermore, "[u]nlike conventional lethal weapons that destroy their targets principally through blast, penetration, and fragmentation, NLW employ means other than gross physical destruction to prevent the target from functioning. NLW are intended to have relatively reversible effects on personnel or materiel."[4]

Key ideas contained in the definition are that the aim of NLW is temporary incapacitation and non-permanent or reversible effects on either personnel or material. NLW are meant to offer a more humane option for neutralizing or disabling a target and reducing death and severe injury of noncombatants.[5] NLWs are, in the Pentagon definition, distinct from information warfare (the use of propaganda) and electronic warfare (electromagnetic jamming).[6] While nonlethality is the intended effect, people attacked with NLW can still die because of NLW usage if they were particularly vulnerable because of age, medical conditions, or other factors, or if a NLW was used incorrectly or inappropriately. The lethal potential of NLW was acknowledged by the US government as early as 1972.[7] Therefore, NLW are sometimes referred to as "less lethal weapons" rather than "nonlethal weapons."

The US military has been interested in nonlethal capabilities since at least the late 1940s when the US Army and the CIA started to investigate chemical incapacitants such as hallucinogens for a broad attack on an enemy population.[8] US Army chemist Wilson Greene argued that "through the techniques of psychochemical warfare, to conquer an enemy without the wholesale killing of his people or destroying his property."[9] The label of "nonlethal weapons" began to be used by policymakers and law enforcement officials in the 1960s to refer to a range of weapons that were used for riot control purposes.[10] The US military started using CS gas in Vietnam from 1965 for riot control and from 1968 also in support of combat operations.[11] In the late 1960s, the US government started to fund the development of new NLWs for law enforcement and riot control. The main NLWs under development at the time were low kinetic impact munitions (rubber bullets or "bean bags") and electrical weapons (tasers).

In the 1970s, the United States and the Soviet Union were also investigating the incapacitating effects of electromagnetic waves, acoustic waves, flicker light, and biochemical agents.[12] Although these technologies were identified for potential development into NLW, it seems that they were given a low military priority in the Cold War context.[13] Only after the 1991 Gulf War did the US military begin to look more seriously into nonlethal capabilities in the context of UN peacekeeping operations, which require less lethal force.

Lieutenant General Anthony Zinni used a range of new NLWs in support of the US withdrawal from Somalia in 1995, including sticky foam, rubber bullets, and laser dazzlers.[14] In July 1996, the Department of Defense issued Directive 3000.3. It called for the establishment of a joint services organization tasked with the development and employment of NLW, which became the DoD Joint Non-Lethal Weapons Program (JNLWP) launched in 1997.[15] The JNLWP had only very modest funding of $25 million to $30 million per year.[16] In May 2020, the JNLWP was renamed Joint Intermediate Force Capabilities Office (JIFCO) to reflect a change in its mission. The term currently preferred by the Department of Defense is "intermediate force," which is "[t]he application of force to deliver effects below lethal intent, when the presence and threat of force is insufficient, and the application of lethal force is unsuitable or undesirable, in order to temporarily impair, disrupt, delay, or neutralize targets across all domains."[17] Intermediate force can be used in the context of so-called "gray zone conflict," where adversaries engage in hostile activities deliberately designed to remain below the threshold of an act of war.[18]

Applications for NLW

There are many reasons why it is sometimes preferable to produce nonlethal rather than lethal effects that makes NLW technology desirable. The original purpose of NLW was riot control and policing, which continues to be an important aspect driving NLW development. The US military has used NLW in the context of peacekeeping, stability, and counterinsurgency operations, which require a minimal use of force for success. As early as 1970, the US government think tank Institute for Defense Analysis advocated for nonlethal technologies in low-intensity conflict.[19] The JNLWP reasoned in 1997 that "any conflict has associated political objectives, and the accomplishment of these objectives is often enhanced by minimizing non-combatant casualties and collateral damage."[20] Modern militaries have to often operate among the people and NLW, which makes it inappropriate, if not illegal, to use heavy firepower associated with conventional military capabilities. NLW can protect civilian lives in situations where civilians and combatants are difficult to distinguish or are co-located.

According to Robert Mandel, "in the aftermath of the terrorist attacks of September 11, 2001, the nonlethal weaponry issue emerged front and center."[21] In 2002, the Russian special services used a chemical incapacitant to facilitate the storming of a Moscow theater that had been occupied by Chechen terrorists armed with automatic weapons and explosives.[22] The episode seemed to suggest that NLW can be effective in hostage liberation situations, even though tragically 129 of the over 800 hostages had died from the effects of the used chemical incapacitant.[23] One year later, the US military was tasked with the occupation of Iraq and with fighting an insurgency that erupted in summer 2003. For well over a decade, the US military fought counterinsurgency campaigns in both Iraq and Afghanistan, which provided an opportunity to test new nonlethal capabilities in battle. NLW have also been used to fight pirates, for crowd control, and for securing checkpoints and facilities.

More recently, the strategic focus of the US military shifted from counterinsurgency and counterterrorism operations in developing countries to fighting major contingency operations against near-peer competitors Russia and China. Since 2013, American strategists have been concerned about so-called "gray zone conflict," which relies on ambiguous, deniable, and indirect actions below the threshold of war.[24] This change was reflected in the 2017 National Security Strategy, which stated that "China and Russia challenge American power, influence, and interests, attempting to erode American security and prosperity."[25] The 2022 National Security Strategy even warned that "[t]he risk of conflict between major powers is increasing" and that "[m]ore capable competitors and new strategies of threatening behavior below and above the traditional threshold of conflict mean we cannot afford to rely solely on conventional forces and nuclear deterrence."[26]

The new focus on near-peer competitors and gray zone conflict has also made nonlethal capabilities more relevant again. Analysts from the think tank RAND have argued that "in 'gray-zone' confrontations short of war with other powers, they can be used to demonstrate resolve while limiting the risk of unwanted escalation" and that "NLWs can be particularly useful when another party's intent is unclear."[27] Nonlethal capabilities would allow the US military to credibly respond to the gray zone actions of adversaries with a lesser risk of escalation. The Joint Chiefs of Staff suggested that "[k]ey to credibility are military capabilities that enable joint forces to counter threats below the level of traditional armed conflict with lethal or intermediate force. When challenged, the Joint Force must impose a cost on adversaries' unacceptable coercive and subversive activities."[28]

The US military has also used the term "non-kinetic effects" to describe military capabilities that do not rely on physical destruction, which include electronic warfare, cyber warfare, and information warfare. Some overlap with NLWs and capabilities is apparent. Robert McCreight has proposed the term "non-kinetic threats," which would "consist of silent, largely undetectable technologies capable of inflicting damaging, debilitating, and degrading physical and neural effects on its unwitting targets. This covert threat is best understood as something to be invoked via rapid surprise attack or as a stealthy forerunner to a **massive kinetic** follow-on attack."[29] In other words, non-kinetic and nonlethal capabilities could be covertly used to soften up an unsuspecting target in preparation for an all-out lethal attack.

Some Ethical and Legal Considerations

While nonlethality is usually praised as a more humane way of conducting conflict, there are also many unresolved ethical and legal issues that make the use of NLWs very controversial. First, NLWs may be used to make subsequent lethal attacks more effective, hence subverting the idea of reducing the number of deaths in war. Eliot Cohen pointed out that "[s]ome of these weapons (blinding lasers) may not kill, but have exceedingly nasty consequences for their victims. And in the end a disabling weapon only works if it leaves an opponent more vulnerable to full-scale deadly force."[30] Nonlethal capabilities are considered an adjunct and not a replacement for lethal capabilities.[31] Since NLWs could make lethal attacks more effective, they could overall make warfare more deadly rather than less deadly.[32]

Secondly, having a supposed nonlethal option may encourage the overuse of the option since it is perhaps wrongly assumed that no permanent damage would occur. Law enforcement officers have used tasers on people with heart conditions, causing them to die, and they may have used tasers in situations that did not call for the use of force.[33] Military commanders may be tempted to indiscriminately target civilians with NLW because they incorrectly assume that the effects would be mild. Even if effects were mild, this still violates the Geneva Conventions, which prohibit the deliberate targeting of civilians with military force, regardless as to whether it is lethal or nonlethal force.[34] There is also a concern that NLW could be used deliberately as instruments of torture.[35]

Fourthly, certain types of NLW may violate existing international treaties. Nonlethal chemical and biological agents could run afoul of other international laws, most importantly the Chemical Weapons Convention and the Biological and Toxin Weapons Convention, which do not make exceptions for nonlethal uses.[36] So-called bioregulators, which are biochemicals produced by the body and which regulate body functions, are under development despite international prohibitions.[37] Some weapons that have less lethal effects may not have effects that are reversible and may be inherently inhumane. The UN worked on the prohibition of inhumane weapons in the 1970s, which led to the Convention on Certain Conventional Weapons of 1980.[38] It specifically outlaws non-detectable fragments, booby traps, incendiary weapons, blinding lasers, and explosive remnants of war.[39] Any weapon that may cause "superfluous injury or unnecessary suffering" in principle violates the conventions of war. Among the factors for establishing whether a weapon causes superfluous injury and unnecessary suffering are: (1) "specific disease, specific abnormal physiological state, specific abnormal psychological state, specific and permanent disability or specific disfigurement," (2) "field mortality of more than 25% or a hospital mortality of more than 5%," (3) "Grade 3 wounds as measured by the Red Cross wound classification," and (4) "effects for which there is no well recognized and proven treatment." A weapon that could cause Havana Syndrome very likely would fall under this international prohibition (even if it was used against combatants) since it causes arguably excessive suffering and excessive injury (it causes a specific permanent disability and there is no available treatment).

Fifthly, as Michael Gross has pointed out, "[h]uman testing is essential for assessing the effects and effectiveness of all nonlethal weapons."[40] NLW development may require the active participation of the medical profession, which in itself raises serious ethical questions. Human experimentation would be needed to determine the precise weapons' effects and to establish safe thresholds for exposure. Obtaining this kind of data may violate the principles established in the Nuremberg Code, which includes not only the requirement of informed consent but also "[t]he experiment should be so conducted as to avoid all unnecessary physical and mental suffering and injury," and the experimental subject must be protected "against even remote possibilities of injury, disability, or death."[41] The US government conducted unethical human experiments during the Cold War period, also in relation to NLW development (hallucinogenic and psychoactive drug testing on unwitting test subjects).[42] It is possible that unethical human experimentation for the purpose of NLW development may still happen in some countries.

Finally, because of their sometimes-questionable status under international law and the close connection to human experimentation and the need to perform unethical experimentation for NLW development, these weapons technologies tend to be secret. There is also the argument that NLW development programs must be classified since adversaries could develop countermeasures to nonlethal technologies.[43] Steven Aftergood suggested that "[b]ecause most non-lethal weapons programs are classified, they are shielded from the democratic process. Such secrecy precludes informed public discussion of the most basic policy issues as well."[44] Some of the NLW under development in the United States are so-called Special Access (SAPs) programs that are not subject to the normal oversight and accountability mechanisms that apply to other government spending. Relatively few people in the US government are "read into" SAPs and even know that these projects exist.[45] Since many nonlethal technologies and potential existing weapons are shielded by secrecy, there is great uncertainty as to how these technologies would work, whether they would work, and whether there would be any long-term risks. Neil Davison has argued that "[t]he associated ethical issues [of NLWs] are profound, especially due to the potential for social control if such weapons were actually realised and used either in policing or warfare."[46] This consideration may motivate government secrecy since it prevents public criticism or a public debate about these weapons and the potential for government abuses.

Directed Energy Weapons

Directed energy is a disruptive or revolutionary technology that could make kinetic weapons (bombs and bullets) completely obsolete in the long-term. The US military has defined DEWs "as electromagnetic systems capable of converting chemical or electrical energy to radiated energy and focusing it on a target, resulting in physical damage that degrades, neutralizes, defeats or destroys an adversarial capability."[47] DEWs offer numerous advantages over projectile weapons and explosives, which is the reason why so many militaries around the world are investing heavily in the R&D of DEWs. The US military is spending over $1 billion per year on the development of DEWs.[48] There are different types of DEWs that can be used for different types of applications and missions. DEWs include acoustic weapons, millimeter wave weapons, high-powered microwaves, EMP weapons, lasers, laser dazzlers, and particle beam weapons. DEWs can range in size from small handheld devices to systems that are so heavy and large that they can only be placed on warships like destroyers. DEWs are extremely versatile, precise, cheap per shot fired, and easy to support logistically (once the support infrastructure is created).

Speed of Light and Long Range

In war, it is preferable to produce effects as quickly as possible to prevent the adversary from taking evasive action or shooting first. DEWs theoretically allow almost instant effects on a target, making any response by the target to an attack impossible and thereby increasing the likelihood that the target will be destroyed or disabled. Lasers can hit a target at near light speed, which is 186,000 miles per second. Even a hypersonic missile with a speed of 4,000 miles per hour is a lot slower than a laser.[49] Faster speed of engagement is also accompanied by longer range. High-powered laser weapons can have effective ranges of hundreds of kilometers, but microwave weapons would only have a range of hundreds of meters.[50] The long range of laser weapons makes it possible to place them on aircraft or even on an orbiting satellite to attack aerial targets well beyond visible range, targets on the ground, or the surface of the earth.

Precision Strikes

DEWs tend to be more precise than projectile weapons as they have a flat trajectory and are somewhat less affected by atmospheric conditions, wind, and air resistance.[51] Lasers have demonstrated that they can be pointed with very high precision at fast-moving targets such as ballistic missiles and destroy them in flight. According to a Center for Strategic and Budgetary Assessments report, "[f]uture laser weapons could be very precisely focused to permit U.S. troops to engage targets surgically, even in very close proximity to friendly forces or noncombatants."[52] Many DEWs allow targeting objects with a narrow beam that will not cause damage to anything outside the beam, which reduces collateral damage. For example, "[a] future gunship aircraft with a suitable laser system may be capable of striking high-value targets with little risk of unwanted collateral damage, a novel capability that would be especially important during operations in urban terrain against irregular forces."[53]

Deep Magazines

A DEW can keep firing as long as its supply of energy is not exhausted. In theory, a DEW could keep firing indefinitely if the energy it uses was continuously generated, for example, by a nearby power plant. Deep magazines extend the mission times of platforms, as pointed out by DoD's Center for Strategic and Budgetary Assessment: "Electric-powered DE weapons could increase the mission duration of air-refuelable aircraft that currently carry expendable air-to-air and air-to-surface munitions. Similarly, DE weapons could increase the time-on-station of deployed naval vessels, since their 'magazines' would not require periodic replenishment at a port facility."[54] Any type of DEW only needs one type of munition, which is energy or electricity. This simplifies logistics, as there is no need for producing, stockpiling, and supplying in the field different types of munitions needed for different types of weapons.

Variable Effects from Nonlethal to Lethal

The same DEW can potentially produce both nonlethal and lethal effects, which could be adjusted for a given mission or purpose. They can be used both against material and against personnel with scalable or variable effects as needed. The Lexington Institute has argued that a

> related feature is that the effects of directed-energy weapons can be tailored to achieve a range of results, lethal or nonlethal, destructive or disruptive. This is achieved primarily by adjusting the amount of energy that is deposited on targets or the wavelengths at which the energy is delivered. For example, radio-frequency weapons can generate waves at particular frequencies and power levels to accomplish the temporary upset of certain types of electronic devices while leaving other types unscathed.[55]

The main factors for the type of effect produced by a DEW are "the time on target, the distance to the target, and even the part of the target on which the DEW is focused."[56] In other words, a lower output may just temporarily disable/incapacitate a target while a higher output may destroy/kill it.

Deniable Attacks

The practice of warfare is shifting toward the application of force that is covert or deniable. It is a long-term trend that was already recognized in a research report by the Department of Justice and DoD from 1997, which suggested that

> [i]ncreasingly, the military finds itself conducting operations such as peacekeeping, in which it is confronted by an absolute mandate to apply force discreetly and then to use only the minimum amount of force necessary to accomplish a particular mission. . . . A further consideration that affects how the military and law enforcement apply force is the greater presence of members of

> the media or other civilians who are observing, if not recording, the situation. Even the lawful application of force can be misrepresented to or misunderstood by the public. More than ever, the police and the military must be highly discreet when applying force.[57]

DEWs allow the military and law enforcement to be discreet in the application of force as they do not leave behind many traces and may not produce effects that can be easily attributed to a DEW attack. Electromagnetic or acoustic waves or lasers are not visible to the naked eye and typically they are silent too.[58] There is no projectile that is left behind or an explosion that leaves behind chemical traces of the explosives and bomb fragments. People who are targeted could be incapacitated in a manner that prevents them from doing harm and that is not apparent to others around them, which sidesteps thorny issues related to how the use of force would be perceived by the public in a specific situation.

Acoustic Weapons

Initially, there was media speculation that the Havana Syndrome weapon may have been an unknown "sonic" or "acoustic" weapon, which had been conceptionalized since at least the 1960s. Acoustic weapons are a special type of DEWs that use sound as a mechanism for incapacitation or injury. Sound requires a medium (air) in which it propagates a mechanical wave, which can affect a receiving object by way of mechanical vibrations.[59] The specific effects depend on "frequency, sound pressure level, and duration."[60] In principle, an acoustic weapon may use audible sound in the frequency range above 20 Hz and below 20,000 Hz, or inaudible sounds in the low frequency range of 1 Hz to 20 Hz (infrasound) and the high frequency range above 20,000 Hz (ultrasound).[61] Sound pressure relates to the intensity of the sound (loudness or volume) and is measured in decibels (dB). Some sound pressure (above 0 dB) is necessary for the human ear to hear, but higher levels cause discomfort (above 120 dB) and become painful above 140 dB, although hearing damage can already occur at already 85 dB at prolonged exposure.[62] The longer the duration of exposure to loud noise, the more likely it becomes that hearing loss occurs.

Audible Sound

Loud audible sounds have been known since ancient times to have destructive effects. According to a biblical story, the Israelites brought down the walls of Jericho through loud cries and trumpets.[63] Loud noises can distract and cause stress or discomfort. One example of how this can be weaponized is flashbang grenades that are meant to stun people for several seconds with loud noise and bright light. Militaries have used loud sounds and music for psychologically manipulating enemies. Loudspeakers are used on the battlefield for psychological operations, including appeals to enemy forces to surrender or desert, noises that are meant to increase fear, and noises that are meant to distract or deceive enemy forces.[64] Loudspeakers and directed audible sound devices can also be used for issuing specific commands to others over a distance, for example, not to approach or to lay down their weapons. However, it might not make sense to characterize loudspeaker systems as weapons if their use was limited to appealing to or commanding others over distance.[65] A weapon must be able to cause harm or inflict damage. However, there is little doubt that audible sound devices can do that.

According to John B. Alexander, audible sound acoustic devices should be included in NLWs as they can force people out of an area such as the perimeter of an embassy. He argued:

> The objective of antipersonnel acoustic weapons is not to create untenable sound, but rather to vibrate the targeted people physically. To establish barriers or to cause people to move from a restricted area, it is necessary to do more than make loud noises. . . . Acoustic weapons will range from 120 dB to as high as 170 dB. At levels above 150 dB, internal injury can occur.[66]

Neil Davison suggested that ear pain occurs at 140 dB, that vestibular effects (balance), effects on respiratory organs, and permanent hearing loss from short exposure occur at 150 dB, and that the eardrum ruptures at 160 dB.[67] At 200 dB, which can be generated by blast waves from explosions, the lungs rupture, and at 210 dB death would occur.[68]

The US Navy started to develop an audible sound acoustic weapon after the attack on the U.S.S. *Cole* in Yemen in 2000. The American Technology Corporation Inc. (ATC) was awarded in 2002 a contract to build an acoustic weapon now known as the Long-Range Acoustic Device (LRAD).[69] The company name has since changed to Genasys, which offers many different versions of their LRAD system for applications in defense, law enforcement, fire and rescue, homeland and border security, critical infrastructure protection, and maritime safety. The models range in size from very small (15 lbs) to large (208 lbs) and in terms of sound pressure and range from 600 meters and 140 dB for the portable system to 3,000 meters and 155 dB for the truck-mounted system.[70] LRAD can project loud noise or speech over long distances in a directional narrow beam, "using a short wavelength ultrasonic carrier, modulated by speech or other signal."[71] However, LRAD has not been classified as a weapon, although it can cause discomfort, pain, and hearing loss to those exposed, depending on intensity, duration, and distance.[72] From September 2005, over 350 LRAD systems were deployed with US forces in Iraq.[73]

Infrasound

Infrasound relates to sound waves in the 0 Hz to 20 Hz range, and it is produced by natural phenomena such as thunder, sea waves, wind turbulence, and volcanic eruptions.[74] Since infrasound uses the same frequency range as brain waves, there have been long-term suspicions that it could interfere with brain function and human well-being.[75] In a well-documented instance (the Dyatlov incident), infrasound generated by wind passing through the Ural mountain ridges may have disoriented a group of hikers in 1959 so much that they ran in the middle of the night, lightly dressed from their camp and perished.[76] There has been a lot of speculation with respect to the weaponization of infrasound as some authors have claimed that it could cause severe effects on humans and structures, but these claims still lack independent scientific confirmation.

The myth of lethal infrasound was apparently started by the French acoustician Vladimir Gavreau in the 1960s.[77] Gavreau made his discovery accidentally by noticing physiological effects on himself and others around him, seemingly caused by a defective ventilation system in his office building, which emitted inaudible infrasound at around 7 Hz. Their eardrums were sometimes painfully compressed by the infrasound waves, which gave him the idea that infrasound could be weaponized.[78] He decided to build an infrasound weapon that he called an "acoustic gun," which produced infrasound at 196 Hz and at 160 dB and which was reportedly able to produce "very nearly lethal" effects.[79] Ever since, there have been claims in the literature on NLWs and in government reports that infrasound could induce effects such as nausea, vomiting, and uncontrolled defecation.

A US Air Force Academy reference work on NLWs and related technologies assembled by Robert Bunker suggested the following about the effects of infrasound:

> Very low-frequency sound which can travel long distances and easily penetrate most buildings and vehicles. Transmission of long wavelength sound creates biophysical effects; nausea, loss of bowels, disorientation, vomiting, potential internal organ damage or death may occur. Superior to ultrasound because it is "in band" meaning that it does not lose its properties when it changes mediums such as from air to tissue. By 1972 an infrasound generator had been built in France which generated waves at 7 hertz. When activated it made the people in range sick for hours.[80]

Alexander similarly suggested that infrasound can disorient people and even damage buildings at sufficiently high intensity.[81] A DoD literature review of nonlethal technologies suggested that experiments with human subjects indicated the following effects of low audible and infrasound: nystagmus (involuntary eye movement where a person sees their own surroundings turn) and vestibular effects (loss of balance) occurred in a lab at five to ten second exposures at 125 dB in the 200–500 Hz range, or at 140 dB at 1,000 Hz, or at 155 dB at 200 Hz.[82] The British military may have developed an infrasound weapon in 1973 called the "squawk box" that emitted two near ultrasound frequencies and combine them to produce a 2 Hz infrasound frequency that was intolerable.[83]

Jürgen Altmann, who is a physicist specialized in acoustics has conducted experiments to investigate claims made by NLW proponents, suggested that the supposed effects of infrasound have been greatly exaggerated. According to Altmann, "Contrary to several articles in the defence press, high-power infrasound has no profound effect on humans. The pain threshold is higher than in the audio range, and there is no hard evidence for the alleged effects on inner organs, on the vestibular system, for vomiting, or uncontrolled defecation up to levels of 170 dB or more."[84] He also suggested that infrasound weapons may be impractical: a transmitter would need to be very large (perhaps 3 meters in diameter) and the effective distance would be less than 50 meters.[85] It has been therefore argued that although strong infrasound generators are feasible, they may be impractical since they require banks of large specialized speakers with high-powered amplifiers, which would also require a specialized large cooling system.[86]

Ultrasound

Ultrasound uses frequencies above 20,000 Hz, and it has different characteristics than infrasound. Ultrasound can penetrate body tissue and is used in medicine for diagnostic imaging, for the destruction of kidney stones, and even for transcranial brain stimulation. According to a report by Scientific Applications and Research Associates produced for the US Army in 1996, high audible sound and ultrasound could at frequencies of 5,000 to 30,000 Hz heat the body temperature to lethal levels, cause tissue burns, dehydration, and micro-lesions in tissue.[87] Altmann mentioned that in the 1950s, there were concerns that ultrasound produced by jet engines could cause headaches, nausea, and fatigue in people exposed.[88] However, where these effects were observed, it was also the case that infrasound and audible sound were present too. Ultrasound at 160–165 dB is known to cause a tickling sensation in the nose and mouth, as well as a sensation of heating. In theory, above 180 dB with an exposure time of fifty minutes, overheating the body would cause death.[89]

The practicality of an ultrasonic weapon seems questionable. Alexander suggested that "the high frequencies involved do not propagate as well as the lower frequencies and can easily be blocked. I am not aware of any attempt to develop weapons in the ultrasonic range."[90] However, ultrasound is used for making sound directional and to project audible sound in a narrow beam that could not be perceived by people outside of the beam. This makes it possible to talk to individuals over distance without others in close proximity hearing the sound, which could be useful for clandestine communication or psychological operations.[91] However, ultrasound is difficult to transmit through walls or closed windows.[92]

An article published by William Thomas online alleged that the US military was secretly using sonar systems in Iraq to pacify the Iraqis. The devices were called "poppers" or "domes" and consisted of transmitters derived from naval equipment for undersea communication and sonars that were generating signals in the ULF, VLF, and UHF frequency ranges.[93] These transmitters were placed in Baghdad to irradiate entire neighborhoods with the supposed effect of constant exposure of making exposed people "stupid for two or three days."[94] Constant exposure would feel like a low-pressure weather system that dampens the energy and the mood of people. No further confirmation of this information could be found.

Subliminals

Subliminals can be visual or acoustic, and they can be weaponized to manipulate people. The main idea behind subliminals is that it is perceptual information that is registered by the brain subconsciously and hence is not consciously perceived by the mind. The subliminal information can still influence perceptions, beliefs, and behavior and has therefore great utility in marketing, political campaigns, and psychological operations. Although the effectiveness or use of subliminals in psychological operations has never been officially acknowledged, rumors that the US military has operationally used subliminals have been circulating for decades.

According to a story by British TV station ITV from 1991, US psyops units broadcast subliminal messages with an FM radio transmitter at the same frequency as an Iraqi radio station.[95] The audible transmissions contained patriotic and religious music, but the inaudible ultrasound subliminal messages were meant to demoralize the Iraqi soldiers in Kuwait listening in. ITV reported, "[a]lthough completely silent to the human ear, the negative voice messages placed on the tapes alongside the audible programming by PSYOPS psychologists were clearly perceived by the subconscious minds of the Iraqi soldiers and the silent messages completely demoralized them and instilled a perpetual feeling of fear and hopelessness in their minds."[96] According to Judy Wall, the ultrasound signal altered the brain waves of the Iraqi soldiers and could induce specific emotions even without the subliminal message. She suggested that the technology was based on an invention by Oliver Lowery called Silent Sound Spread Spectrum or "S-quad."[97] The patent filed by Lowery in 1989 claimed the following:

> A silent communications system in which nonaural carriers, in the very low or very high audio frequency range or in the adjacent ultrasonic frequency spectrum, are amplitude or frequency modulated with the desired intelligence and propagated acoustically or vibrationally, for inducement into the brain, typically through the use of loudspeakers, earphones or piezoelectric transducers. The modulated carriers may be transmitted directly in real time or may be conveniently recorded and stored on mechanical, magnetic or optical media for delayed or repeated transmission to the listener.[98]

The description of the technology does fit the description of its potential use during the 1991 Gulf War. Messages that use inaudible sound could theoretically be picked up by the brain subconsciously and induce emotions and shape behaviors. However, the ultrasound source would have to be in close proximity to the target.

Electromagnetic Weapons

Research into the uses of electromagnetic waves for nonlethal weaponry goes back to the Second World War when Japan was trying to develop a "death ray."[99] Electromagnetic weapons are primarily discussed in the literature on NLW in terms of anti-material weapons: they can disrupt any kind of electric or electronic device or machinery. Well known is the concept of the electromagnetic pulse (EMP), which can destroy electronic components by overcharging the transistors, which will physically destroy them.[100] Less known and far more controversial are the potential antipersonnel applications of electromagnetic weaponry.

High-Powered RF and Microwaves

Microwaves are electromagnetic waves in the frequency range of 300 MHz to 300 GHz, and they have short wavelengths between 1 mm and 1 meter. Microwaves can be continuous wave (CW) or pulsed. If pulsed, they can have different pulse widths or duration of a pulse and different pulse repetition frequencies. They can also have different amplitudes and different power outputs. This means that the characteristics of microwaves vary greatly, as do the effects that they might cause on a target. According to an Air War College paper by John Geis, "[t]his is why an 800-watt (illegal) Citizen's Band radio booster amplifier at 20 MHz is harmless, but watching one's dinner cook from inside an 800-watt (typical) microwave oven would be fatal."[101] It follows that "[d]esigning an HPM is strongly influenced by the electromagnetic properties of the target. The great complexity of real systems makes this basically an experimental problem."[102] HPMs are known to cause three different categories of effects, namely heating effects, bioeffects, and effects on electronics.[103]

The heating effects are well understood and have been mentioned before: heating the brain by 1°C can cause disruption of working memory and disorientation with an onset time of fifteen minutes to thirty minutes. Prolonged hyperthermia (heating above 41°C) will cause brain damage and death.[104] The main challenge is to achieve a high enough power output for a heating effect, which means that it would not be a portable system, but it could be used in the form of a truck-mounted system with a directional antenna that could be hidden inside a larger vehicle.

Since the 1980s, there have been efforts by the superpowers to weaponize the microwave heating effect for antipersonnel applications. The Soviet

Union reportedly developed a short-range tactical RF weapon that could kill a goat from a distance of 1 kilometer.[105] It was reported by *Spotlight* magazine in 1996 that the Pentagon had awarded a contract for the development of "high-power electromagnetic generators to interfere with human brain waves," but there is no independent confirmation of the claim.[106] The bioeffects of HPMs are insufficiently understood as there is not enough physiological data.[107] The only area where actual weapons have been developed and are acknowledged to exist is the use of HPMs for interfering with or destroying electronics.

HPMs are feasible as a weapons technology with respect to their use against electronics. According to David Guyatt, it is known since 1943 that engines of cars can be remotely turned on or off by tuned waves and that internal organs can be damaged by waves in the RF range between 60 cm and 2 meters.[108] The US Air Force Research Laboratory (AFRL) has funded the Counter-electronics High-Power Microwave Advanced Missile (CHAMP) project built by Boeing. As of 2019, the US Air Force has deployed at least twenty CHAMP missiles, which are air-launched cruise missiles that can be carried by B-52 bombers and which are able to disable electronic devices and equipment in a target area.[109] In theory, the CHAMP missile could knock out the electricity in a city or disable a missile site. The AFRL has also developed a system called Tactical High-Power Operational Responder (THOR), which is designed to destroy drones with HPMs. The system has the size of a shipping container and uses a large disc-shaped antenna that is positioned on top of the container. Several other countries, including Russia, China, and Cuba, have been working on HPM weapons.[110]

According to Edl Schamiloglu, an engineer and defense scientist at the University of New Mexico, HPMs tend to use a lot of power but do so in the form of extremely short (in the range of nanoseconds) repeated pulses that do not cause direct heating. Schamiloglu suggested that such HPMs could have been used in potential attacks on US personnel that caused the Havana Syndrome, even though there were no reported effects on electronics. This would suggest that the power densities were simply lower than those needed for attacks on electronics.[111] It would follow that a weapon that used HPMs may not need to be as big as a shipping container but could be a lot more compact since it required far less power to operate (and hence no large cooling system).

Active Denial System

The ADS was developed by the US AFRL from 1997 at a cost of $51 million, of which $9 million was spent on assessing its safety (as of 2005).[112] Its existence was publicly revealed in 2000. The ADS has been called a millimeter wave rather than a microwave weapon, although the 95 GHz frequency it uses still falls into the microwave range that goes up to 300 GHz. The narrow beam of about 1.5 meters generated by the ADS can penetrate about 0.3 mm to 0.4 mm of the skin to heat it to 45°C to 55°C.[113] A pain sensation occurs within seconds on exposed skin, and the threshold for tissue damage is 25 seconds of exposure.[114] The approximate range of the ADS is 1,000 meters.[115] The main idea of the ADS is to cause a burning sensation on exposed skin that forces people instinctively to move outside of the weapon's beam. The main application of the weapon is crowd control and removing people from, or denying people access to, secure areas and checkpoints.[116]

The ADS was considered for deployment to Iraq in 2005 and was briefly deployed to Afghanistan in 2010, but it was reportedly never used against humans in an operational setting. According to Sharon Weinberger, the reason for the reluctance of the US military to use an NLW that they deemed to be safe was a combination of logistical issues that made it impractical and low effectiveness in adverse weather conditions. The ADS is truck-mounted and requires its own support vehicle, and it takes sixteen hours to cool the microwave generators to 4 kelvins before it can be used.[117] Furthermore, moisture in the air absorbs some of the energy of the microwaves, and hence what was meant to be an unbearable burning sensation becomes some pleasant warming on a cold rainy day.[118] There are also continuing concerns about potential damage to eyes (if a person was looking directly into the beam) and about the possibility that people may not be able to move away from the beam because they are disabled, wounded, or unconscious, which could cause much more serious damage to exposed skin.[119]

The original version of the ADS (System 0) weighed 7.5 tons and was hence difficult to move, but a lighter truck-mounted two-ton version was built for the Marine Corps. Neil Davison has claimed that the US military was working (as of 2008) on several different smaller versions of the ADS, including a HUMVEE-mounted version (100 kW power), an airborne version (larger and more powerful for a C-130 with 3 kilometers range), a portable version on a tripod (400 W power), and even a handheld version (no further details provided).[120]

The US Army developed a new version of the ADS that they call Solid State Active Denial Technology (SS-ADT), which is smaller, lighter, and easier to support logistically.[121] Hambling claimed in 2013 that Raytheon was working on a smaller version of the ADS for law enforcement and maritime security, to be placed on buildings, prisons, and on ships.[122]

ELF, VLF, and Low Power Microwaves

Ever since the 1960s, it has been suggested in some military and journalistic sources that serious incapacitating bioeffects could be achieved at power levels far below the threshold for heating biological tissue, and there have been rumors that such weapons have been developed and may be secretly in use by different governments. There are specific concerns about radiofrequency in the ELF and VLF ranges, as these are close to the frequency range for the brain. Robert O. Becker claimed that ELF waves that "[t]he interaction of abnormal magnetic fields with the brain is now evident . . . there may be direct effects of ELF fields on the nerve cells themselves. These effects are competent to produce behavioral disturbances and learning disabilities."[123]

Defense journalist David Hambling raised the question: "Could new weapons stun or paralyze with a beam of radio energy?"[124] It is hard to give a definitive answer as so little weapons research in this area is public. Hambling cites research carried out at the University of Nevada, which suggests that "a correctly tuned beam of microwaves (possibly pulsed or modulated) would be able to interfere with skeletal muscles."[125] Eldon Byrd, who was the engineer in charge of the Marine Corps Electromagnetic Weapon research program from 1980 to 1983, claimed that he could use very low frequency (VLF) electromagnetic waves to cause the brain to release biochemicals that regulate behavior. He stated: "We could put animals into a stupor. . . . We got chick brains—in vitro—to dump 80 percent of the natural opioids in their brains. . . . These fields were extremely weak. They were undetectable. . . . The effects were nonlethal and reversible. You could disable a person temporarily."[126] According to Byrd, his lab would have been able to develop a stun gun based on this discovered mechanism within a year, but for some reason, the project was cancelled, which could suggest that it was moved into a more classified program.[127]

Lasers

Laser stands for Light Amplification by Stimulated Emission of Radiation and the main difference from microwaves is the much shorter wavelength.[128] The development of lasers goes back over a hundred years, and lasers have been evaluated for military applications since the 1960s. A stepping stone toward the development of lasers was the "maser" built by Charles Townes in 1958, which intensifies microwaves and emits them in a narrow and coherent (identical wavelengths) beam. Lasers work similarly but use the much higher wave frequency spectrum of visible light. A laser focuses light in a very narrow beam that can transmit energy to a target and, with sufficient power, can heat it.

The first laser was built by Theodore Maiman at the Hughes Research Laboratory in Malibu in 1960.[129] Lasers are now widely used by militaries for range finding and target designation, with a few operational uses for air and missile defense and as NLWs (laser dazzlers). They are divided into four classes based on their energy output: class 1 and class 2 lasers have very low-energy output (0.1 mW or less), class 3 has medium-energy output (1–500 mW), and class 4 has high-energy output (everything above 500 mW). Heating is for lasers the main mechanism for injury, although lasers can also cause damage through chemical alterations of tissue and through a mechanical-acoustical effect on tissue when a laser is pulsed at extremely short intervals (1 nanosecond to 0.1 nanoseconds).[130] Obviously, the greater the energy output of the laser, the more harmful or destructive the effects would be. Class 3b lasers (5–500 mW) can cause permanent damage to eyes, while class 4 lasers can cause eye damage and damage to the skin.[131]

Air and Missile Defense Lasers

High-energy lasers (HEL) used by the military for destroying missiles or drones have energy outputs in the tens of thousands of Watts and even millions of Watts, which is powerful enough to burn holes through metals and structures.[132] The Reagan administration funded laser research in connection with its Strategic Defense Initiative (SDI), which was announced in 1983. The idea was to have ground-based or spaceborne lasers that could shoot down incoming ICBMs. Despite the immaturity of the technology in the 1980s, military high-energy laser development continued in the 1990s, which led to several experimental technology platforms such as the Airborne Laser (ABL) testbed. The ABL project was launched in 1996 and was terminated in 2009 because of its high cost—over $5 billion was spent on the development of a chemical oxygen-iodine laser (COIL) carried by a modified Boeing 747 to shoot down enemy missiles in the boost stage (shortly after launch) more than 50 miles from the launch site.[133] Alongside the ABL development, the Pentagon also pursued an Advanced Tactical Laser (ATL) that had a reusable COIL and could be operated from a smaller aircraft such as a C-130. The ATL weighs about 20 tons, fits into a C-130, and has a power output in the 100 kW range, which allows it to engage targets over a distance of 10 kilometers to 20 kilometers.[134] A test demonstrated that the ATL could hit a target as small as a truck from a distance of 10 kilometers.

The US Army developed a Mobile High-Energy Laser (MEHEL), which can be placed on a Stryker armored vehicle. It has an energy output of 5 kW, which is sufficient for destroying small drones. A more powerful system is under development called Ground-Based Air Defense on the Move (GBAD OTM), which uses a 30 kW laser and which would also be vehicle-based with potentially two support vehicles: one with a radar and one with the computerized control system.[135] These systems could be used for air defense, including shooting down artillery and mortar rounds. In theory, they could also be used against enemy personnel, for example, to blind pilots of targeted aircraft. In 2003, there was an incident where two US Army helicopters were illuminated with a strong laser near the demilitarized zone in South Korea. It was believed that the North Koreans had used a Chinese ZM 87 antipersonnel laser.[136]

Dazzling Lasers

Although blinding lasers have been banned under international law since 1995, it is permissible to use dazzling lasers that have sufficiently low power output that they will (probably) not cause permanent damage to eyes. The issue is that dazzling lasers could cause permanent damage when used at a closer than safe distance or when a person keeps staring into a laser beam for several seconds.[137] During the 1980s, the US Army developed a Close Combat Laser Assault Weapon that was designed to damage optics and windscreens, and the US Air Force developed a blinding laser called Coronet Prince, but both programs were cancelled by the early 1990s.[138] The US military brought the Saber 203 dazzler to Somalia in 1995, which fits into a 40 mm grenade launcher and can disorient a person for several seconds with a range of about 300 meters. Reportedly, the US military decided not to use the dazzlers in Somalia over humanitarian concerns.

The Saber 203 program was cancelled in 1998 due to concerns over eye safety.[139] Laser dazzlers can cause eye damage at less than 10 meters from the target and should only be used at 70 meters from the target.[140]

The JNLWP has also developed a laser rifle called the Personnel Halting and Stimulation Response (PHaSR) weapon that has a range finder that allows for the correct power output for temporarily dazzling a person at any distance.[141] Davison suggested that the PHaSR can use two wavelengths, the visible for dazzling, and a mid-infrared wavelength for heating skin/repelling people.[142] In other words, the PHaSR could also function as a pain ray, similar to the ADS. A Pentagon document on bioeffects of some NLW suggests:

> Some high-power lasers can cause antipersonnel effects by deposition of thermal energy. These lasers must operate at a wavelength that is readily absorbed by the skin or the cornea. These generally include the far- and mid-IR region (10 to 12 microns and 3 to 5 microns) as well as the ultraviolet region (<0.4 microns). . . . Although relatively modest amounts of far-IR laser power are required to produce superficial bums on the skin at short ranges, and efforts to design rheostatically lethal laser weapons are ongoing.[143]

This means that lasers with a moderate power output (class 3b) could be used for producing other effects than just dazzling or blinding a targeted person, but also causing heating of tissue, burns, and lesions from a distance of perhaps hundreds of meters. As indicated in the PHaSR concept, this could be a rifle-like handheld device.

Conclusion

Militaries have been interested in less lethal or nonlethal technologies since at least the 1950s, generally with a view of using them against civilian populations or in situations where it is difficult to distinguish between combatants and noncombatants. NLWs have been discussed in the West since the 1960s and the initial directions were rubber bullets, tear gas, and electrical weapons (tasers). Since the 1970s, there has been research into new types of NLWs that use acoustics and electromagnetic waves for disorienting or stunning individuals, seemingly inspired by speculations of Soviet breakthroughs in psychotronic weaponry. It is difficult to evaluate the various claims that have been made with respect to the effects of infrasound, ultrasound, or electromagnetic waves on people, since no antipersonnel weapons of these types are known to exist. However, there has been a lot of speculation that such weapons have been secretly developed and may have been secretly used. The secrecy surrounding nonlethal technologies is not actually surprising, considering how controversial such weapons are, given the likelihood that they will sometimes produce irreversible damage or substantial suffering if vulnerable individuals are targeted or if they are used incorrectly or recklessly. There are concerns that NLWs such as tasers could be used as torture instruments, precisely because they do not leave behind characteristic traces or marks that would serve as evidence. In any case, NLWs that do not produce temporary and reversible incapacitation but cause permanent injury are prohibited under international law, which is another reason why any nation that has developed such weapons would keep them secret.

Notes

1 John B. Alexander, *Future War: Non-Lethal Weapons in Twenty-First-Century Warfare* (New York: St. Martin's Griffin, 1999), 59–123.
2 Steven Aftergood, "The Soft-Kill Fallacy," *The Bulletin of Atomic Scientists* 50, no. 5 (1994): 42–3.
3 US Department of Defense, "Directive Number 3000.03E: DoD Executive Agent for Non-Lethal Weapons (NLW), and NLW Policy," April 25, 2013, Part 2: Definitions.
4 US Department of Defense, "Directive Number 3000.03E," 2.
5 Robert Mandel, *Security, Strategy, and the Quest for Bloodless War* (Boulder: Lynne Rienner Publishers Inc., 2004), 103.
6 US Department of Defense, "Directive Number 3000.03E."
7 Neil Davison, *'Non-Lethal' Weapons* (New York: Palgrave Macmillan, 2008), 1.
8 Davison, *'Non-Lethal' Weapons*, 107.
9 Quoted from: H. P. Albarelli, *A Terrible Mistake: The Murder of Frank Olson and the CIA's Cold War Experiments* (Walterville: TrineDay, 2009), 61.
10 Davison, *'Non-Lethal' Weapons*, 12.
11 Davison, *'Non-Lethal' Weapons*, 17.
12 John D. LaMothe, "Controlled Offensive Behavior—USSR," Defense Intelligence Agency, July 1972.
13 Nick Lewer and Steven Schofield, *Non-Lethal Weapons: A Fatal Attraction? Military Strategies and Technologies for the 21st Century* (London: Zed Books, 1997), 34–5.

14 David A. Koplow, *Non-Lethal Weapons: The Law and Policy of Revolutionary Technologies for Military and Law Enforcement* (Cambridge: Cambridge University Press, 1996), 28.
15 US Department of Justice, "Department of Defense Non-Lethal Weapons and Equipment Review: A Research Guide for Civil Law Enforcement and Corrections," National Institute of Justice, July 2002, 2.
16 US National Research Council, *An Assessment of Non-Lethal Weapons Science and Technology* (Washington, DC: The National Academies Press, 2003), 4.
17 US Joint Chiefs of Staff, "Joint Concept for Competing," February 10, 2023, Glossary.
18 Michael J. Mazarr, *Mastering the Gray Zone: Understanding a Changing Era of Conflict* (Carlisle: US Army War College Press, 2015), 4.
19 J. Coates, *Nonlethal and Non-Destructive Combat in Cities* (Washington, DC: Institute for Defense Analysis, 1970).
20 Quoted from: Mandel, *Security, Strategy, and the Quest for Bloodless War*, 103.
21 Mandel, *Security, Strategy, and the Quest for Bloodless War*, 89.
22 Koplow, *Non-Lethal Weapons*, 100–4.
23 Koplow, *Non-Lethal Weapons*, 104.
24 Mazarr, *Mastering the Gray Zone*, 4.
25 US White House, "National Security Strategy of the United States," December 2017, 2.
26 US White House, "National Security Strategy of the United States," October 2022, 6 and 22.
27 Scott Savitz and Krista Romita Grocholski, "Revealing the Impact of Non-Lethal Weapons," *RAND Commentary*, July 15, 2022, available at: https://www.rand.org/pubs/commentary/2022/06/revealing-the-impact-of-non-lethal-weapons.html.
28 US Joint Chiefs of Staff, "Joint Concept for Competing," 31.
29 Robert McCreight, "Non-Kinetic Threats and the Threshold Spectrum of Strategic Endgame Warnings," *Mad Scientist Laboratory blog*, May 11, 2023, available at: https://madsciblog.tradoc.army.mil/444-non-kinetic-threats-and-the-threshold-spectrum-of-strategic-endgame-warnings/.
30 Eliot Cohen, "The Mystique of U.S. Airpower," *Foreign Affairs* 73, no. 1 (1994): 121.
31 Aftergood, "The Soft-Kill Fallacy," 42.
32 Davison, *'Non-Lethal' Weapons*, 3.
33 Davison, *'Non-Lethal' Weapons*, 206.
34 Pauline Kaurin, "With Fear and Trembling: An Empirical Framework for Non-Lethal Weapons," *Journal of Military Ethics* 9, no. 1 (2010): 105.
35 Davison, *'Non-Lethal' Weapons*, 62.
36 Aftergood, "The Soft-Kill Fallacy," 44.

37 Davison, *'Non-Lethal' Weapons*, 214.
38 Davison, *'Non-Lethal' Weapons*, 37.
39 United Nations, "The Convention on Prohibitions or Restrictions on the Use of Certain Conventional Weapons Which May Be Deemed to Be Excessively Injurious or to Have Indiscriminate Effects," October 10, 1980, available at: https://disarmament.unoda.org/the-convention-on-certain-conventional-weapons/.
40 Michael L. Gross, "Medicalized Weapons & Modern War," *Hastings Center Report*, January–February 2010, 38.
41 Evylene Schuster, "Fifty Years Later: The Significance of the Nuremberg Code," *The New England Journal of Medicine* 337, no. 20 (1997): 1436–40.
42 Cheryl Welsh, "Cold War Nonconsensual Experiments: The Threat of Neuroweapons and the Danger It Will Happen Again," *Essex Human Rights Review* 9, no. 1 (2012): 3.
43 Davison, *'Non-Lethal' Weapons*, 52.
44 Aftergood, "The Soft-Kill Fallacy," 42–3.
45 Marc Ambinder and D. B. Grady, *Deep State: Inside the Government Secrecy Industry* (Hoboken: Wiley, 2015), 166.
46 Davison, *'Non-Lethal' Weapons*, 184.
47 US Navy, "Directed Energy Weapons: Counter Directed Energy Weapons and High Energy Lasers," Office of Naval Research, available at: https://www.onr.navy.mil/organization/departments/code-35/division-353/directed-energy-weapons-cdew-and-high-energy-lasers.
48 US General Accountability Office, "Science & Tech Spotlight: Directed Energy Weapons," GAO 23-106717, May 25, 2023, available at: https://www.gao.gov/assets/gao-23-106717.pdf.
49 Louis A. Del Monte, *War at the Speed of Light: Directed Energy Weapons and the Future of Twenty-First Century Warfare* (Lincoln: Potomac Books, 2022), 4.
50 Doug Beason, *The E-Bomb: How America's New Directed Energy Weapons Will Change Future Wars Will Be Fought* (Cambridge: Da Capo Press, 2005), 57.
51 Del Monte, *War at the Speed of Light*, 44.
52 Mark Gunzinger, "Changing the Game: The Promise of Directed Energy Weapons," Center for Strategic and Budgetary Assessments, 2012, 45.
53 Gunzinger, "Changing the Game," 63–4.
54 Gunzinger, "Changing the Game," 43.
55 Lexington Institute, "Directed-Energy Weapons: Technologies, Applications and Implications," Directed-Energy Program, 2003, 5.
56 U.S. General Accountability Office, "Science & Tech Spotlight."
57 US Department of Justice and US Department of Defense, "Joint Technology Program: Second Anniversary Report," National Institute of Justice, February 1997.

58 Del Monte, *War at the Speed of Light*, 43.
59 Juliette Volcler, *Extremely Loud: Sound as a Weapon* (New York: The New Press, 2013), 7.
60 Davison, *'Non-Lethal' Weapons*, 186.
61 Volcler, *Extremely Loud*, 9.
62 Volcler, *Extremely Loud*, 14.
63 Volcler, *Extremely Loud*, 91.
64 Volcler, *Extremely Loud*, 94–105.
65 Jürgen Altmann, "Non-Lethal Weapons Technologies—The Case for Independent Scientific Analysis," *Medicine, Conflict, & Survival* 17, no. 3 (2001): 234.
66 Alexander, *Future War*, 97.
67 Davison, *'Non-Lethal' Weapons*, 187.
68 Jürgen Altmann, "Acoustic Weapons—A Prospective Assessment," *Science & Global Security* 9, no. 3 (1999): 191.
69 Davison, *'Non-Lethal' Weapons*, 196.
70 Genasys, "LRAD Overview & Product Guide," available at: https://genasys.com/wp-content/uploads/2024/03/LRAD-Product-Guide-2024.pdf.
71 Geoff Leventhall, "Big Noise in Baghdad," *Noise & Vibration Worldwide* 35, no. 6 (2004): 27.
72 Davison, *'Non-Lethal' Weapons*, 198.
73 Davison, *'Non-Lethal' Weapons*, 197.
74 Altmann, "Acoustic Weapons," 192.
75 Ryszard Panuszka, Zbigniew Damijan, Cezary Kasprzak, and James McGlothlin, "Infrasounds and Biorhythms of the Human Brain," *Acoustical Society of America Journal* 111, no. 5 (2002): 2335–6.
76 Donnie Eichar, *Dead Mountain: The Untold True Story of the Dyatlov Pass Incident* (San Francisco: Chronicle Books, 2013), 248.
77 Volcler, *Extremely Loud*, 24.
78 Volcler, *Extremely Loud*, 25.
79 Quoted from Volcler, *Extremely Loud*, 26.
80 Robert Bunker, "Nonlethal Weapons: Terms and References," *U.S. Air Force Academy Institute for National Security Studies Occasional Paper* 15 (1997): 2–3.
81 Alexander, *Future War*, 97.
82 US Department of Defense, "Bioeffects of Selected Nonlethal Weapons," February 17, 1998, 13.
83 Jürgen Altmann, "Acoustic Weapons—A Prospective Assessment: Sources, Propagation, and Effects of Strong Sounds," *Cornell University Peace Studies Program Occasional Paper* 22 (1999): 4, 6.
84 Altmann, "Acoustic Weapons," 202.

85 Altmann, "Acoustic Weapons—A Prospective Assessment: Sources, Propagation, and Effects of Strong Sounds," 46–7.
86 D. V. Giri, *High-Power Electromagnetic Radiators: Nonlethal Weapons and Other Applications* (Cambridge, MA: Harvard University Press, 2004), 141.
87 Referenced by Altmann, "Acoustic Weapons—A Prospective Assessment: Sources, Propagation, and Effects of Strong Sounds," 7.
88 Altmann, "Acoustic Weapons—A Prospective Assessment: Sources, Propagation, and Effects of Strong Sounds," 27.
89 Altmann, "Acoustic Weapons—A Prospective Assessment: Sources, Propagation, and Effects of Strong Sounds," 28.
90 Alexander, *Future War*, 97–8.
91 Volcler, *Extremely Loud*, 121–2.
92 Nicole Chavez, "Using Sound to Attack: The Diverse World of Acoustic Devices," *CNN*, September 27, 2017, available at: https://www.cnn.com/2017/08/10/health/acoustic-weapons-explainer/index.html.
93 William Thomas, "Microwaving Iraq: 'Pacifying' Rays Pose New Hazards to Iraqi," January 25, 2005, available at: https://rense.com/general62/mciro.htm.
94 Thomas, "Microwaving Iraq."
95 ITV, "High Tech Psychological Warfare Arrives in the Middle East," *ITV News*, March 23, 1991, available at: https://bibliotecapleyades.net/CIENCIA/ciencia_nonlethalweapons05.htm.
96 ITV, "High Tech Psychological Warfare Arrives in the Middle East."
97 Judy Wall, "PSYOPS Weaponry Used in the Persian Gulf War," *Nexus Magazine* 5, no. 6 (1998): 13–18.
98 Oliver Lowery, "Silent Subliminal Presentation System," Patent No. US5159703A.
99 David Guyatt, "Anti-Personnel 'Soft Kill' Weaponry," *World Affairs* 9, no. 2 (2005): 41.
100 Beason, *The E-Bomb*, 107.
101 John P. Geis, "Directed Energy Weapons on the Battlefield: A New Vision for 2025," *Center for Strategy and Technology Air War College Occasional Paper* 32 (2003): 7–8.
102 Giri, *High-Power Electromagnetic Radiators*, 56.
103 Giri, *High-Power Electromagnetic Radiators*, 66.
104 US Department of Defense, "Bioeffects of Selected Nonlethal Weapons," 2–5.
105 Douglas Pasternak, "Wonder Weapons: The Pentagon's Quest for Nonlethal Weapons Is Amazing. But Is It Smart?," *U.S. News & World Report* 123, no. 1 (1997): 38–44.
106 Guyatt, "Anti-Personnel 'Soft Kill' Weaponry," 53.
107 Giri, *High-Power Electromagnetic Radiators*, 68.

108 Guyatt, "Anti-Personnel 'Soft Kill' Weaponry," 41–2.

109 John Keller, "Air Force Deploys B-52 Missiles That Could Disable Enemy Military Electronics with High-Power Microwaves," *Military & Aerospace Electronics*, May 17, 2019, available at: https://www.militaryaerospace.com/rf-analog/article/14033453/air-force-deploys-b-52-missiles-that-could-disable-enemy-military-electronics-with-high-power-microwaves.

110 Edl Schamiloglu, "Scientists Suggest US Embassies Were Hit With High-Power Microwaves—Here's How the Weapons Work," *The Conversation*, December 10, 2020.

111 Schamiloglu, "Scientists Suggest US Embassies Were Hit With High-Power Microwaves—Here's How the Weapons Work."

112 Davison, *'Non-Lethal' Weapons*, 167.

113 Davison, *'Non-Lethal' Weapons*, 167.

114 Gross, "Medicalized Weapons & Modern War," 38.

115 US Department of Defense, "Active Denial System," *Join Intermediate Force Capabilities Office* website, https://jnlwp.defense.gov/About/Frequently-Asked-Questions/Active-Denial-System-FAQs/ (accessed July 24, 2024).

116 Susan LeVine, "The Active Denial System: A Revolutionary, Non-Lethal Weapon for Today's Battlefield," Center for Technology and National Security Policy National Defense University, June 2009, 1.

117 Sharon Weinberger, "Wasted Energy: Despite 50 Years of Research on High-Power Microwaves, the US Military Has Yet to Produce a Usable Weapon," *Nature* 489, no. 7415 (2012): 200.

118 Weinberger, "Wasted Energy," 198.

119 PHR and INCLO, "Lethal in Disguise: The Health Consequences of Crowd Control Weapons," Physicians for Human Rights/ International Network of Civil Liberties Organizations, April 2014, available at: https://www.aclu.org/wp-content/uploads/publications/lethal_in_disguise_inclo_single_page.pdf.

120 Davison, *'Non-Lethal' Weapons*, 171.

121 Lauren Poindexter, "ARDEC Engineers Develop Solid State Active Denial Technology for Nonlethal Crowd Control," *US Army* website, *October 16, 2016, available at:* https://www.army.mil/article/176579/ardec_engineers_develop_solid_state_active_denial_technology_for_non_lethal_crowd_control.

122 David Hambling, "Pain Ray: The U.S. Military's Agony Beam Weapon," *New Scientist*, May 8, 2013, available at: https://www.newscientist.com/article/mg21829162-300-pain-ray-the-us-militarys-new-agony-beam-weapon/.

123 Robert O. Becker, *Cross Currents: The Perils of Electropollution* (New York: Penguin, 1990), 216.

124 David Hambling, "US Bioelectromagnetic Weapon Research," *Military.com*, November 26, 2006, available at: https://www.military.com/defensetech/2006/11/26/us-bioelectromagnetic-weapons-research.
125 Hambling, "US Bioelectromagnetic Weapon Research."
126 Pasternak, "Wonder Weapons: The Pentagon's Quest for Nonlethal Weapons Is Amazing. But Is It Smart?"
127 Pasternak, "Wonder Weapons: The Pentagon's Quest for Nonlethal Weapons Is Amazing. But Is It Smart?"
128 Beason, *The E-Bomb*, 53.
129 Beason, *The E-Bomb*, 62.
130 US Department of Defense, "Bioeffects of Selected Nonlethal Weapons," 15–16.
131 Davison, *'Non-Lethal' Weapons*, 145.
132 Davison, *'Non-Lethal' Weapons*, 145.
133 Jason Sherman, "Boeing's Phantom Works Tapped to Design Airborne Laser in New MDA Tech Effort," *Inside the Pentagon's Inside Missile Defense* 23, no. 25 (2017): 1–9.
134 Lewis Page, "Boeing Announces 'Laser Gunship' Completion," *The Register*, December 11, 2007, available at: https://www.theregister.com/2007/12/11/boeing_atl_advanced_tactical_laser_fitted/.
135 David Axe, "Laser-Armed Trucks Are Coming to Shoot Drones Out of the Sky," *Daily Beast*, April 13, 2017, available at: https://www.thedailybeast.com/laser-armed-trucks-are-coming-to-shoot-drones-out-of-the-sky.
136 UPI, "Report: N. Korea Fired Laser at Troops," *UPI.com*, May 13, 2003, available at: https://www.upi.com/Odd_News/2003/05/13/Report-N-Korea-fired-laser-at-troops/31591052808827/.
137 Laura Eggertson, "Military Claims Laser Dazzlers Have 'Negligible' Risk," *Canadian Medical Association Journal* 180, no. 11 (2009): 1099.
138 Davison, *'Non-Lethal' Weapons*, 148.
139 Davison, *'Non-Lethal' Weapons*, 148.
140 Davison, *'Non-Lethal' Weapons*, 153.
141 US Air Force, "Personnel Hatling and Stimulation Response (PHaSR) Fact Sheet," *Air Force Research Laboratory*, April 2006.
142 Davison, *'Non-Lethal' Weapons*, 154.
143 US Department of Defense, "Bioeffects of Selected Nonlethal Weapons," 16.

5

The Havana Syndrome

The Havana Syndrome consists of a set of symptoms that was first observed in United States and Canadian diplomats and intelligence personnel working in Havana, Cuba, with unclear causes or origins. Since the first cases appeared in Cuba in late 2016, there have been numerous reports from around the world of primarily US diplomats, intelligence officers, other officials, and their close family members falling ill for no apparent reason. Over 1,500 individuals have been diagnosed by medical doctors with Havana Syndrome as of 2024 if one includes the dependents of US government employees.[1] There could be many more individuals with no connection to the US government who have the same symptoms but who are not included in the US government investigations. Havana Syndrome has been officially referred to by the US Department of State as "Anomalous Health Incidents" (AHIs) or "Unexplained Health Incidents" (UHIs). Many of the affected individuals seem to recover from the symptoms within weeks, but there is also a sizable segment that suffers from permanent damage to their health that appeared after the initial symptoms had disappeared. The Havana Syndrome sufferers who decided to speak out and give public interviews are generally convinced that their condition was caused by some kind of covert attack. These attacks purportedly occurred in residencies, hotels, offices, on the street, in public parks, and other public places. However, over 90 percent of 200 reported incidents (as of 2021) occurred indoors.[2] The victims have only received limited support from the government, and there has been a lot of disagreement within the government and among experts as to whether Havana Syndrome is the result of some sort of attack or whether it is only a psychological phenomenon caused by stress, anxiety, and social contagion. This chapter reviews the publicly available information as to how the story of the Havana Syndrome unfolded in the media and political debates from mid-2017.

The History of the Havana Syndrome

Since the first reports of a potential "sonic weapon" that may have been used against US and Canadian diplomats in August 2017, there has been steady media reporting on a continuously growing list of cases, as well as on various investigations and expert commentary. There are hundreds of newspaper articles, many TV interviews and documentaries, and many studies and academic papers on this topic. From the publicly available information, it seems that there were only a few locations with individuals reporting Havana Syndrome in 2016–18, namely Cuba, China, and Russia. In 2019 and 2020, some officials inside the United States were identified as potential Havana Syndrome cases. There was a flurry of cases all over the world in 2021, but between 2022 and 2024, the media reporting became scarcer because of claims by the IC and the Biden administration that a deliberate attack as a cause for the Havana Syndrome was "very unlikely."[3]

Possible Havana Syndrome Cases before 2016

Although Havana Syndrome became only publicly discussed from mid-2017 onwards, it is possible that US diplomats and intelligence officers have been targeted much earlier than that. Former NSA officer Michael Beck has claimed that he was targeted with a DEW when he visited an unnamed hostile country in 1996.[4] He and his colleague Charles Gubete were sent to the country to make sure the US embassy under construction there was not bugged.[5] They discovered a technical threat and reported it, but were warned by a translator that the host country authorities were not happy. Beck felt dizzy the next day and returned to the United States. Ten years later, he had an unexplained health incident in the UK, which was diagnosed as Parkinson's disease. His colleague, Gubete, suffered from the same condition around the same time, which seems to be an unlikely coincidence.[6] Beck had to leave the country and eventually recovered from his symptoms.

A NSA document declassified in 2014 and obtained by national security lawyer Mark Zaid stated: "There is intelligence information from 2012 associating the hostile country to which Mr. Beck traveled in the late 1990s with a high-powered microwave system weapon that may have the ability to weaken, intimidate, or kill an enemy over time and without leaving evidence."[7] According to this document, "[t]he 2012 intelligence information indicated that this weapon is designed to bathe a target's living quarters in microwaves, causing numerous physical effects, including a damaged nervous system."[8] The document also stated that the NSA had no knowledge of the existence of such a weapon, which makes the previous statement more ambiguous. According to Zaid, who represents Beck as his lawyer, "[t]he fact is that this mystery has its origins and answers within the Intelligence Community, and most information remains classified. . . . Until the classified info is pried loose, there will be little more than conspiracies and allegations dominating the discussion."[9]

Another pre-2016 case may have occurred in Frankfurt, Germany, in early 2014, which was shortly before the Russian annexation of Crimea. A US government employee identified as "Taylor" was working out of the US consulate in Frankfurt when he was seemingly knocked unconscious by a directed energy beam, according to a report by *The Insider*.[10] *The Insider* article stated that "the symptoms began as an intense feeling of pressure, which started in the torso and radiated up to the head and neck. Then there was nausea, followed by a 'high-pitched squeal.' Taylor [a pseudonym] raced to a bathroom to vomit before collapsing unconscious on the floor."[11] Taylor received a diagnosis of vestibular neuronitis by German physicians and a diagnosis of traumatic brain injury in an American hospital.

Early Cases in Havana, Cuba

The early cases may be the ones that possibly provide the best indications as to what may be behind the Havana Syndrome in terms of causation and potential perpetrators and motives. They are also the cases with some of the most publicly available details. Starting in November 2016, several US diplomats in Havana suffered from inexplicable health conditions, with the first medical visits occurring in December 2016.[12] The *Associated Press* was first to report on Havana Syndrome in August 2017. They claimed that "[i]n the fall of 2016, a series of U.S. diplomats began suffering unexplained losses of hearing" and that this was "attributed to a covert sonic device."[13] Some of them heard a very loud high-pitched chirping sound when they suffered from symptoms, and a recording produced by one of the embassy workers was later published online by *Associated Press*.[14] Six of them had to be flown from Cuba to Miami for emergency medical treatment.

One of the affected diplomats was Tina Onefur, who stated in an *NBC News* interview that one night in March 2017, she suffered sudden pain when she was washing the dishes, standing close to the kitchen window. She stated: "It was gripping—it was like I'd been seized by some invisible hand, and I couldn't move."[15] As of 2021, Onefur was still suffering from "excruciating headaches . . . losing my balance . . . [and] vision degradation."[16] Some of the most common symptoms experienced by US personnel in Cuba included headaches, dizziness, insomnia, ear pain, temporary loss of hearing, weakened sense of balance, diminished memory, inability to regulate emotion, and indications of traumatic brain injury and concussion.[17] The attacks that started sporadically in late March continued until April and then appeared to stop. Two more confirmed cases occurred in late August 2017.[18] At least twenty-one American diplomats in Cuba suffered symptoms by September 2017.[19] Altogether twenty-five US Havana embassy staffers were evacuated in 2017, many of whom actually did not want to leave Cuba because of the contacts they had made and their belief in the importance of the mission.[20]

The Canadian Cases

When the Havana Syndrome story broke in the summer of 2017, there were reports that, apart from the American diplomats in Cuba, several Canadian diplomats also complained about similar symptoms.[21] From April 2017, Canadian diplomats reported Havana Syndrome, and the affected individuals were flown out of Cuba to receive medical treatment. A Canadian diplomat identified in a news report as "Allen" stated that in late winter 2017, he and his until then healthy family suffered inexplicable symptoms such as nosebleeds, headaches, irritability, and hearing high-pitched noises. Only at that point did an American colleague in Havana inform Allen about other incidents that had affected American diplomats.[22] The Canadian Global Affairs Office (their State Department) did not, unlike the State Department, reduce its diplomatic presence in Cuba or take any punitive measures against the Cuban government.

The Canadian government has been far more skeptical about the reality of Havana Syndrome and has provided less support to the individuals who believe they have been exposed to some kind of DEW. In 2019, five of the Canadian diplomats and their family members (fourteen in total) decided to sue the Canadian government for $21 million in damages for knowingly exposing them to "extremely serious and debilitating attacks" and for actively preventing them from getting appropriate medical care.[23] The lawsuit stated: "Throughout the crisis, Canada downplayed the seriousness of the situation, hoarded and concealed critical health and safety information, and gave false, misleading and incomplete information to diplomatic staff."[24]

The Canadian government contracted Dalhousie University's Brain Repair Centre to test the afflicted diplomats. Altogether, twenty-five individuals participated in the study.[25] Some of the diplomats who are suing the Canadian government claim that the government failed to disclose at least three more cases of Havana Syndrome that occurred in 2019 and 2020. The Canadian government asked the court to dismiss the lawsuit, stating that "there is no definitive medical diagnosis of any medical condition, illness or disease called Havana Syndrome, notwithstanding the use of this term by the Plaintiffs."[26]

Havana Syndrome in Russia, China, Europe, Australia, and Taiwan

The first AHI after the series of incidents in Cuba was a USAID official and his wife, who fell ill in Tashkent, Uzbekistan, in September 2017 and had to be flown out of the country. At the time, State Department spokesperson Heather Nauert denied that there was an incident in Uzbekistan, and the Russian government also denied that it had any role in it. However, the location and timing of the incident are suspicious since Uzbekistan was considering rejoining the Collective Security Treaty Organization it had withdrawn from in 2012.[27]

In December 2017, CIA officer Marc Polymeropoulos was on a routine trip to Moscow to discuss counterterrorism issues with Russian officials.[28] Polymeropoulos was at that time the deputy chief of operations for the Europe/Eurasia Mission Center, which made him very senior in the CIA.[29] In the middle of the night, he experienced severe ear-ringing, vertigo, a sudden onset of nausea, and paralysis in his Moscow hotel room. He recovered and suffered a second attack two days later in a Moscow restaurant.[30] He then left Russia and again recovered. Several weeks later, in February 2018, "he started feeling an intense and painful pressure that started in the back of his head and radiated forward into his face."[31] This suggests that he may have been attacked a third time when he was back in the United States. Polymeropoulos was subsequently diagnosed with brain damage, which forced him to retire from his CIA career of twenty-six years in 2019.[32]

Several diplomats in Guangzhou, China, suffered from Havana Syndrome symptoms, including hearing strange noises and brain injury.[33] It started with one embassy employee hearing sounds and getting sick in late 2017. Department of Commerce employee Catherine Werner claimed to have been attacked during the night, which prompted the US Department of State to medically evaluate 300 employees, of which 15 showed Havana Syndrome symptoms.[34] More cases appeared in April 2018, one of which was Mark Lenzi, a security engineer at the consulate, who had to be flown out of China together with his family.[35] He later stated in a *CBS* interview that he was targeted because of his work detecting electronic threats to the embassy and that "[t]his was a directed standoff attack against my apartment . . . it was a weapon. . . . I believe it's RF, radio frequency energy, in the microwave range."[36] The Chinese government claimed that they had conducted an investigation but that they could not determine any cause.

At least one other AHI occurred in Europe during 2018. CIA analyst Erika Stith was on an assignment in an unnamed European country when she suffered what she believed to be a directed energy attack. Initially, Stith believed that the intense symptoms of nausea, headaches, blurred vision, balance, and memory issues were the consequence of a prior concussion that she had suffered. Only when Stith's mother made her aware of Havana Syndrome later did she think that this was perhaps the cause. Stith claimed during a *CBS* interview that her "brain is broken" and that she was not sure whether she could ever work again.[37]

Several more incidents occurred in Europe in 2019. A CIA officer suffered an AHI first in Poland in Spring 2019 and a second AHI in Tbilisi, Georgia in Fall 2019.[38] Another case occurred in London in 2019, which affected at least two White House officials in a hotel room, one of whom was accompanying National Security Advisor John Bolton. The incident started with one staffer suffering from sudden painful ringing in the ears and migraines. According to a story by *GQ*, "she suddenly felt a tingling in the side of her head that was facing the window. The intense pressure in her head was accompanied by a tinning in her ears. When she left the room, the symptoms stopped."[39] When a second staffer entered the room, they both suffered the same symptoms which endured until their return to the United States.[40] The staffer reported the incident to the Secret Service.

The incident in London is similar to one that occurred in Australia in Fall 2019 and that affected two CIA officers while they were staying in their hotel rooms. They heard a strange sound, suffered from pressure in their heads, migraines, and ear-ringing. Both continued to travel to Taiwan and suffered the same symptoms again while they were in their hotel rooms. One of the officials was among the five most high-ranking CIA officials.[41]

Havana Syndrome Cases Inside the United States

Several media reports have suggested that potential attacks causing Havana Syndrome have not only occurred in overseas locations but even inside the United States, including near the White House. Critics have been dismissive of the US-based Havana Syndrome cases, citing the much greater security in places like Washington, DC, and the improbability that an adversary would take the risk of conducting attacks on US soil. Nevertheless, some individuals who claim to have been attacked in the United States have come forward and given interviews to tell their story.

At least two White House staffers reported Havana Syndrome, one of them claiming to have been attacked close to the White House. One of them is Olivia Troye, who was a homeland security and counterterrorism advisor to Vice President Pence. She stated on *CBS News* that she suffered an attack when she was walking down the stairs of the Executive Building on her way to the White House in the summer of 2019. In the interview, she described it as a "piercing feeling on the side of my head . . . on the right side of the head . . . vertigo . . . I felt nauseous, I was somewhat disoriented."[42] She had a second episode one year later, again near the White House walking to her car, where she experienced vertigo, dizziness, and a lack of depth perception.

The second case was Miles Taylor, who was at the time chief of staff of the Department of Homeland Security and who experienced similar symptoms as Troye. Taylor was in his Washington, DC apartment near Capitol Hill during a night in April 2018 when he woke up to a loud chirping noise that sounded like "a cricket or digital sound." He looked out of the window and saw a parked white van speeding away.[43] Although the incident lasted only ten minutes, Taylor was unable to work the next morning because of concussion-like symptoms.

On Thanksgiving in 2019, an unnamed White House staffer reported that she was attacked while walking her dog in a Virginia suburb. First, her dog was seizing up, and then she suffered "a high-pitched ringing in her ears, an intense headache, and a tingling on the side of her face."[44] This was a potential second attack as she may have already suffered one in August 2019 after she had accompanied National Security Advisor John Bolton on a trip to London.

One senior intelligence officer suffered Havana Syndrome symptoms when he was in Boston in late 2019, and a second intelligence officer in Northern Virginia reported symptoms in 2020.[45] Both reportedly worked on issues related to Russia. No further details were reported.

Robyn Garfield worked for the Department of Commerce in Shanghai, China, where he claimed to have been covertly attacked several times. He had to be brought to the United States for treatment in June 2018.[46] After his and his family's return from China, they were undergoing treatment in Philadelphia, where they were suffering from new attacks. One night, the whole family woke up because of "strange vibrations in our bodies, and a sound."[47] Garfield's children suffer from unexplained balance issues, stuttering, and problems with their vision that they did not have before the incidents started in China.

An unnamed FBI agent identified as "Carrie" claims to have been covertly attacked in Key West, Florida, in 2020.[48] She was at the time investigating a suspected Russian spy, identified as "Vitali," who was arrested on June 16, 2020, after a high-speed car chase.[49] "Vitali" carried a device to erase the car's computer data, including the GPS data.[50] Later the Russian individual was identified in a joint *The Insider/Der Spiegel* investigation as Vitalii Kovalev, who reportedly was a member of Russia's military intelligence organization GRU (now GU).[51] "Carrie" was one of the FBI agents who interviewed Kovalev for an extended period of time. Several months after the interview with Kovalev, "Carrie" developed symptoms consistent with Havana Syndrome. She stated: "It was like a high pitched, metallic drilling noise, and it knocked me forward at, like, a 45-degree angle this way. Immediately [I] felt pressure, and pressure and pain started coursing from inside my right ear, down my jaw, down my neck, and into my chest, while that sound was concentrated inside my right ear."[52] A second attack occurred a year later after Carrie had a new posting in California.

Later Cases in Austria, Germany, and Vietnam

The media reporting on Havana Syndrome became sparser from 2021, which seemed to indicate that either the media had become more skeptical of the phenomenon or that the AHIs no longer happened. However, there are some important cases that occurred from 2021 to 2023, some of which only surfaced with some delay. In the first six months of 2021, there were over two dozen Havana Syndrome cases reported in Vienna, Austria, making it the location with the most Havana Syndrome victims after Cuba.[53] This included diplomats, intelligence officers, and their spouses and children.[54] According to Adam Entous, the Biden administration decided not to publicize the Vienna cases over concerns that this could hamper ongoing investigations.[55] The US ambassador to Austria and the CIA chief of station were seemingly skeptical about the cases and failed to respond more quickly, which resulted in the station chief being recalled in late summer 2021.[56]

There was at least one suspected Havana Syndrome case in Berlin in July 2021, with two more US officials, who required medical treatment for suspected Havana Syndrome in August 2021.[57] In October 2021, the German magazine *Der Spiegel* reported that several members of the CIA in Berlin were affected by Havana Syndrome and that the Berlin state police had launched an investigation into the matter in August 2021.[58]

There were two separate incidents that took place in Hanoi in August 2021, affecting altogether eleven Americans, of whom two were US embassy officials and the remaining nine were part of a team of the Department of Defense, who arrived in Hanoi ahead of Vice President Kamala Harris' visit to Vietnam.[59] The arrival of Vice President Harris was delayed for several hours as one US diplomat affected by Havana Syndrome had to be flown out of the country. Harris was there to discuss with Vietnamese leaders Chinese expansionism in the South China Sea and Covid-19 pandemic responses.[60] A later *60 Minutes* investigation found a source in Vietnam that claimed the Vietnamese were given by the Russians a technology for spying on the American delegation, which without their knowledge may have inflicted harm on the American officials. An email obtained by journalist Christo Grozev to the Russian Security Council indicated that the Russian government had authorized the transfer of a Russian version of LRAD and a short-wave device for scanning the human body.[61]

Other Locations

Havana Syndrome cases have been reported in many locations around the world, covering almost every continent (see table 5.1). The general patterns seem to be similar, but media reporting after 2018 has been sketchier with respect to the specific details of individual cases, focusing more on the potential general explanations for the phenomenon. A CIA operations officer, his wife, and child suffered an AHI inside his apartment in Tashkent, Uzbekistan, in December 2020, which resulted in their evacuation from the country and their hospitalization at Walter Reed National Military Medical Center.[62] Three Americans working in the Geneva consulate reported Havana Syndrome symptoms in summer 2021, one of whom had to be flown back to the United States for medical treatment. Shortly after the incidents in Geneva, another case was reported by the US embassy in Paris.[63] In September 2021, CIA Director William Burns travelled

Table 5.1 List of Reported Havana Syndrome Cases

Location	Time Frame	Approximate Cases	Victims	Characteristics
United Kingdom	2006	2	2 NSA officers	May have started in 1999, victims developed cancer
Frankfurt	Early 2014	1	1 US official	Concussion symptoms
Havana, Cuba	November 2016–April 2017	35	21 US diplomats and intelligence officers and 14 Canadian diplomats	High-pitched sound, headaches, ear-ringing, concussion symptoms
Tashkent, Uzbekistan	September 2017	2	1 USAID official and wife	State Department denied that it was a Havana Syndrome case
Guangzhou, China	December 2017–April 2018	15	15 US diplomats	Strange noises, brain injury
Moscow, Russia	December 2017	1	1 senior CIA official	Severe ear-ringing, vertigo, nausea, dizziness, paralysis
Moscow, Russia	July 2018	1	1 US member of Congress	Loss of hearing in one ear and loss of balance
Washington, DC	April 2018 and summer 2019	2	2 White House staffers	Piercing feeling on the side of the head, vertigo, blurred vision, chirping noise, concussion symptoms
Poland	Spring 2019	1	1 CIA officer	No further details
Tbilisi, Georgia	Fall 2019	1	1 CIA officer	The same officer who was targeted in Poland was also targeted in Tbilisi
Northern Virginia	November 2019	1	1 White House staffer	Second attack on the same staffer who was attacked in London
Boston	Late 2019	1	1 US intelligence officer	No further details
Northern Virginia	2020	1	1 US intelligence officer	No further details
Key West, Florida	June 2020	1	1 FBI agent	High-pitched noise, pressure and pain in the right ear

Tashkent, Uzbekistan	December 2020	3	1 CIA officer, wife, and child	No further details
California	2021	1	1 FBI agent	The same FBI agent who was attacked in Florida suffered a second attack one year later in California
Vienna, Austria	Summer 2021	26	US intelligence officers and families	No further details
Berlin, Germany	July/August 2021	3	3 US officials	No further details
Hanoi, Vietnam	August 2021	11	2 US embassy officials and 9 DoD employees	No further details
Geneva, Switzerland	Summer 2021	3	3 US diplomats	Evacuated from country
Paris, France	Summer 2021	1	1 US official	No further details
Delhi, India	September 2021	1	1 CIA officer	The officer accompanied CIA Director William Burns on this trip
Serbia	September 2021	1	1 CIA officer	No further details
Bogotá, Colombia	September 2021	6	6 US diplomats and family members of which one was a child	At least one family was flown out of the country for treatment
Tbilisi, Georgia	September 2021	1	1 wife of a US diplomat	Powerful sound, piercing headache, vomiting
Vilnius, Lithuania	July 2023	1	1 US official	No further details
Total number of cases listed here		**123**		

to Delhi, India, where he witnessed one of his staff members fall sick from a suspected Havana Syndrome attack.[64] This was followed by another case where a CIA officer, who had been recently posted to Serbia, developed Havana Syndrome symptoms.[65] Just a few days later, the *Washington Post* reported that "[a]t least five families with links to embassy staffers were afflicted" in Bogotá, Colombia.[66] Secretary of State Anthony Blinken, whose trip to Colombia coincided with the reported AHIs, spoke to the affected families at the US embassy. At least one family member of a US diplomat had to be evacuated from Colombia for treatment.[67]

In September 2021, the wife of a US diplomat in Tbilisi, Georgia, was at home, waiting for her son to return from school when she experienced a powerful sound wave through the window, causing her a terrible headache.[68] She said that "[i]t just pierced my ears, came in my left side, felt like it came through the window, into my left ear. . . . I immediately felt fullness in my head, and just a piercing headache," prompting her to vomit.[69] She called her husband to immediately come back home, and while waiting, she saw a young well-dressed man next to a black Mercedes just outside her gate. When she took a picture of him and the car, he quickly stepped into the car and drove off.

A more recent incident occurred in Lithuania. A senior US Department of Defense official attended the NATO summit in Vilnius in July 2023, when he suffered an attack.[70] The official was travelling alone and was not part of Secretary of Defense Lloyd Austin's delegation. The incident was confirmed to have happened and to be subject to an IC investigation by Pentagon press secretary Sabrina Singh on April 1, 2024, but no further details were provided.[71]

US Government Responses to Havana Syndrome

The responses of different parts of the US government to the AHIs were mixed, ranging from overly cautious to outright skeptical. Here it is important to understand the political context during which Havana Syndrome emerged. Relations with Russia were clearly worsening because of the 2014 Ukraine crisis, and there was perhaps a new Cold War paranoia that may have influenced the way US national security officials and politicians perceived the reported incidents.

US Department of State Responses

In spring 2017, the State Department issued multiple protests to the Cuban government in connection to the AHIs. In a tit-for-tat response for the US embassy personnel, who had to be flown home for treatment, two Cuban diplomats were expelled from the Washington, DC, embassy in May 2017.[72] From summer 2017, all diplomats deploying to Cuba were given a medical briefing on the threat and were encouraged to undergo a pre-deployment medical screening.[73] On September 14, 2017, the Trump administration expelled two members of the Cuban delegation to the UN, claiming that they had conducted "influence operations," while restricting the travel for the rest of the Cuban delegation to Manhattan. Fifteen more Cuban diplomats were expelled from the Washington, DC, embassy in the same month.[74] Two weeks later, on September 29, Secretary of State Rex Tillerson decided to remove all nonessential personnel from the Havana embassy to protect US diplomats.[75]

Tillerson ordered in January 2018 an independent Accountability Review Board (ARB) study to determine the cause of the AHIs and to determine the adequacy of security procedures. Ambassador Peter Bodde chaired the review board, consisting of five members. They conducted interviews with 116 individuals and reviewed all the available information on AHIs, covering twenty-four cases that occurred in Cuba.[76] The report was completed on June 7, 2018. The report claimed that "we know 24 Embassy Havana Community members have been medically confirmed to have sustained brain injuries while serving in Havana with the severity of injury ranging from mild impairment to injuries in a few patients so severe they may never be able to return to their previous jobs."[77] Its main findings were that there was no single State Department entity or official to which incidents could be reported, that interagency coordination needed to be enhanced, that there were insufficient resources to support individuals affected by the long-term conditions of Havana Syndrome, and that the training of security personnel needed to be improved.[78]

On May 23, 2018, the State Department established the Health Incidents Response Task Force (HIRTF) to serve "as the coordinating body for Department and interagency activities, including identification and treatment of affected personnel and family members, investigation and risk mitigation, messaging, and diplomatic outreach" with "interagency partners, such as the Departments of Health and Human Services, Commerce, Justice, Defense and Energy, as well as other members of the foreign affairs community."[79] In summer 2023,

Secretary of State Anthony Blinken incorporated the HIRTF permanently into the departmental structure of the State Department under the Deputy Secretary for Management and Resources. Ambassador Jonathan Moore was appointed as the task force coordinator and Ambassador Margaret Uyehara was appointed as senior care coordinator.[80]

US Intelligence Community Responses

The FBI's Criminal Investigative Division opened a case file in May 2017 and sent a team to Havana to investigate the potential attacks, which included interviewing victims and witnesses and examining the locations where the attacks were believed to have occurred.[81] The FBI looked at the possibility that air pressure waves or infrasound were used to hurt American personnel but found no evidence.[82] The FBI's Behavioral Analysis Unit reviewed the case files and concluded that the cause of Havana Syndrome was likely "psychogenic illness." The conclusions were later criticized based on the FBI's use of a flawed methodology: the Behavioral Analysis Unit did not talk to any of the victims and did not do any medical examinations.[83] In 2021, the FBI acknowledged for the first time that some of their agents have been afflicted with Havana Syndrome and stated that they would be working with the intelligence community to identify the causes.[84]

The CIA also investigated Havana Syndrome early on from 2017. The CIA sent one of its senior medical officers to Havana to investigate the potential attacks on US personnel in April 2017. In an interview that he gave on CNN with Sanjay Gupta, the CIA officer, introduced as "Dr Paul Andrews," stated that in the early morning after his arrival in Havana he was awakened by "severe pain in his right ear, nausea and a terrible headache."[85] The attack occurred in his hotel room and caused him to be seriously disoriented for the rest of the day. He believed he and his colleagues were under surveillance. Andrews left Cuba and sought help from a doctor in Miami, who had examined other Havana Syndrome victims (most likely Dr. Michael Hoffer).

Initially, the CIA was particularly alarmed about the Havana Syndrome incidents. A report by Tim Golden and Sebastian Rotella stated:

> The suspicious fact that CIA officers seemed to have been struck first and disproportionately by the strange sounds and illnesses—at least four people connected to the small Havana station reported symptoms, as well as a CIA

> employee who came to the island on temporary duty later on—led agency officials to assume that the incidents were some kind of harassment or electronic-monitoring effort directed at intelligence officers.[86]

Many senior CIA officials became convinced that deliberate attacks were occurring, and CIA officials made the case in interagency meetings that the Cuban security forces or Russian intelligence could be responsible. CIA Director Michael Pompeo decided to close the CIA station in Havana in September 2017.[87]

In December 2020, CIA Director Gina Haspel, who was not convinced about the merits of the issue, decided to establish a new Havana Syndrome task force to investigate the causes or origins of the AHIs. It was reported by the *New York Times* that "[t]he task force will be made up of medical experts, human resources specialists and intelligence officers, some on a full-time basis."[88] The CIA has since released a number of skeptical statements about Havana Syndrome, as they were unable to back up any of the incidents with evidence for an attack. In January 2022, the CIA released a statement summarizing their interim report on Havana Syndrome. The report suggested that it was unlikely that there was "a sustained worldwide campaign" by Russia or another foreign power targeting US personnel and that they would continue to look into "whether any device or mechanism plausibly could cause the symptoms reported."[89] The wording is eerily similar to the summary of the intelligence assessment published by ODNI in March 2023.

US Department of Defense Responses

The Pentagon seems to have been slow to respond to the potential threat posed by Havana Syndrome, perhaps because few of their own personnel were affected by it before 2021. The acting secretary of defense (Chris Miller) established the Emerging Threats Cell (ETC) in the Office of the Under Secretary of Defense for Policy.[90] In August 2021, when Vice President Harris was making a visit to Vietnam, at least nine Department of Defense personnel were affected by Havana Syndrome. Soon thereafter, in September 2021, Secretary of Defense Lloyd Austin encouraged, in a memo sent to all 2.9 million Department of Defense personnel worldwide to report AHIs to superior officers, counterintelligence, and medical providers.[91] The memo stated:

> Over the course of the last several years, and predominantly overseas, some DoD personnel have reported a series of sudden and troubling sensory events

> such as sounds, pressure, or heat concurrently or immediately preceding the sudden onset of symptoms such as headaches, pain, nausea, or disequilibrium (unsteadiness or vertigo). As part of a government-wide effort, the Department is committed to finding the cause and the source of these AHI and ensuring that affected individuals receive appropriate medical care as quickly as possible when needed.[92]

In addition to asking DoD employees to report AHIs, the Pentagon also initiated a program to provide healthcare to employees and dependents affected by AHI through a cross-functional team (CFT) established in February 2022, which seemingly replaced the earlier ETC. The CFT had, in 2023, eleven full-time employees attached to it.[93] The purpose of the CFT is primarily to oversee the implementation of DoD policies in relation to AHIs.[94] There is an official Pentagon health page dedicated to reporting AHIs called "patient registry," which also includes a section with Frequently Asked Questions that contains some more information. It states: "The purpose of the AHI registry is to collect patient medical data related to reported health incidents for the purpose of analysis so that knowledge and characteristics of these incidents can be expanded for further advancements in the diagnosis, treatment, and outcomes of AHI-affected individuals."[95] DoD established a Care Coordination Cell to assist AHI patients with getting care. As of July 2024, altogether 334 individuals with Havana Syndrome qualified for care in the military healthcare system, of which 35 percent (117) belonged to DoD.[96]

The Pentagon is also conducting its own research projects to determine the potential causes of the AHIs and whether a new type of weapon was used by adversaries against US personnel. They intended to spend altogether $15 million on investigating AHIs in FY 2023.[97] Several Pentagon research laboratories are testing weapons to determine how Havana Syndrome is caused.[98] One of the research projects was a $750,000 research grant awarded by the US Army to fund animal research at Wayne State University to "develop and test a novel laboratory animal model to mimic mild concussive head injury."[99] The main idea behind the experiments was to expose ferrets to radio waves to determine whether they could produce injury, which seems reminiscent of experiments conducted by the CIA and DARPA in the 1960s. This research program was reportedly cancelled in August 2023, possibly over the negative publicity of potentially cruel animal experiments.[100]

The DoD Inspector General conducted a review of DoD policies and implementation related to AHIs in March 2023. According to the redacted published report, the DoD improved its centralized management of AHIs but still needs to improve the timeliness of responding to reported AHIs, as this had taken four to six weeks in the past. The report also claimed that the CFT was "Unable to Integrate or Execute the DoD's Intelligence and CI Responses to AHIs."[101] Among the organizational issues is the inability of the CFT to initiate investigations since only the Military Department CI organizations are permitted to do so. It was also claimed in the report that CFT members were not fully informed about all the research, development, evaluation, and testing programs conducted within DoD in relation to AHIs.[102] AHI-related information was over-classified, which created challenges for sharing it with relevant parties. The picture that emerged from the Inspector General report is that there was, in 2023, still not enough coordination to manage well AHI reporting, response, investigation, and research across DoD.

US Congress Responses

Committees in both the House of Representatives and the Senate held hearings with expert witnesses to determine the causes of the AHIs, the steps that need to be taken to help afflicted individuals, and potential options for preventing or deterring future incidents. Congress also passed a law called the HAVANA Act to provide financial assistance to US government employees who have been diagnosed with Havana Syndrome. Congress continues to fund research related to Havana Syndrome despite the skeptical IC assessment. It even seems possible that some members of Congress could be covertly targeted with DEWs. For example, Senator Ron Johnson from Wisconsin, who previously served on the Senate Foreign Relations Committee, was evaluated for Havana Syndrome when he lost his hearing and balance simultaneously after a trip to Moscow in 2018.[103] It is not known whether any other members of Congress may have been affected.

On January 2018, the Senate Foreign Relations Committee Hearing held a hearing discussing "The Attacks on US Diplomats in Cuba: Response and Oversight," chaired by Senator Bob Corker. In his opening statement, Senator Marco Rubio pointed out that there were twenty-four cases out of eighty evaluated that had been medically confirmed by the State Department Bureau of Medical Services, who had concluded that "[t]he patterns of injury were most likely related to trauma from a non-natural source."[104] Among the witnesses who testified was Dr. Charles Rosenfarb, the Medical Director of the Bureau of Medical Services. He stated that in some patients, the symptoms resembled a mild traumatic brain injury or concussion. Senator Rubio asked Rosenfarb about the possibility of mass hysteria being a plausible explanation, which Rosenfarb denied:

> 24 people have had symptoms and findings consistent with what looks like a mild traumatic brain injury. The objective tests that were done were not ones that could be basically easily faked. There are exact findings that our experts have determined. That being said, you know, no etiology, no cause has been fully rolled out [*sic*], and we are—there are doctors who are looking at everything. But the findings suggest that this is not an episode of mass hysteria.[105]

The Deputy Director of Diplomatic Security Brown conceded that he was not aware of any technology that could cause the observed symptoms and that there was no precedent for Havana Syndrome. Senator Rubio concluded the hearing by stressing that it was highly improbable for anyone to conduct any attack on US personnel in Cuba without the Cuban government knowing about it since Cuba was a surveillance society or police state.[106]

In April 2021, members of the House Armed Services Committee received a classified briefing from Pentagon's two senior officials about Havana Syndrome. The briefers were Jennifer Walsh, Under Secretary of Defense for Policy, and Griffin Decker, the director of the ETC.[107] *Politico* reported that there was an "urgent threat of directed-energy attacks on US troops in the Middle East and elsewhere" and that Russia was a "likely culprit."[108] According to *Politico*, "[t]he briefers said they were concerned about the growing frequency of apparent attacks around the world, but noted that they are especially concerned about the vulnerability of U.S. personnel in the U.S. Central Command area of operations, which includes combat zones from Syria and Iraq to Afghanistan."[109] It also was pointed out that members of the armed forces may have been hurt by Havana Syndrome, although no further details were reported.

On May 8, 2024, the Homeland Security Subcommittee on Counterterrorism, Law Enforcement, and Intelligence, chaired by Representative August Pfluger, conducted a hearing on Havana Syndrome with three experts who gave their testimony on the issue: Christo Grozev, a journalist for *The Insider* and who was part of the *60 Minutes* investigation into Havana Syndrome; Greg Edgreen, a retired Lieutenant Colonel and current Pentagon consultant; and Mark Zaid, a lawyer representing several Havana Syndrome victims.[110] Christo pointed out that there were at least sixty-eight Havana Syndrome cases that could not be explained away with preexisting conditions and psychosomatic symptoms.

He claimed that a GRU (Russian military intelligence) Unit 29155, specializing in sabotage and assassination, was connected to the Havana Syndrome incidents through the way of members of this unit having been in or near those locations. According to Christo, the GRU had shown interest in the development of acoustic weaponry, and that the St. Petersburg Institute for Experimental Medicine had conducted research in this area on behalf of the GRU.[111]

Edgreen, who previously led the DIA's investigation into the AHIs, emphasized that "America's best men and women in national security are being targeted and neutralized around the world in a global campaign." Edgreen claimed that the top 5 percent to top 10 percent of the DIA's personnel had been targeted and that everything would indicate that Russia was responsible.[112] Zaid stated that he represented more than two dozen AHI victims from the CIA, ODNI, NSA, DIA, FBI, Department of State, and Department of Commerce. Zaid pointed at publicly available information on DEW research, including recent patents on a "non-lethal and non-destructive electromagnetic personnel interdiction control stun type weapon system."[113] Zaid claimed that overwhelming evidence was available in the intelligence community that Havana Syndrome was caused by deliberate attacks with DEW. He also pointed at the inconsistency with which the HAVANA Act was implemented across the different agencies and the inadequacy of the low to provide help to the victims.[114]

The Legislative Actions

The S.1828 "Helping American Victims Afflicted by Neurological Attacks" or HAVANA Act was first introduced by Senator Susan Collins and coauthored by Senator Jeanne Shaheen in May 2021.[115] The gist of the law is to provide financial compensation to affected current or former US government employees and their dependents. The bill was signed into law by President Biden in October 2021 and became Public Law 117–46 on October 8, 2021. The law provides between $100,000 to $200,000 in compensation to affected government employees and their dependents for a "qualifying injury" of the brain.[116] Although the HAVANA Act seems like a step in the right direction, the compensation seems insufficient for individuals who are financially burdened by medical expenditures and the loss of a career. There are further concerns that there are no clear eligibility criteria, that the diagnosis itself is difficult to establish with hard evidence, and that different agencies may be more or less willing to recommend HAVANA Act compensation for affected individuals.[117] However, the HAVANA Act represents up to now the most substantive response by Congress to the alleged worldwide attacks on US personnel.

There have been a few other legislative proposals by different members of Congress. Representative Michael McCaul introduced the bill H.R. 4914 "Havana Syndrome Attacks Response Act" cosponsored by twenty-three other members of the House of Representatives in August 2021. The bill makes a couple of assertions, saying that "United States personnel have suffered persistent brain injuries after being targeted in attacks that have been increasing in number, geographic location, and audacity"; that "[t]he number and locations of these attacks have significantly expanded and, according to press reporting, as of May 2021 there have been more than 130 possible cases that have occurred in Asia, in Europe, and in the Western Hemisphere, including within the United States"; and that "[t]he continuing and expanding scope of these attacks has become a serious security concern that is also undermining the morale of United States personnel, especially those posted at overseas diplomatic missions."[118] The objective of the proposed law is to "detect, deter, and punish clandestine attacks that cause persistent brain injury in United States personnel" by implementing sanctions against any nation found responsible. The bill has not passed, and there has not been any further action since January 2022.

More recently, Representatives Brad Wenstrup and Abigail Spanberger introduced H.R. 7305 in the House Armed Services Committee, which seeks to improve the reporting to Congress of AHI and require the secretary of defense to develop a strategy for protecting DoD employees.[119] Under this legislative proposal, the secretary of defense would be required to

> provide to the Committees on Armed Services of the Senate and House of Representatives a report and briefing on—(1) anomalous health incidents affecting members of the Armed Forces and civilian employees of the Department of Defense; (2) any ongoing efforts carried out by the Secretary to protect such members and employees from the effects of anomalous health incidents; and (3) the extent and nature of engagement by the Secretary with the heads of other Federal departments and agencies regarding anomalous health incidents affecting the employees of such other departments and agencies.[120]

Spanberger released the following statement on the legislative proposal that she cosponsored: "I've spoken directly with public servants, including from Virginia, impacted by anomalous health incidents. These Americans include

US diplomats, servicemembers, intelligence officers, and civilian personnel. As a former CIA case officer and member of the US House Permanent Select Committee on Intelligence, I believe that lawmakers and the Pentagon must better understand the extent of these incidents and develop a strategy to address the issue."[121] As of July 2024, no further actions have been taken in connection with this proposal.

Conclusion

Cases of US intelligence officers having suffered Havana Syndrome may go back to the late 1990s, as is indicated by the case of former NSA officer Michael Beck. The first time the US government became aware of incidents in Cuba was in January 2017, when the first individuals were examined by US State Department medical doctors who had fallen ill in December 2016. There was a second wave of cases in March and April 2017, prompting initial investigations by the FBI and the CIA. The Havana Syndrome was first reported in the news in August 2017. The original theory was that an unknown acoustic or sonic weapons had been used because of most of the victims hearing a high-pitched sound, suffering imbalance, and suffering from hearing damage. The US government was (and seemingly remains) divided on the critical issue as to whether Havana Syndrome was caused by deliberate attack with some sort of weapon or surveillance device, or whether it was/is a case of mass hysteria. More cases were reported in 2017 and 2018 in Russia and China, with some cases that occurred inside of the United States, some of which were reported in close proximity to Congress and the White House. The State Department seemed most convinced that an attack was occurring and that its personnel were at risk. The FBI was skeptical from the start, and the CIA became increasingly dismissive of the AHI issue. Congress has conducted a few high-profile hearings with expert witnesses and it passed the HAVANA Act of 2021. Other proposed legislation that threatened sanctions for any foreign power that was attacking US personnel covertly has failed so far. The next chapter will discuss the main studies that have been conducted by US agencies and academics and contractors, which have attempted to provide some much-needed clarity as to what Havana Syndrome is and what may be the cause of it.

Notes

1 Lewis Regenstein, "The Havana Syndrome: The History Behind the Mystery," *Foreign Policy Research Institute*, April 1, 2024, available at: https://www.fpri.org/article/2024/04/havana-syndrome-the-history-behind-the-mystery/.

2 JASON, "An Analysis of Data and Hypotheses Related to the Embassy Incidents," "An Analysis of Data and Hypotheses Related to the Embassy Incidents," *MITRE Corporation*, October 16, 2021, 3.

3 Julian Barnes and Adam Entous, "Foreign Adversaries 'Very Unlikely' to Blame for Havana Syndrome, Intelligence Review Finds," *New York Times*, March 1, 2023.

4 Julian Borger, "Havana Syndrome: NSA Officer's Case Hints at Microwave Attacks Since 1990s," *The Guardian*, May 2, 2021, available at: https://www.theguardian.com/world/2021/may/02/havana-syndrome-nsa-officer-microwave-attacks-since-90s.

5 The new US embassy in Moscow was under construction from 1979, but construction was halted when it was discovered that the walls contained numerous bugs. The construction was halted in 1985, but resumed in 1994. The new embassy was opened in May 2000. It hence seems likely that the "hostile country" in Michael Beck's account was Russia.

6 Borger, "Havana Syndrome."

7 Quoted from: Peter Kornbluh, "The Secrets of the So-Called 'Havana Syndrome,'" *The Nation*, November 17, 2021, available at: https://www.thenation.com/article/world/havana-syndrome-attacks-cia/.

8 Quoted from Borger, "Havana Syndrome."

9 Josh Ledermann and Brenda Breslauer, "Legal, Financial Fights Mount as 'Havana Syndrome' Goes Unsolved," *NBC News*, December 22, 2021, available at: https://www.nbcnews.com/politics/national-security/legal-financial-fights-mount-havana-syndrome-goes-unsolved-n1286399.

10 Roman Dobrokhotov, Christo Grozev, and Michael Weiss, "Unraveling Havana Syndrome: New Evidence Links the GRU's Assassination Unit 29155 to Mysterious Attacks on U.S. Officials and Their Families," *The Insider*, March 31, 2024, available at: ttps://theins.ru/en/politics/270425.

11 Dobrokhotov, Grozev, and Weiss, "Unraveling Havana Syndrome."

12 US Congress, "Attacks on U.S. Diplomats in Cuba: Response and Oversight, Senate Subcommittee on the Western Hemisphere, Transnational Crime, Civilian Security, Democracy, Human Rights and Global Women's Issues," January 9, 2018, 2, available at: https://www.govinfo.gov/content/pkg/CHRG-115shrg40253/html/CHRG-115shrg40253.htm.

13 Matthew Lee and Michael Weissenstein, "Hearing Loss of US Diplomats in Cuba Blamed on Covert Device," *Associated Press*, August 9, 2017, available at: https://apnews.com/article/51828908c6c84d78a29e833d0aae10aa.
14 Josh Lederman and Michael Weissenstein, "Dangerous Sound? What Americans Heard in Cuba Attacks," *Associated Press*, October 13, 2017, available at: https://apnews.com/article/88bb914f8b284088bce48e54f6736d84.
15 Alex Hammer, "US Diplomats Struck by 'Havana Syndrome' Share Agonizing Symptoms of the Condition Which Left Them BRAIN DAMAGED and Destroyed Their Careers, as They Tearfully Refute Claims Illness Doesn't Exist," *Daily Mail*, October 14, 2021, available at: https://www.dailymail.co.uk/news/article-10091839/Diplomats-struck-Havana-Syndrome-say-destroyed-careers.html.
16 Hammer, "US Diplomats Struck by 'Havana Syndrome' Share Agonizing Symptoms of the Condition Which Left Them BRAIN DAMAGED and Destroyed Their Careers."
17 F. Robles and K. Semple, "U.S. and Cuba Baffled by 'Health Attacks' on American Envoys in Havana," *New York Times*, August 12, 2017, A6.
18 US Congress, "Attacks on U.S. Diplomats in Cuba: Response and Oversight."
19 Amanda Erickson, "All the Theories What's Happening to the Diplomats in Cuba: At Least 21 Americans Have Reported a Bizarre Rash of Symptoms," *Washington Post blogs*, September 30, 2017, available at: https://www.washingtonpost.com/news/worldviews/wp/2017/09/30/all-the-theories-about-whats-happening-to-the-diplomats-in-cuba/.
20 Carol Morello, "U.S. Declares Reduced Staffing Levels 'Permanent' at Embassy in Havana: The State Department Also Extended an Advisory Urging Americans to Reconsider Travel to Cuba for Months After 24 U.S. Diplomats Suffered Unexplained Injuries," *Washington Post*, March 2, 2018.
21 Erickson, "All the Theories About What Is Happening to the Diplomats in Cuba."
22 Elizabeth Payne, "The Havana Syndrome: Why Canadian Diplomats Have Accused Their Government of Abandoning Them," *Ottawa Citizen*, February 25, 2019, available at: https://ottawacitizen.com/news/national/our-men-women-and-children-in-havana-how-a-dream-posting-became-a-nightmare.
23 Vanessa Romo, "Canadian Diplomats Suing Government for $28 Million Over Mysterious Illness," *NPR*, February 7, 2019, available at: https://www.npr.org/2019/02/07/692548213/canadian-diplomats-suing-government-for-28-million-over-mysterious-illness.
24 Payne, "The Havana Syndrome."
25 Josh Lederman, "Canadian Diplomats Say Their Government Is Withholding Info on More 'Havana Syndrome' Brain Injury Cases," *NBC News*, April 28, 2021, available at: https://www.nbcnews.com/politics/national-security/canadian

-diplomats-say-their-government-withholding-info-more-havana-syndrome-n1265702.

26 Brian Platt, "In Court Filing, Canadian Government Argues Diplomats Exaggerated 'Havana Syndrome' Claims Behind $28 Million Lawsuit," *National Post*, November 26, 2019, available at: https://nationalpost.com/news/politics/in-court-filings-canadian-government-argues-havana-syndrome-claims-are-exaggerated-by-diplomats.

27 Steve Dorsey, "Uzbekistan Incident Raises Suspicions of Russian Involvement in Cuba Attacks," *CBS News*, November 28, 2017, available at: https://www.cbsnews.com/news/uzbekistan-incident-raises-suspicions-of-russian-involvement-in-cuba-attacks/.

28 60 Minutes Australia, "Havana Syndrome: Is Russia Behind the Mysterious Illness?," *60 Minutes Australia*, April 28, 2024, available at: https://www.youtube.com/watch?v=aq7dTOPMViI.

29 Ken Dilanian, Andrea Mitchell, and Brenda Breslauer, "CIA Officer Suffered Crippling Symptoms in Moscow. What Is 'Havana Syndrome'?" *NBC News*, December 7, 2020, available at: https://www.nbcnews.com/news/world/cia-officer-suffered-crippling-symptoms-moscow-was-it-havana-syndrome-n1250177.

30 Julia Ioffe, "The Mystery of the Immaculate Concussion," *GQ Magazine*, October 20, 2020, available at: https://www.gq.com/story/cia-investigation-and-russian-microwave-attacks.

31 Ioffe, "The Mystery of the Immaculate Concussion."

32 Dilanian, Mitchell, and Breslauer, "CIA Officer Suffered Crippling Symptoms in Moscow."

33 H. Gardiner, "25th Person at U.S. Embassy Is Mysteriously Sickened," *New York Times*, June 21, 2018, available at: https://www.nytimes.com/2018/06/21/us/politics/us-diplomat-cuba-embassy-illness.html.

34 Amanda Erickson, "Another Diplomat Was Diagnosed with 'Havana Syndrome'. Here Is What We Know," *Washington Post*, December 3, 2018.

35 S. L. Meyers and J. Perlez, "U.S. Diplomats Evacuated in China as Medical Mystery Grows," *New York Times*, June 6, 2018.

36 Will Croxton, "5-Year Havana Syndrome Investigation Finds Evidence Who Might Be Responsible," *CBS News*, July 7, 2024, available at: https://www.cbsnews.com/news/5-year-havana-syndrome-investigation-finds-new-evidence-of-who-might-be-responsible-60-minutes/.

37 Nate Burleson, Catherine Herridge, and Gayle King, "Struggling with Havana Syndrome," *CBS Morning News*, March 31, 2022.

38 Ioffe, "The Mystery of the Immaculate Concussion."

39 Ioffe, "The Mystery of the Immaculate Concussion."

40 Adam Entous, "Are U.S. Officials Under Silent Attack?," *The New Yorker*, May 24, 2021, available at: https://www.newyorker.com/magazine/2021/05/31/are-us-officials-under-silent-attack.

41 Ioffe, "The Mystery of the Immaculate Concussion."

42 Scott Pelley, "Havana Syndrome: High-Level National Security Officials Stricken with Unexplained Illness on White House Grounds," *CBS News*, June 26, 2022, available at: https://www.cbsnews.com/news/havana-syndrome-white-house-cabinet-60-minutes-2022-06-26/.

43 Pelley, "Havana Syndrome."

44 Ioffe, "The Mystery of the Immaculate Concussion."

45 Olivia Gazis, "U.S. Intensifies Efforts to Address 'Havana Syndrome', But Answers Remain Elusive," *CBS News*, July 27, 2021, available at: https://www.cbsnews.com/news/havana-syndrome-efforts-united-states/.

46 Christopher Eberhart, "CIA Evacuates Intelligence Officer from Serbia as 'Havana Syndrome' Attacks on American Spies and Diplomats Continue to Grow," *Daily Mail*, September 28, 2021, available at: https://www.dailymail.co.uk/news/article-10038159/CIA-evacuates-intelligence-officer-Serbia-result-Havana-Syndrome.html.

47 Pelley, "Havana Syndrome."

48 US Congress, "Silent Weapons: Examining Foreign Anomalous Health Incidents Targeting Americans in the Homeland and Abroad: Written Testimonies," House Homeland Security Subcommittee on Counterterrorism, Law Enforcement, and Intelligence, May 8, 2024, 8, available at: https://homeland.house.gov/wp-content/uploads/2024/05/2024-05-08-CTI-HRG-Testimony.pdf.

49 Nora Gamez Torres, "An FBI Agent Was Victim of a Havana Syndrome 'Attack' in Key West, Lawyer Tells Congress," *Miami Herald*, May 8, 2024, available at: https://www.miamiherald.com/news/nation-world/world/americas/cuba/article288423243.html.

50 Bradford Betz, "Florida Car Chase in 2020 May Be Linked to Havana Syndrome: Report," *New York Post*, April 1, 2024, available at: https://nypost.com/2024/04/01/us-news/florida-car-chase-in-2020-may-be-linked-to-mysterious-havana-syndrome/.

51 The Insider Staff, "Undercover Chef: How the FBI Interrogator of a Russian Spy Arrested in Florida Later Came Down with Havana Syndrome," *The Insider*, April 1, 2024, available at: https://theins.ru/en/politics/270450.

52 The Insider, "Undercover Chef."

53 Adam Entous, "Vienna Is the New Havana Syndrome Hotspot," *The New Yorker*, July 16, 2021, available at: https://www.newyorker.com/news/news-desk/vienna-is-the-new-havana-syndrome-hotspot.

54 John Hudson and Shane Harris, "CIA Chief in Vienna Recalled Amid Criticism of Management and Handling of Mysterious 'Havana Syndrome' Incidents," *Washington Post*, September 24, 2021.
55 Entous, "Vienna Is the New Havana Syndrome Hotspot."
56 Hudson and Harris, "CIA Chief in Vienna Recalled Amid Criticism of Management and Handling of Mysterious 'Havana Syndrome' Incidents."
57 Bojan Pancevski, "U.S. Officials in Germany Hit by Havana Syndrome," *Wall Street Journal*, August 18, 2021.
58 Der Spiegel Staff, "Berliner Landeskriminalamt ermittelt wegen Havana Syndrom," *Der Spiegel*, October 10, 2021, available at: https://www.spiegel.de/politik/deutschland/berliner-landeskriminalamt-ermittelt-wegen-havanna-syndrom-a-637fbcd2-8229-447e-956b-350e34b4174c.
59 RFA Vietnamese, "Report: US Officials Had Sudden Symptoms Before Harris' Hanoi Visit," *Radio Free Asia*, April 3, 2024, available at: https://www.rfa.org/english/news/vietnam/hanoi-havana-syndrome-report-04032024152734.html.
60 RFA Vietnamese, "Report: US Officials Had Sudden Symptoms Before Harris' Hanoi Visit."
61 Brit McCandless Farmer, "Havana Syndrome in Vietnam: Possible Russian Role in Attack on Americans, According to New Evidence," *CBS News*, July 7, 2024, available at: https://www.cbsnews.com/news/havana-syndrome-in-vietnam-possible-russian-role-in-attack-on-americans-new-evidence-60-minutes/.
62 Dobrokhotov, Grozev, and Weiss, "Unraveling Havana Syndrome."
63 Vivian Salama, "U.S. Diplomats in Geneva, Paris Struck with Suspected 'Havana Syndrome,'" *Wall Street Journal*, October 12, 2021.
64 Olivia Gazis, "CIA 'Havana Syndrome' Task Force Rules Out Foreign Attacks in Most Reported Cases in Interim Report," *CBS News*, January 20, 2022, available at: https://www.cbsnews.com/news/havana-syndrome-cia-task-force-foreign-attacks-rule-out/.
65 Warren P. Strobel, "Havana Syndrome Attacks Widen with CIA Officer's Evacuation from Serbia," *Wall Street Journal*, September 28, 2021.
66 Ellen Francis, "Colombia Aware of 'Havana Syndrome' Cases Reported at U.S. Embassy in Bogotá," *Washington Post*, October 13, 2021.
67 Salama and Ferero, "Havana Syndrome Hits at Least Five U.S. Families Connected to Embassy in Colombia."
68 Dobrokhotov, Grozev, and Weiss, "Unraveling Havana Syndrome."
69 Dobrokhotov, Grozev, and Weiss, "Unraveling Havana Syndrome."
70 Tara Copp, "U.S. Defense Department Official Had 'Havana Syndrome' Symptoms During a 2023 NATO Summit, the Pentagon Confirms," *PBS News Hour*, April 1, 2024, available at: https://www.pbs.org/newshour/politics/u-s-defense-official

-had-havana-syndrome-symptoms-during-a-2023-nato-summit-the-pentagon-confirms.

71 Anne Faherty, "Senior DoD Official Experienced 'Havana Syndrome' Symptoms at NATO Summit in July, Pentagon Says," *ABC News*, April 1, 2024, available at: https://abcnews.go.com/Politics/senior-dod-official-experienced-havana-syndrome-symptoms-nato/story?id=108714952.

72 Anne Gearan, "U.S. Expelled Two Cuban Diplomats After Embassy Employees Developed Ailments," *Washington Post*, August 9, 2017.

73 US Congress, "Attacks on U.S. Diplomats in Cuba: Response and Oversight," Senate Hearing 115-783, January 9, 2018.

74 Matt Spetalnick, "U.S. Expels Cuba's UN Diplomats, Citing 'Influence Operations,'" *Reuters*, September 19, 2019, available at: https://www.reuters.com/article/idUSKBN1W42W1/.

75 Elise Labott and Patrick Oppman, "State Department Orders Nonessential Diplomats and Families Out of Cuba Following Mysterious Attacks," *CNN*, September 29, 2017, available at: https://www.cnn.com/2017/09/29/politics/us-cuba-sonic-attacks-pulls-out-diplomats/index.html.

76 Peter Kornbluh, ed., "U.S.-Cuba: Secrets of the 'Havana Syndrome,'" *National Security Archive*, February 10, 2021, available at: https://nsarchive.gwu.edu/briefing-book/cuba/2021-02-10/secrets-havana-syndrome-how-trumps-state-department-cia-mishandled-mysterious-maladies-cuba.

77 US Department of State, "Havana, Cuba: Accountability Review Board," June 7, 2018, available at: https://nsarchive.gwu.edu/document/20672-havana-cuba-accountability-review-board-june-2018, 1.

78 US Department of State, "Cuba Accountability Review Board," *Office of the Spokesperson*, August 30, 2018, available at: https://2017-2021.state.gov/cuba-accountability-review-board/.

79 Michael Pompeo, "Establishment of the Health Incidents Response Task Force," *US Department of State Press Statement*, June 5, 2018, available at: https://2017-2021.state.gov/establishment-of-the-health-incidents-response-task-force/.

80 US Department of State, "Health Incident Response Task Force," *Deputy Secretary of State for Management and Resources*, available at: https://www.state.gov/health-incident-response-task-force/.

81 US Congress, "Attacks on U.S. Diplomats in Cuba: Response and Oversight."

82 US Congress, "Attacks on U.S. Diplomats in Cuba: Response and Oversight."

83 Sean Power and Michael Miner, "Report—Havana Syndrome: Americans Under Attack," *Belfer Center for Science and International Affairs*, Harvard University, November 4, 2021, available at: https://www.belfercenter.org/publication/report-havana-syndrome-american-officials-under-attack.

84 Emily Crane, "FBI Acknowledges Agents May Have Had 'Havana Syndrome' Symptoms," *New York Post*, November 24, 2021, available at: https://nypost.com/2021/11/24/fbi-acknowledges-agents-may-have-had-havana-syndrome-symptoms/.
85 Katie Bo Lillis, "CIA Doctor Hit by Havana Syndrome Says He Was in 'Disbelief' as He Suffered What He Was Investigating," *CNN*, September 25, 2022, available at: https://edition.cnn.com/2022/09/25/politics/havana-syndrome-cia-doctor-cnn-special/index.html.
86 Tim Golden and Sebastian Rotella, "The Strange Case of American Diplomats in Cuba: As the Mystery Deepens So Do Divisions in Washington," *ProPublica*, November 9, 2018, available at: https://www.propublica.org/article/the-strange-case-of-american-diplomats-in-cuba-as-the-mystery-deepens-so-do-divisions-in-washington.
87 Golden and Rotella, "The Strange Case of American Diplomats in Cuba."
88 Julian Barnes, "C.I.A. to Expand Inquiry Into Mysterious Health Episodes Overseas," *New York Times*, March 4, 2021.
89 Katie Bo Lillis, "CIA Assesses It's Unlikely Havana Syndrome Is Due to 'Sustained Worldwide Campaign' by a Foreign Country in Interim Report," *CNN Wire Service*, January 20, 2022.
90 US Department of Defense, "Evaluation of the DoD's Response to Anomalous Health Incidents, or 'Havana Syndrome,'" Office of the Inspector General, March 9, 2023, 1, available at: https://media.defense.gov/2023/Mar/28/2003187716/-1/-1/1/DODIG-2023-054_REDACTED.PDF.
91 Julian E. Barnes, "Pentagon Asks Personnel About Health Anomalies," *New York Times*, September 16, 2021.
92 US Department of Defense, "Memorandum for All Department of Defense Employees," Secretary of Defense, September 15, 2021, available at: https://irp.fas.org/news/2021/09/dod-ahi.pdf.
93 US Department of Defense, "Evaluation of the DoD's Response to Anomalous Health Incidents, or 'Havana Syndrome,'" 7.
94 US Department of Defense, "Evaluation of the DoD's Response to Anomalous Health Incidents, or 'Havana Syndrome,'" 2.
95 US Department of Defense, "AHI Patient Registry FAQs," Military Health System, available at: https://www.health.mil/Reference-Center/Frequently-Asked-Questions/AHI-Patient-Registry?query=ahi (accessed July 30, 2024).
96 General Accounting Office Staff, "Havana Syndrome—Americans Affected by Mysterious Symptoms May Struggle to Get Care," *General Accounting Office*, July 29, 2024, available at: https://www.gao.gov/blog/havana-syndrome-americans-affected-mysterious-symptoms-may-struggle-get-care.

97 US Department of Defense, "Defense Health Program Budget," Office of the Comptroller, March 2022, available at: https://comptroller.defense.gov/Portals/45/Documents/defbudget/fy2023/budget_justification/pdfs/09_Defense_Health_Program/25-Vol_II_Sec_7-RDTE_Budget_Item_Justification_DHP_PB23.pdf.

98 Ken Klippenstein, "Pentagon Requests $36 Million for Havana Syndrome," *The Intercept*, April 20, 2023, available at: https://theintercept.com/2023/04/20/pentagon-budget-havana-syndrome/.

99 Lara Seligman, "The Pentagon Is Funding Experiments on Animals to 'Recreate Havana Syndrome,'" *Politico*, March 9, 2023.

100 PETA Staff, "Victory! Army Ends Brain-Damage Testing on Ferrets at Wayne State Following PETA Pressure," *PETA Press Release*, November 16, 2023, available at: https://www.peta.org/media/news-releases/victory-army-ends-brain-damage-testing-on-ferrets-at-wayne-state-following-pressure-from-peta/.

101 US Department of Defense, "Evaluation of the DoD's Response to Anomalous Health Incidents, or 'Havana Syndrome,'" 8.

102 US Department of Defense, "Evaluation of the DoD's Response to Anomalous Health Incidents, or 'Havana Syndrome,'" 9.

103 Steve Schuster, "Alleged CIA Developed Havana Syndrome Energy-Weapon, Attorney Says One Possible Theory for Cover-Up," *Wisconsin Law Journal*, April 10, 2024, available at: https://wislawjournal.com/2024/04/10/cia-developed-havana-syndrome-energy-weapon-attorney-says-possible-reason-for-coverup-2/.

104 US Congress, "Attacks on U.S. Diplomats in Cuba: Response and Oversight."

105 US Congress, "Attacks on U.S. Diplomats in Cuba: Response and Oversight."

106 US Congress, "Attacks on U.S. Diplomats in Cuba: Response and Oversight."

107 Lara Seligman, Andrew Desiderio, and Erin Banco, "U.S. Probing Suspected Directed-Energy Attack on Government Personnel in Miami," *Politico*, April 29, 2021, available at: https://www.politico.com/news/2021/04/29/directed-energy-attack-probe-485086.

108 Lara Seligman, Andrew Desiderio, and Betsy Woodruff Swann, "U.S. Troops Increasingly Vulnerable to Directed-Energy Attacks, Pentagon Tells Lawmakers," *Politico*, April 22, 2021, available at: https://www.politico.com/news/2021/04/22/troops-directed-energy-attacks-484246.

109 Seligman, Desiderio, and Woodruff Swan, "U.S. Troops Increasingly Vulnerable to Directed-Energy Attacks, Pentagon Tells Lawmakers."

110 US Congress, "Chairman Pfluger Opens 'Havana Syndrome' Hearing: 'It Is Paramount That We Acknowledge the Gravity of the Situation,'" House Homeland Security Committee, May 8, 2024, available at: https://homeland.house.gov/2024/05/08/chairman-pfluger-opens-havana-syndrome-hearing-it-is-paramount-that-we-acknowledge-the-gravity-of-the-situation/.

111 US Congress, "Testimony of Christo Grozev," Homeland Security Committee, May 8, 2024, available at: https://homeland.house.gov/wp-content/uploads/2024/05/2024-05-08-CTI-HRG-Testimony.pdf.
112 US Congress, "Testimony of Greg Edgreen," Homeland Security Committee, May 8, 2024, available at: https://homeland.house.gov/wp-content/uploads/2024/05/2024-05-08-CTI-HRG-Testimony.pdf.
113 US Congress, "Testimony of Mark Ziad, Esq," Homeland Security Committee, May 8, 2024, 2, available at: https://homeland.house.gov/wp-content/uploads/2024/05/2024-05-08-CTI-HRG-Testimony.pdf.
114 US Congress, "Testimony of Mark Ziad, Esq," 2.
115 US Congress, "S.1828—HAVANA Act of 2021," Congress.gov, introduced May 25, 2021, available at: https://www.congress.gov/bill/117th-congress/senate-bill/1828/text.
116 John Hudson and Shane Harris, "U.S. to Give Some 'Havana Syndrome' Victims Six-Figure Compensation," *Washington Post*, June 23, 2022.
117 Hudson and Harris, "U.S. to Give Some 'Havana Syndrome' Victims Six-Figure Compensation."
118 US Congress, "H.R. 4914—Havana Syndrome Attacks Response Act," House Foreign Affairs Committee, August 3, 2021.
119 US Congress, "H.R. 7305—IIR on AHI Act," House Armed Services Committee, February 7, 2024.
120 US Congress, "H.R. 7305—IIR on AHI Act," Section 2a.
121 Brandi Vincent, "Lawmakers Question How 'Havana Syndrome' Is Affecting DoD," *Defensescoop.com*, February 12, 2024, available at: https://defensescoop.com/2024/02/12/lawmakers-question-how-havana-syndrome-is-affecting-dod/.

6

The Investigations

The US government has conducted numerous investigations into the possible causes of Havana Syndrome, some of which are still ongoing. The different studies vary greatly in their methodologies and conclusions. Some of the investigations suggest that Havana Syndrome is unlikely to be the result of a deliberate act but may have other causes that explain the health incidents. Other investigations that have looked more at the potential mechanisms for causing Havana Syndrome suggest that a deliberate attack cannot be ruled out based on the alleged impossibility of a Havana Syndrome weapon (see table 6.1). This chapter seeks to provide an overview of the government-sponsored research into Havana Syndrome to the extent it has been released. Obviously, a lot more information can be assumed to exist in the classified realm, which may or may not provide a better answer to the phenomenon.

Clinical Studies on AHIs

The State Department commissioned several academic studies to determine whether US diplomats had suffered measurable brain injuries because of some kind of exposure. The University of Pennsylvania's Center for Brain Injury and Repair produced two studies, which were published in the JAMA in February 2018 and July 2019.[1] These two studies were instrumental in lending academic credibility to the assertions of the State Department and the individuals affected by AHIs that they had been covertly attacked with a new type of DEW. However, in March 2024, JAMA published an NIH study that refuted many of the findings of the earlier two studies.[2]

Table 6.1 Government Investigations and Studies

Government Investigation	Year	Methodology	Conclusions	Comments
FBI investigation	2017	Investigation of the AHIs in Cuba	No detection of adversarial activity in Cuba	Report not published
FBI Behavioral Analysis Unit study	2018	Review of case files for behavioral analysis	Mass psychogenic illness	Did not interview victims or consider medical diagnoses—report not released to the public
JASON study 1	2018	Analysis of sound and video recordings from Cuba	Sounds likely caused by crickets	Only investigated recorded sounds
State Department Accountability Review Board study	2018	Review of case files and medical data of the first 24 AHIs in Cuba, interviews with some AHI patients	The board determined that the cases were security related but mechanism and perpetrators remained unknown	The report relied largely on the medical data to reach the conclusion
CDC study	2019	Reviewed 95 medical records	Unable to determine mechanism of injury	Purpose of the study was the development of a diagnosis
National Academies of Sciences study	2020	Review of medical records, interviewing of victims, consultation of experts	Most likely mechanism of injury is pulsed microwaves	NAS team had only limited access to classified information
CIA investigation	2021	Detection of signs of adversarial activity at the time when AHIs occurred	No detection of adversarial activity related to AHIs	The CIA's interim assessment on AHI's remains classified
IC Expert Panel	2022	Review of 1,000 classified documents by experts and interviewing of victims	Most likely mechanism of injury is electromagnetic directed energy	Report has been declassified in redacted form
ODNI assessment	2023	Intelligence assessment by the IC, review of foreign weapons and research, medical analysis	Highly unlikely that foreign adversaries were responsible for AHIs	Only a summary has been publicly released to the public

First JAMA Study

The first study led by Randel Swanson was based on the medical examination of twenty-one individuals (ten men and eleven women) who had been afflicted by Havana Syndrome, as determined by medical doctors from the State Department.[3] The twenty-one individuals had to undergo multiple tests conducted by a multidisciplinary team using different methodologies. "Neuropsychological test batteries included assessment of the following domains: (1) auditory attention, (2) auditory and visual working memory, (3) auditory and visual memory, (4) visual-spatial perception, (5) visual-motor construction, (6) motor function, (7) language function, (8) executive function, (9) processing speed, (10) academic achievement, (11) reasoning, (12) mood functioning, and (13) effort."[4] There were vestibular evaluations using an MRI, oculomotor evaluations to test saccadic speed and accuracy, auditory evaluations, and imaging evaluations.

The study indicated that almost all individuals experienced a rapid onset of symptoms, and that these symptoms lasted for longer than three months. In six individuals who had undergone complete neuropsychological testing, there were measurable impairments "in executive function (n = 6), motor function (n = 5), auditory and visual memory (n = 4), visual-spatial perception and visual-motor construction (n = 4), auditory attention and working memory (n = 3), language (n = 3), processing speed (n = 4), and reasoning (n = 1)."[5] The study found that nine out of twenty-one suffered from persistent hearing reduction, that eighteen suffered from sleep problems, that eighteen developed headaches and sixteen suffered from persistent headaches, and that the neuroimaging findings were inconclusive. The authors argued that the discovered findings indicated a "novel clinical entity, which appears to have resulted from a widespread brain network dysfunction (i.e., cognitive, oculomotor, and central vestibular) as seen in mild traumatic brain injury, or concussion, as well as injury to the peripheral vestibular system in some cases."[6] The authors claimed that "[s]everal of the objective manifestations consistently found in this cohort (such as oculomotor and vestibular testing abnormalities) could not have been consciously or unconsciously manipulated."[7] They hence rejected the possible diagnosis of a mass psychogenic illness as a cause, pointing out that there was great variance in age among the affected individuals (untypical for mass psychogenic illness) and a desire to return to work (even against the advice of their physicians).

There were a number of limitations to the study. First, the study was undertaken on average 203 days after the onset of the AHIs, which could have affected the results or the physical evidence for an attack.[8] Because of the sensitive nature of the work of the individuals, various details about the cases could not be included in the publication. Not every patient underwent the full set of tests. There remained uncertainty as to how many individuals were affected since some with milder symptoms may not have reported them, which would make it more difficult to determine the necessary exposure for acute or chronic symptoms.[9] Critics have pointed out several flaws in the study. For example, Sergio Della Sala and Roberto Cubelli from the University of Edinburgh claimed that the study "represents a case of neuropsychology," which was "clinically inappropriate and methodologically improper."[10] Sala and Cubelli argued that the study set the bar too low for the threshold of impaired performance, which meant that there would be "no evidence that the people assessed present with any cognitive deficit (to be linked or not with their stay in Cuba)."[11]

Critics also claimed that the physical evidence for a concussion or brain trauma was weak, which was somewhat acknowledged by the lead author, Randel Swanson: "If you took any one of these patients and put them into a brain injury clinic, and you didn't know their background, you would think that they had a traumatic brain injury from being in a car accident or a blast in the military. . . . It's like a concussion without a concussion."[12] In other words, the determination that the individuals suffered a concussion is subjective since there was no evidence of a blunt trauma that caused cognitive impairment measured by the psychometric tests. Furthermore, the article did not discuss what exactly caused the condition experienced by the individuals, other than alleging that it was induced by some kind of harmful exposure.

Second JAMA Study

The second University of Pennsylvania study was led by Ragini Verma and was a neuroimaging study conducted on altogether forty patients (including twenty of the twenty-one patients from the 2018 study) to determine whether there were any brain changes possibly connected to some kind of harmful exposure. The study was supposed to provide hard scientific evidence of brain damage suffered by individuals with Havana Syndrome. The results of the MRI scans were compared with two control cohorts with similar characteristics (age, education, health, and status) to the test cohort.[13]

The brain scans were examining the following: brain tissue volume maps, which mapped white matter and gray matter volumes; tissue microstructural integrity maps, which measured water diffusion in the brain; and functional connectivity, which used imaging data to map auditory, visuospatial, and executive control subnetworks.[14] The researchers hypothesized that there would be differences in overall white matter and gray matter volume, in tissue microstructural integrity, and in the functional connectivity between the control and the test group.[15] The brain imagery analysis was supported by statistical modeling to establish a baseline normality, adjust for age and sex, and interpret results of the imaging.

Among the findings were that "[w]hole brain white matter volume of patients was significantly smaller than that of controls," and that "there were widespread voxel-wise differences in the brains of patients compared with controls in the voxel-wise analysis, both in white matter and gray matter."[16] The "[m]icrostructural tissue metrics of the gray matter exhibited nonnormal residuals," and "indicated lower mean diffusivity and axial diffusivity in the anterior limb of the internal capsule, inferior colliculi, superior cerebral peduncle, and occipital white matter" for the patient group.[17] Although "[t]here was no significant difference in the executive control subnetwork, . . . [a]nalysis of the secondary hypothesis revealed lowered interregional functional connectivity within the visuospatial subnetworks of patients vs controls."[18] The study concluded:

> Among US government personnel in Havana, Cuba, with potential directional phenomena exposure, compared with healthy controls, advanced brain MRI techniques revealed significant neuroimaging differences in whole brain white matter volume, regional gray and white matter volume, cerebellar tissue microstructural integrity, and functional connectivity in the auditory and visuospatial subnetworks but not in the executive control subnetwork.[19]

The researchers acknowledged that it was difficult to match the patient group with a control group that was sufficiently similar, that there was a small heterogenous sample of patients, which makes it possible that "the findings represent group-level statistical differences as opposed to individual changes that may be highly variable . . . it cannot be determined whether the differences among the patients are due to individual differences between patients or differences in level and degree of exposure to an uncharacterized directional phenomenon."[20] In other words, it is possible that observed differences in the imaging results could be accounted for by individual variation.[21]

National Institutes of Health Study

In March 2024, the NIH published a neuroimaging study in JAMA that seemed to refute the findings of the earlier neuroimaging study conducted at the University of Pennsylvania. Essentially, the NIH team conducted a very similar study to the University of Pennsylvania study, where the brain scans of an AHI patient group were compared with a control group composed of individuals with similar characteristics as the patient group. The findings of the study were widely reported in the press as showing "no evidence of 'Havana Syndrome' in brain scans."[22] It seemed that the results of previous studies showing indications of brain changes in AHI patients were wrong. A closer look at the study reveals a somewhat different conclusion.

The NIH team conducted MRI brain scans of 81 AHI patients and compared them to MRIs of a control group of 48 healthy individuals with some similar characteristics such as age, sex, and profession. The mean age for the AHI patients was 42, with 40 female and 41 male patients. The study lists the symptoms experienced by the AHI patients during or after the incidents as: headache (60), sleep dysfunction (47), depression (18), vision changes (30), PTSD (7), imbalance (43), cognitive dysfunction (55), and dizziness (32). They also received the following diagnoses during or after the incidents: migraine headache (32), tinnitus (45), peripheral neuropathy (11), cranial neuropathy (6), headache, unspecified (13), cancer (5), strabismus (vision disorder) (3), seizure disorder (1), functional neurologic disorder (20), new daily persistent headache (20), current cataract (21), benign paroxysmal positional vertigo (3), and tension-type headache (2).[23] The study confirmed the existence of symptoms in the AHI group, most of which were experienced only during or after the incidents by the AHI group.

The neuroimaging sought to determine whether there were significant differences in the brains of the AHI patients compared to a healthy control group, which could indicate some kind of brain damage that may cause the experienced symptoms. The study authors stated that "[t]he majority of the brain MRI scans were unremarkable as read by clinical neuroradiologists" and that the AHI patients had a slightly lower amount of white matter abnormality (gliosis) compared to the control group.[24] They concluded that "there were no significant differences between participants with AHIs and control participants for any MRI modality . . . [and] there was no evidence of widespread brain lesions in the AHI group."[25]

The NIH team acknowledged some limitations of their study, which indicate that they do not refute the existence of symptoms in the AHI patients group or the possibility of environmental factors being causative for the symptoms. The sample size was still relatively small, the brain scans in the AHI patients group occurred at a minimum 14 days after the incident and at a maximum of 1,505 days, and the MRI scans were limited to standard protocols. They stated that "[t]hese findings suggest that the current criteria used by the Intelligence Community Experts Panel to identify cases of interest do not correspond to distinct MRI patterns. That this study did not identify a neuroimaging signature of brain injury in this AHI cohort does not detract from the seriousness of the clinical condition."[26] In other words, they acknowledge that the symptoms experienced by the AHI patient group were real, but they could not be connected to some abnormal brain condition indicated in the MRI scans. Hence, the NIH study did not disprove the existence of Havana Syndrome or the possibility that it was externally induced through some sort of harmful exposure. In an interesting twist, NIH has now ended their research into Havana Syndrome after complaints that some study participants had been unethically coerced by their employers.[27]

The JASON Reports (2018 and 2021)

JASON is an independent scientific advisory group to DoD that is contracted from time to time to weigh in on military technology issues such as the feasibility of a new weapons system without the bias that results from dealing directly with defense companies or individuals within the government.[28] They are leading US scientists who offer their expertise on a variety of important topics relevant to DoD. The JASONs were consulted with respect to Havana Syndrome, and they produced two studies that have since been declassified.

The First JASON Report

One theory to explain the sounds heard by the diplomats affected by the Havana Syndrome is that they actually heard crickets rather than anything caused by a DEW. Sounds were recorded by some affected diplomats in Havana, and one recording was released by the *Associated Press*.[29] The high-pitched sounds heard by the diplomats in Cuba could be related to a sonic weapon causing disorientation and/or some kind of brain damage. The JASONs were asked to "[e]valuate possible sources for the generation of the acoustic and other sensations experienced by personnel (and their families) . . . [and to] [s]uggest ways to protect personnel in their residencies to avoid medical consequences from any similar future events."[30] For this purpose, the JASONs reviewed audio and video recordings produced by US personnel in Cuba and some medical records, and they spoke to one affected individual, who had recorded some of the video evidence. The report was finished in November 2018 but was only declassified and released in a heavily redacted form in 2021.

The JASON report states that many individuals who suffered AHIs reported hearing unusual sounds at the time of the onset, although some did not hear any sound. They also pointed out that audible sound at the observed sound intensity pressure level and duration would not be harmful in itself. The report examined the possible external causes for the medical conditions of the twenty-one US embassy personnel affected by AHIs in Cuba, including audible sound, infrasound, ultrasound, radiofrequency waves, microwaves, as well as the possibility of biological and chemical attacks, and of mass psychogenic illness.

The JASONs claimed that "[t]he recorded audio signal is, with high confidence, not produced by the nonlinear detection of high-power radiofrequency or ultrasound pulses. . . . We judge as highly unlikely the notion that pulsed RF mimics acoustic signals in both the brain (via the Frey effect) and in electronics (through RF interference/pickup)."[31] They concluded: "We believe the recorded sounds are mechanical or biological in origin. The most likely source is the Indies short-tailed cricket, *Anurogryllis celerinictus*."[32] Incidentally, two biologists, one from the University of California, Berkeley, and the other from the University of Lincoln, UK, analyzed the sounds published by AP and similarly claimed that the recorded sounds matched that of a Caribbean cricket if "played on a loudspeaker and recorded indoors."[33] They also claimed that the cricket species that can be heard in the recording is *Anurogryllus celerinictus* based on the analysis of one recording. The JASONs further alluded that mass psychogenic illness could explain some of the clinical symptoms such as dizziness, noting that "psychogenic effects on vestibular function are common, and the symptoms can be chronic."[34]

There are several limitations in the JASON study that shall be pointed out. First, the study was based on just two audio and one video recording from Havana, Cuba. The sample size for the recordings is just too small, and they cannot account for AHIs that occurred later in locations in which there were no crickets present. The sounds captured may or may not have had any connection to the health incidents. The JASONs suggested that "the use of a 'natural' sound . . . would be for cover or deniability, in which the use of an unusual electronic signal would be too revealing."[35] More than 50 percent of the JASONs' report was redacted, especially the sections that were not discussing crickets, including the conclusion part of the report. It is therefore difficult to draw any meaningful conclusions from the finding that a few recordings of US personnel in Cuba happened to capture cricket sounds.

The Second JASON Report

JASON produced a second report that is dated November 2021 and revised the earlier conclusions with respect to cricket noises combined with mass psychogenic illness being the most plausible explanation for the Havana Syndrome.[36] The second report was released to the public in early February 2022.[37] What is notable about the released report is that it is largely unredacted apart from sections in the appendix that are marked as classified. The second study is a review of the AHI data and it tests various hypotheses with respect to the potential causes, which include an acoustic attack, an electromagnetic attack, and more benign explanations such as psychogenic illness. JASON tried to fit the available information on the AHI cases in terms of the medical data and specific circumstances of the reported incidents with possible mechanisms of injury based on a systematic review of the available literature.

JASON pointed out that for AHIs having been caused by some kind of attack, the following conditions would need to be met:

> [E]nergy must be able to penetrate into buildings through walls and windows from a distance of several tens of meters, be localized to areas the size of a room or smaller, be generated with equipment that is mobile and covert, lead to audible and/or recordable sounds, cause immediate symptoms of pressure, vertigo, headache, or nausea, and cause long-term vestibular and/or cognitive dysfunction.[38]

JASON found that there were inconsistencies with respect to all the conceivable mechanisms that include audible sound devices, infrasound devices, ultrasound devices, ionizing electromagnetic radiation, and RF/microwave electromagnetic radiation.

They considered infrasound unlikely because existing studies only indicate mild and transient effects on human health.[39] In any case, there is no possibility for infrasound to cause traumatic brain injury or concussion. Audible sound is also unlikely because most of the AHIs occurred within buildings, which dampen the effect. To deliver enough sound intensity inside the building, the emitter would need to be extremely powerful and large, which would mean that a covert attack would be difficult. Ultrasound is, for a similar reason, unlikely since it is even less able to penetrate walls. JASON also noted that "no persistent effects have been reported" with respect to ultrasound at higher exposure intensity.

A large portion of the report discussed the possibility of electromagnetic radiation as a potential cause for AHI. Ionizing radiation is relatively easy to dismiss as a cause as "[t]he combined difficulties of generation, collimation, and penetration of ionizing radiation across the relevant distances renders this attack modality highly improbable with a portable device."[40] The JASONs pointed out that RF energy cannot in principle cause traumatic brain injury "without concomitant sensations of heat and or pain," while also stating that they found "no compelling evidence of TBI to date."[41] They dismiss RF/microwaves below 500 MHz as a mechanism because that would require a very large antenna and any heating of the brain would also be felt on the skin as a heating sensation, which is inconsistent with the AHIs. On the other hand, at the higher-frequency spectrum of 30 GHz and above there would be no ability of the electromagnetic waves to penetrate the body deeper than the skin. Of course, this would also produce a heating sensation on the skin.[42] This leaves the frequency range between 1 GHz and 10 GHz as the most likely mechanism of injury and it would also be most consistent with the Frey effect for explaining auditory sensations reported in many AHIs. However, there were also several inconsistencies with the AHIs in the authors' view, as it would cause a heating sensation on the skin, the ability to penetrate buildings would be limited, and a medium-sized antenna would be needed.[43]

The report concludes that

> [r]egarding adversarial intent, it is not possible to conclude at this time that the events reviewed by JASON are the result of intentional attacks that cause physical harm. However, it is not possible either, to rule out mechanisms that do not cause any physical harm but which might constitute harassment and lead to health conditions and functional disorders, for example through unpleasant sounds or pressure sensations.[44]

They noted that "85–90% of the reported incidents are consistent with common and known symptoms of pathophysiological or environmental origins; the remainder appear more complex and defy a straightforward explanation at present."[45] JASON suggested that "no single hypothesized mechanism can explain all of the incidents" and they hence proposed identifying the most relevant criteria for AHIs in order to remove cases from the AHI data that have other more plausible explanations.[46]

What becomes clear from this report is that the AHIs are very heterogenous, which suggests that there could be a range of different causes or mechanisms at play. It is conceivable that if the 10–15 percent of more mysterious cases were caused by a deliberate attack, then perhaps different types of weapons with different mechanisms were used against different individuals. The JASON report was dismissive of the idea of nonthermal effects of electromagnetic energy, which, as previously noted, is not well-researched in the published Western literature (see table 6.2).

Table 6.2 Comparison of Symptoms in Three Havana Syndrome Studies

Subjective Symptoms	**JAMA 2018 (%)**	**CDC 2019 (%)**	**NIH 2024 (%)**
Cognitive and behavioral			
Combined	81	39	64
Difficulty remembering	76	-	-
Mental fog	76	-	-
Difficulty concentrating	71	-	-
Feeling slowed	67	-	-
Irritability	67	-	-
Feeling more emotional	52	-	-
Disorientation	-	6	-
Depression	-	-	22
Balance and vestibular			
Combined	71	40	53
Balance problems	67	-	-
Dizziness	62	-	37
Nausea	33	21	-
Vision and ocolumotor			
Combined	86	25	37
Visual problems	76	-	-
Light sensitivity	62	-	-
Difficulty reading	57	-	-
Eye strain	52	-	-

(*Continued*)

Table 6.2 (Continued)

Subjective Symptoms	JAMA 2018 (%)	CDC 2019 (%)	NIH 2024 (%)
Auditory			
Combined	68	34	-
Sound sensitivity	67	-	-
Tinnitus	57	-	55
Hearing reduction	43	-	-
Ear pressure	38	-	-
Sleep			
Combined	86	-	60
Drowsiness or fatigue	76	-	-
Decreased sleep duration	71	-	-
Trouble falling asleep	67	-	-
Headache			
Combined	76	37	70
With cognitive tasks	62	-	-
With therapy	52	-	-
Due to photophobia	43	-	-
Due to phonophobia	29	-	-
Head pressure	-	12	-
Migraine headache	-	-	39
Other diagnoses			
Cancer	-	-	6
Strabismus	-	-	4
Seizure disorder	-	-	1
Functional neurologic disorder	-	-	25
Current cataract	-	-	26

The National Academy of Sciences Report (2020)

The Department of State tasked the National Academies of Sciences (NAS) with investigating the possible causes of the AHIs by reviewing the known cases and by finding potential mechanisms of injury. The NAS established a committee of nineteen experts chaired by David Relman, a professor of medicine at Stanford University. Relman has substantial credentials in the area of national security: he was vice-chair of the National Research Council that reviewed the FBI's anthrax investigation, he was chair of the National Academies of Sciences Forum on Microbial Threats, he is a current member of the Intelligence Community Studies Board, he is a founding member of the National Science and Advisory Board on Biosecurity, and he was a member of the White House Working Group on Biodefense for the president.[47] The committee members consisted of scientists in the fields of medicine, neuroscience, biostatistics, epidemiology, public health, medical ethics, physics, toxicology, bioeffects of directed energy, psychiatry, and electrical and computer engineering. The committee held two in-person meetings in 2019 and 2020 and one virtual meeting in 2020.[48] The committee published their final report in December 2020. The report is notable because of its conclusion that directed pulsed radio frequency energy was the most likely cause for the AHIs.[49]

Methodology

The primary method used by the committee was a review of the clinical data produced by the two teams at the University of Miami and the University of Pennsylvania. They also reviewed clinical data from the affected Canadian diplomats (data from Dalhousie University). The committee met with eight of the individuals suffering from Havana Syndrome, who had been posted to Cuba and China. Furthermore, the committee heard expert opinions on the different possible mechanisms of injury, such as chemical exposure and exposure to radiofrequency. The committee had access to information from the Department of State Bureau of Medical Services and to their employees.

The report suggested that

> [t]he most distinctive clinical aspects of the illnesses described in DOS Havana personnel are the nature of the onset and the initial features: the sudden onset of a perceived loud sound, a sensation of intense pressure or vibration in the head, and pain in the ear or more diffusely in the head. Most individuals reported that the sound or these other sensations seemed to originate from a particular direction and that they were perceived only when the individual was in a specific physical location. Different numbers of individuals also reported sudden onset of tinnitus, hearing loss, dizziness, unsteady gait and visual disturbances.[50]

The report argued that the possible explanations for the acute symptoms experienced by individuals who suffered AHIs could be explained "by directed RF energy, as well as toxic, infectious, and psychological processes."[51]

The committee considered the possible exposure of affected personnel to organophosphates (nerve agents), which are used in insecticides. The report pointed out that some AHIs coincided with the spraying of insecticides to combat the spread of Zika virus, a mosquito-borne disease. The Canadian fumigation study that had been carried out at the University of Dalhousie concluded that exposure to organophosphates could explain the acute symptoms in the affected Canadian diplomats. The NAS team rejected the conclusion by arguing that residues of insecticides were not discovered in affected US diplomats and only in a smaller subsection of the affected Canadian diplomats.[52] Furthermore, they pointed out that "the clinical history of affected US Embassy personnel is not consistent with acute OP poisoning."[53]

The NAS committee considered the possibility that AHIs in Havana and China may have been caused by an exotic infectious disease such as Zika virus, dengue, and chikungunya, which are all transmitted by mosquitoes. Although Zika virus was present in Cuba at the time of the AHIs, very few people were infected, and complications of Zika that could have caused some of the Havana Syndrome symptoms occur only in less than one in a thousand, while some of the more common symptoms associated with Zika were not experienced at all by affected US personnel in Cuba.[54] All of this makes it unlikely that the Zika virus was the cause of AHIs.

Psychological and social factors, such as traumatic stress and social contagion, could have conceivably caused some of the symptoms, especially the more generic chronic symptoms. Acute auditory and vestibular symptoms could have been hallucinations or delusions. The report stated that "the committee did conclude that delusional disorders could not explain the full range of symptoms reported by the entire group of patients."[55] Mass psychogenic illness should be resolved within months and some of the experienced AHI symptoms such as hearing directional would not match other cases of psychogenic illness.[56]

The NAS committee considered directed radiofrequency as a potential mechanism of injury. They mainly pointed at the possible nonthermal bioeffects of radiofrequency energy other than cancer, which have been demonstrated in some studies. The report stated:

> [T]he committee finds that many of the acute, early phase symptoms and observations reported by DOS employees are consistent with RF effects, including a perceived clicking sound within the head even when the ears were covered, a perceived force/pressure sensation within the head and on the face, perceived spatial localization and directionality of these perceived phenomena and other loud sounds, hearing loss, tinnitus, impaired gait and loss of balance,

> as well as the absence of heating sensation and absence of observed disruption of electronic devices in the immediate environment. In addition, many of the chronic, nonspecific symptoms are also consistent with known RF effects, such as dizziness, headache, fatigue, nausea, anxiety, cognitive deficits, and memory loss.[57]

The reports cite studies and reviews of studies on nonthermal bioeffects of RF energy that were undertaken in the Soviet Union during the Cold War, as well as some newer studies that suggest the influence of RF energy on the central nervous system, cognitive and behavioral effects, effects on sleep, and auditory effects. They mentioned the Frey effect, which could explain the loud noises heard by some affected individuals. The committee found that both the acute symptoms and the chronic symptoms would be most consistent with harmful RF exposure. They suggested that "[i]t is not necessary for RF energy sources to produce gross structural damage to cause symptoms. Rather, as with the Frey effect or potential thermoelastic pressure waves, RF sources may trigger symptoms by transiently inducing alterations in brain functioning."[58]

Limitations

Although the NAS committee made a good case for pulsed RF energy as a likely cause for at least some of the AHIs, the study has some major limitations, which have invited a lot of criticism. The committee acknowledged that the AHI cases were too heterogenous to identify a single causal mechanism, that there is "no consistent picture of brain injury," and that they did not have access to all relevant data, which meant that "follow-up studies on this topic [should] be undertaken by subject-matter experts with proper clearance."[59] Bartholomew and Bahoh called the findings of the NAS committee "perplexing" and alluded that the committee was politically biased against the more obvious conclusion of mass psychogenic illness since the only expert on it, Simon Wessely, was removed from the team.[60] It is also the case that the NAS team emphasized the directional auditory aspect of the AHIs that may have led them to conclude that the Frey effect and hence pulsed microwave was a main mechanism for the acute and some of the chronic phenomena. These conclusions were derived primarily from fairly outdated open scientific literature and were not informed by classified studies that may have pointed in different directions.

The IC Expert Panel Report

The Biden administration commissioned an additional expert review of the Havana Syndrome, following the increase in cases in late summer 2021. The DNI Avril Haines and CIA Deputy Director David Cohen formed a panel of IC experts, which produced a final report in September 2022. The report was initially classified but was released in redacted form to the public after a Freedom of Information Act request by the James Madison Project in March 2023. What is different about the earlier studies is that the IC Expert Panel utilized a larger number of classified sources, which were not available to the JASON group or the NAS committee. The panel was composed of experts from within the government and from outside of the government with expertise in science, medicine, and engineering.[61] The panel met periodically with members of the JASON group that produced the 2021 report.[62]

Methodology

The objective of the study was to determine the causal mechanisms for the AHIs and to make recommendations on how to move forward. The panel had access to "more than 1,000 classified documents on scientific, medical, and intelligence topics," as well as "sensitive intelligence reporting, AHI event descriptions and trend analyses. . . . Affected individuals also shared their personal experiences and portions of their medical records."[63] The panel considered the following mechanisms: (1) acoustic signals, (2) chemical and biological agents, (3) ionizing radiation, (4) psychosocial, medical, and other natural and environmental factors, and (5) radiofrequency and other electromagnetic energy. The panel tested each hypothesis against the available data to determine the most likely causal mechanism and draw further conclusions as to what needs to be done to prevent future AHIs.

The panel identified four core characteristics of the AHIs:

> (1) the acute onset of audiovestibular sensory phenomena, including sound and/or pressure, sometimes in only one ear or on one side of the head; (2) other nearly simultaneous signs and symptoms such as vertigo, loss of balance, and ear pain; (3) a strong sense of locality or directionality; and (4) the absence of known environmental or medical conditions that could explain the reported signs and symptoms.[64]

The panel pointed out, similarly to the NAS committee, that the AHI cases were heterogenous in terms of symptoms and circumstances, which makes it likely that there could be different or multiple mechanisms responsible. The most common symptoms would be "a sudden sense of pressure or loud, unpleasant sound, and the signs and symptoms are most commonly pain, nausea, dizziness, and cognitive impairment" with "[a] subset of incidents also reports very distinctive events including the sensation of locality or directionality."[65] The long-term or chronic symptoms included "persistent new headache, worsening of migraine headache, sleep disorders, imbalance, a sense of dizziness, tinnitus, and the loss of high-level cognitive abilities in the memory and executive function domain."[66] All of this would amount to a unique neurosensory syndrome.

The panel suggested that "the disturbance of the auditory or vestibular components of the ear" could be explained by "[a]n external stimulus that can cause small pressure waves or changes in electric potentials could create symptomatology in the inner ear, without distinct symptoms elsewhere in the brain or body."[67] They suggested that disruptions of the blood-brain barrier could lead to leakage of blood proteins and cause oxidative stress and an inflammatory response, which could cause cognitive impairment, while "[l]ocal damage to the dura [a membrane that surrounds the brain] has also been associated with cerebrospinal fluid leaks, which can cause headaches, dizziness and vertigo, a sensation of pressure in the head, tinnitus, and cognitive impairment."[68]

The panel reasoned that "the core characteristics [of the AHIs] cannot be explained by benign natural or environmental factors."[69] It follows that AHIs are more likely caused by some kind of deliberate attack using directed energy. A covert attack as a cause of AHIs would require the following:

> (1) a concealable source that could generate the required stimulus and be difficult to detect; (2) the propagation and delivery of the stimulus to an individual in a way that would be difficult to detect; (3) the coupling of the stimulus to the human body; (4) the ability of the coupling to cause biological effects; and (5) the ability of the biological effects to explain the core clinical signs and symptoms.[70]

Main Findings

The report has a number of interesting findings: "[t]he signs and symptoms of AHIs are genuine and compelling . . . that cannot be explained by environmental or medical conditions . . . [and] [e]lectromagnetic energy, particularly pulsed signals in the radiofrequency range, plausibly explain the core characteristics."[71]

They dismissed bulk heating of the brain as an implausible mechanism because it does not fit with the lack of a heating sensation during AHIs, the fact that there were no effects on electronics, and the existence of metallic barriers during some AHIs.[72] They claimed that "[p]ower levels that are insufficient to cause thermo-acoustic effects may still cause a range of other biological effects" and they suggested that "[t]he lack of biological effects is consistent with the vast majority of research on the Frey effect."[73] The panel argued that extremely low frequency (ELF) waves (below 100 Hz) would be a plausible pathway since "[h]uman biological systems are vulnerable to disruption or influence by external fields and forces that resonate with their naturally occurring patterns, including at low powers."[74] This would mean that by

> [c]ombining a low-frequency modulating signal with a higher-frequency carrier signal produces a modulated signal that exhibits characteristics of both components. The resultant signal will have some of the more effective propagation characteristics of the higher-frequency component, while causing biological effects similar to those produced by the lower-frequency component.[75]

Criticism

The IC Expert Report essentially supported the conclusions of the NAS committee report, adding some more details as to the plausible mechanism of injury. The IC experts also acknowledged the existence of knowledge gaps with respect to the nonthermal bioeffects of RF energy, advising to conduct more research in this area. Interestingly, the main criticism of this report came from the IC itself in the form of a CIA interim report on AHIs, which was reported in the US media in January 2022, and in the form of an ODNI "Updated Assessment on Anomalous Health Incidents," both of which declared that "it is 'very unlikely' a foreign adversary is responsible for the reported AHIs."[76] The CIA's expertise is in HUMINT and their objective differed from the IC Expert Panel in the sense of determining as to whether a foreign power was involved and concluding that there was no evidence for a "sustained global campaign by a foreign power."[77] The 2023 ODNI report uses the very same rationale to come to the same conclusion that the AHIs were not deliberately caused "because the IC has failed to detect some adversaries' activities."[78] Two IC agencies came to the conclusion with moderate to high confidence while three have moderate confidence. The report also questioned whether RF energy would be a plausible mechanism of injury due to a lack of scientific evidence and stated "that there is no credible evidence that a foreign adversary has a weapon or collection device that is causing AHIs."[79]

The Question of a Havana Syndrome Cover-up

The different conclusions of the IC Expert Panel and the CIA/ODNI assessments are quite astonishing, which raises the question as to whether there was some political pressure on the IC to declare the possibility of a deliberate and malicious cause of AHIs as implausible. The *National Review* argued that "at this stage, the possibility that Biden administration officials are downplaying evidence of Russian involvement to avoid forcing Washington into an escalatory confrontation with Moscow is at least as likely to be true as the intelligence community's conclusion that a foreign adversary is probably not involved."[80] Obviously, several groups of experts made an elaborate scientific case that directed energy of some kind could be responsible for many of the common Havana Syndrome symptoms. The latest assessments by the CIA are only available in the form of basic summaries and lack any further information as to how the different agencies reached their conclusions.[81] After the ODNI "Updated Assessment" was published, White House Speaker Karine Jean-Pierre refused to definitively answer a reporter's question as to whether the Havana Syndrome was now "settled," which leaves it open as to what the White House and IC actually think did happen.[82]

Benign Explanations of the Updated Assessment

CIA Director William Burns commented on the "Updated Assessment on Anomalous Health Incidents" that it was based on "one of the largest and most intensive investigations in the Agency's history" and that it "reflects more than two years of rigorous, painstaking collection, investigative work, and analysis by IC agencies, including CIA."[83] An unnamed intelligence official claimed that the two-year IC investigation was "extremely aggressive" and high risk, as "[i]ntelligence officers vigorously studied what happened in the hours, days and weeks surrounding the incidents."[84] Another official said that "[t]here was nothing" in terms of evidence of a foreign power trying to harm US personnel.

What is inconsistent with this explanation is the fact that senior officials did not call into question as to whether individuals affected with severe symptoms of Havana Syndrome were genuinely injured, which leaves a remaining mystery as to how exactly they got injured. DNI Avril Haines made it clear that "these findings do not call into question the very real experiences and symptoms that our colleagues and their family members have reported."[85] Critics of the ODNI report have suggested that the investigation was flawed and may have come to incorrect inclusions because of a poor methodology used or because of a lacking ability to detect potential adversarial activity responsible for the incidents after the incidents had occurred.[86] The alternative explanation would be that the ODNI conclusions were deliberately politicized.

Politicized Intelligence

If the ODNI "Updated Assessment" had been politicized, it would not have been the first time that this happened. Politicization of intelligence is the introduction of a political bias in the analysis and it is a "normal" feature of intelligence in the United States.[87] US intelligence agencies exaggerated the Soviet threat during the "bomber gap" and "missile gap" debates in the 1950s and early 1960s, systematically underestimated enemy strength in Vietnam before the Tet Offensive, and overstated the intelligence for Iraq possessing WMDs prior to the Iraq War.[88] More recently, there has been a debate as to whether US intelligence has become highly politicized in the wake of the Trump presidency with the Russiagate investigation (triggered by an IC Assessment on Russian activities in US elections) and the now infamous letter by fifty-one intelligence officials stating that the Hunter Biden laptop had "the classic earmarks of a Russian information operation," despite the laptop having been proven to have been authentic.[89]

Perhaps more relevant and instructive for understanding the intelligence dimension of the Havana Syndrome is the political and scientific battle over the origins of Covid, which started with President Trump calling SARS-COV-2 the "China virus," which implied Chinese culpability in the pandemic and led to widespread accusations by the political left that Trump's position was xenophobic and racist. The question as to how SARS-COV-2 emerged became so politicized that scientists who dared to question the natural origin hypothesis were subjected to vicious attacks by their colleagues and the press. In a final act of defiance, the Trump State Department released a "fact sheet" that made the case for a possible lab leak from the Wuhan Institute of Virology.[90] The incoming Biden administration ordered an IC assessment on the Covid origins, and the unclassified summary was published on October 29, 2021. Four IC agencies judged with low confidence that Covid emerged by a spillover from animals from the Wuhan wet market, while one agency judged with moderate confidence that the virus leaked from the lab.[91] The Biden administration consistently downplayed the possibility of a lab leak, seemingly out of concerns over retaliation by China.

In September 2023, a CIA whistleblower alleged in a Congressional testimony that six members out of a CIA team of seven intelligence analysts working on the Covid origin problem "were given significant monetary incentive to change their positions."[92] If this allegation is true, it would be the most blatant public case of intelligence politicization in US history. Robert F. Kennedy Jr. has claimed that DNI Avril Haines (who also oversaw the AHI IC Assessment) played a key role in the cover-up of the Covid origins.[93] Kennedy wrote that "Haines, herself, took the lead in deflecting the emerging lab leak hypothesis in the earliest days of the pandemic," and the Biden administration pressured social media companies to censor people promoting the lab leak hypothesis.[94] In the view of Kennedy, the IC Assessment of the Covid origins was a "whitewash" overseen by somebody who had "distinguished herself as the CIA's reigning cover-up impresario," which was an attempt by the IC to kill a serious investigation into the Covid-19 origins.[95] In short, Haines has, according to Kennedy, a history of "sweeping inconvenient truths under the carpet."[96] In this context, the idea that the other major investigation presided over by Haines may have been politically manipulated to show a desirable result is hardly far-fetched.

Potential Motivations for a Cover-up

David Ignatius of the *Washington Post* has pointed out that "dealing with 'Havana Syndrome' is a policymaker's nightmare" since "[y]ou can't accuse another country of warlike assaults without solid facts."[97] These solid facts either seem to be missing or there is a reluctance to acknowledge them in public, even though actions may be taken in secret. The most obvious reason as to why the US government would not want to publicly acknowledge possible attacks on their own personnel by a foreign adversary is that they may be concerned about the risk of escalation. According to the dominant theory as to who the foreign adversary may be, the consequence could be an open conflict with a major nuclear weapons state. If there was some solid evidence that Russia had any part in the covert attacks on US personnel, making that evidence public only increases the pressure on US policymakers to take some decisive action to prevent, punish, and deter. The problem is that there may not be good options for any of these objectives, making it more convenient to publicly deny the issue and act covertly until a better option presents itself.

The US government would also be interested in not acknowledging a serious vulnerability to US national security since this could encourage others to try exploiting it as well. As has been revealed in several investigations, up to now there does not seem to be a good solution available to protect their own personnel against a mode of attack that is insufficiently understood. As could be seen in the earlier Moscow Signal episode, it was demoralizing for the US Moscow embassy personnel to learn later that the State Department had withheld information about potentially harmful microwave radiation from them while secretly trying to determine the intent and possible damage to people. If there was officially acknowledged real harm to US personnel, the government would need to have a viable plan as to how to protect their people to restore confidence. What if there is no such plan yet?

A final motivation, which has been stated by some critics of the ODNI report on AHIs, is that the US government may be fully aware of the weapons technology that can remotely attack the brain and central nervous system of people, but does not want to publicly acknowledge the existence of these weapons to prevent proliferation (if foreign adversaries were aware of the technology, they may want to pursue it themselves) and/or to allow the covert use of this weapons technology by the US government. For example, James Giordano stated in an interview that he was aware of an unnamed country that had developed microwave weapons that could disrupt the brain.[98] An unnamed US intelligence officer stated in an interview with the *Daily Mail* that "[a]nyone in the intelligence community will tell you the US has had these kinds of energy weapons for a while."[99] Journalist Nicky Woolf said in an interview about Havana Syndrome that

> [t]he wildest stuff I think has been when we looked into what kind of research has been going on in this kind of field, and we have heard that not only does America possess devices like the ones that could do this stuff that we saw in Havana, but that they're actively, we've heard they have deployed it in the field.[100]

Woolf said that he had spoken to the CEOs of defense companies, who confirmed to him that weapons that could cause Havana Syndrome would be possible and might exist.[101] It shall also be mentioned that there is a large group of people around the world, including in the United States and Europe, who claim that they are abused for human experiments to test DEW on them.[102] The claims of unethical mind control experimentation and electronic harassment go back to at least the 1980s. The Greenham Common Women Peace Camp (a protest against US deployment of nuclear weapons in the UK) was targeted by authorities with an unknown DEW, which according to David Guyatt, caused the following symptoms: "vertigo, retinal bleeding, burnt face (even at night), nausea, sleep disturbances, palpitations, loss of concentration, loss of memory, disorientation, severe headaches, temporary paralysis, faulty speech coordination, irritability and a sense of panic in non-panic situations."[103]

Conclusion

The published studies on Havana Syndrome make it clear that there is a lot of uncertainty as to what case qualifies as an AHI, whether there is any common cause of AHIs, and what would be the likely mechanisms for injury if AHIs were caused by a covert deliberate attack. Parts of the government seem to be convinced that AHIs were caused by DEW attacks with an unknown weapon used by an unknown adversary, while other parts of the government believe that this is highly unlikely, in part because no adversary was ever caught pointing a DEW at US personnel and in part because they do not believe that covert attacks with DEWs would be even possible. In contrast, experts like Edl Schamiloglu pointed out that there is no real mystery as to how people can be injured remotely with HPMs—"the technology most likely involved comes from textbook physics, and the military powers of the world continue to develop and deploy it."[104] What seems to be indisputable is that a smaller subsection of AHI cases (perhaps sixty-eight of them) cannot be explained away with environmental factors, mass psychogenic illness, or preexisting health conditions.[105] The scientists who believe that some AHIs were caused by DEWs point to the wealth of scientific studies from the Cold War era that indicated harmful effects of radiofrequency energy and acoustic waves, while skeptics point to the absence of hard evidence for the feasibility and existence of such weapons. The idea that DEW and in particular electromagnetic weapons are responsible for the AHIs is sound and based on the extensive history of psychotronic and NLW research of the Cold War era, the studies mentioned above, and some other studies that were not mentioned here because of space constraints.[106] What could explain this lack of evidence for the existence of such weapons is that either Western weapons technology had fallen behind in the critical area of DEW or that the technology is simply so highly classified that only few people in Western governments and militaries know about it. Those that do know about it might be just not willing or able to talk about these weapons as they are sworn to secrecy with serious consequences for them if they violated their secrecy oaths.

Notes

1 Randel L. Swanson, Stephen Hampton, Judith Green-Mackenzie, Ramon Diaz-Arrastia, M. Shawn Grady, Ragini Verma, Rosette Biester, Diana Duda, Ronald L. Wolf, and Douglas H. Smith, "Neurological Manifestations Among US Government Personnel Reporting Directional Audible and Sensory Phenomena in Havana, Cuba," *JAMA* 319, no. 11 (2018): 1125–33; Ragini Verma, Randel L. Swanson, Drew Parker, Abdul Aziz Ould Ismail, Russell T. Shinohara, Jacob A. Alappatt, Jimit Doshi, Christos Davatzikos, Michael Galloway, Diana Duda, H. Isaac Chen, Junghoon J. Kim, Ruben C. Gur, Ronald L. Wolf, M. Sean Grady, Stephen Hampton, Ramon Diaz-Arrastia, and Douglas H. Smith, "Neuroimaging Findings in US Government Personnel with Possible Exposure to Directional Phenomena in Havana, Cuba," *JAMA* 322, no. 4 (2019): 336–47.

2 Carlo Pierpaoli, Amritha Nayak, Rakibuhl Hafiz et al., "Neuroimaging Findings in US Government Personnel and Their Family Members Involved in Anomalous Health Incidents," *JAMA* 331, no. 13 (2024): 1122–34.

3 Swanson et al., "Neurological Manifestations Among US Government Personnel Reporting Directional Audible and Sensory Phenomena in Havana, Cuba," 1125–33.

4 Swanson et al., "Neurological Manifestations Among US Government Personnel Reporting Directional Audible and Sensory Phenomena in Havana, Cuba," 1126.

5 Swanson et al., "Neurological Manifestations Among US Government Personnel Reporting Directional Audible and Sensory Phenomena in Havana, Cuba," 1128.

6 Swanson et al., "Neurological Manifestations Among US Government Personnel Reporting Directional Audible and Sensory Phenomena in Havana, Cuba," 1131.

7 Swanson et al., "Neurological Manifestations Among US Government Personnel Reporting Directional Audible and Sensory Phenomena in Havana, Cuba," 1131.

8 Rita Rubin, "More Questions Raised by Concussion-Like Symptoms Found in US Diplomats Who Served in Havana," *JAMA* 319, no. 11 (2018): 1079.

9 Swanson et al., "Neurological Manifestations Among US Government Personnel Reporting Directional Audible and Sensory Phenomena in Havana, Cuba," 1131–2.

10 Sergio Della Sala and Roberto Cubelli, "Alleged 'Sonic Attack' Supported by Poor Neuropsychology," *Cortex* 103 (2018): 387–8.

11 Sala and Cubelli, "Alleged 'Sonic Attack' Supported by Poor Neuropsychology," 388.

12 Quoted from Rubin, "More Questions Raised by Concussion-Like Symptoms Found in US Diplomats Who Served in Havana," 1079.

13 Verma et al., "Neuroimaging Findings in US Government Personnel with Possible Exposure to Directional Phenomena in Havana, Cuba," 337.

14 Verma et al., "Neuroimaging Findings in US Government Personnel with Possible Exposure to Directional Phenomena in Havana, Cuba," 338.

15 Verma et al., "Neuroimaging Findings in US Government Personnel with Possible Exposure to Directional Phenomena in Havana, Cuba," 338–9.

16 Verma et al., "Neuroimaging Findings in US Government Personnel with Possible Exposure to Directional Phenomena in Havana, Cuba," 340–1.

17 Verma et al., "Neuroimaging Findings in US Government Personnel with Possible Exposure to Directional Phenomena in Havana, Cuba," 342.

18 Verma et al., "Neuroimaging Findings in US Government Personnel with Possible Exposure to Directional Phenomena in Havana, Cuba," 343.

19 Verma et al., "Neuroimaging Findings in US Government Personnel with Possible Exposure to Directional Phenomena in Havana, Cuba," 346.

20 Verma et al., "Neuroimaging Findings in US Government Personnel with Possible Exposure to Directional Phenomena in Havana, Cuba," 346.

21 Robert W. Baloh and Robert E. Bartholomew, *Havana Syndrome: Mass Psychogenic Illness and the Real Story Behind the Embassy Mystery and Hysteria* (Cham: Switzerland: Springer, 2020), 47.

22 Katie Bo Lillis and Jen Christensen, "Despite Symptoms, NIH Research Finds No Evidence of 'Havana Syndrome' in Brain Scans," *CNN*, March 18, 2024, available at: https://www.cnn.com/2024/03/18/health/havana-syndrome-studies/index.html; Deena Beasley, "No Evidence of Havana Syndrome Brain Injury, Study Finds," *Reuters*, March 18, 2024, available at: https://www.reuters.com/world/us/us-study-finds-no-evidence-havana-syndrome-brain-injury-2024-03-18/; Dennis Thompson, "No Brain Injuries Seen Among 'Havana Syndrome' Patients," *US News*, March 19, 2024, available at: https://www.usnews.com/news/health-news/articles/2024-03-19/no-brain-injuries-seen-among-havana-syndrome-patients; Joel Achenbach and Shane Harris, "NIH Probe of 'Havana Syndrome' Finds No Sign of Brain Injuries," *Washington Post*, March 18, 2024; and Julian E. Barnes, "New Studies Find No Evidence of Brain Injury in Havana Syndrome Cases," *New York Times*, March 18, 2024.

23 Carlo Pierpaoli, Amritha Nayak, Rakibuhl Hafiz et al., "Neuroimaging Findings in US Government Personnel and Their Family Members Involved in Anomalous Health Incidents," 1125.
24 Carlo Pierpaoli, Amritha Nayak, Rakibuhl Hafiz et al., "Neuroimaging Findings in US Government Personnel and Their Family Members Involved in Anomalous Health Incidents," 1126.
25 Carlo Pierpaoli, Amritha Nayak, Rakibuhl Hafiz et al., "Neuroimaging Findings in US Government Personnel and Their Family Members Involved in Anomalous Health Incidents," 1132–3.
26 Carlo Pierpaoli, Amritha Nayak, Rakibuhl Hafiz et al., "Neuroimaging Findings in US Government Personnel and Their Family Members Involved in Anomalous Health Incidents," 1132.
27 Jen Christensen, "NIH Cancels 'Havana Syndrome' Research, Citing Unethical Coercion of Participants," *CNN*, September 1, 2024, available at: https://www.cnn.com/2024/08/30/health/nih-havana-syndrome-study/index.html.
28 Ann Finkbeiner, *The Jasons: The Secret History of Science's Postwar Elite* (New York: Viking, 2006), 33.
29 Josh Lederman and Michael Weissenstein, "Dangerous Sound? What Americans Heard in Cuba," *Associated Press*, October 13, 2017, available at: https://apnews.com/article/88bb914f8b284088bce48e54f6736d84.
30 JASON, "Acoustic Signals and Physiological Effects on U.S. Diplomats in Cuba," *The MITRE Corporation*, November 2018, 6.
31 JASON, "Acoustic Signals and Physiological Effects on U.S. Diplomats in Cuba," 8.
32 JASON, "Acoustic Signals and Physiological Effects on U.S. Diplomats in Cuba," 8.
33 Alexander Stubbs and Fernando Montealegre-Zapata, "Recordings of 'Sonic Attacks' on U.S. Diplomats in Cuba Spectrally Matches the Echoing Call of a Caribbean Cricket." bioRxiv, January 2019, 2.
34 JASON, "Acoustic Signals and Physiological Effects on U.S. Diplomats in Cuba," 93.
35 JASON, "Acoustic Signals and Physiological Effects on U.S. Diplomats in Cuba," 71.
36 JASON, "An Analysis of Data and Hypotheses Related to the Embassy Incidents," *The MITRE Corporation*, October 2021.
37 Ken Dilanian, "'Havana Syndrome' Symptoms in Small Group Most Likely Caused by Directed Energy, Says US Intel Panel of Experts," *NBC News*, February 2, 2022, available at: https://www.nbcnews.com/politics/national-security/havana-syndrome-symptoms-small-group-likely-caused-directed-energy-say-rcna14584.
38 JASON, "An Analysis of Data and Hypotheses Related to the Embassy Incidents," 4.
39 JASON, "An Analysis of Data and Hypotheses Related to the Embassy Incidents," 47–50.
40 JASON, "An Analysis of Data and Hypotheses Related to the Embassy Incidents," 62.

41 JASON, "An Analysis of Data and Hypotheses Related to the Embassy Incidents," 79, 2.
42 JASON, "An Analysis of Data and Hypotheses Related to the Embassy Incidents," 97–8.
43 JASON, "An Analysis of Data and Hypotheses Related to the Embassy Incidents," 99.
44 JASON, "An Analysis of Data and Hypotheses Related to the Embassy Incidents," 5.
45 JASON, "An Analysis of Data and Hypotheses Related to the Embassy Incidents," 6.
46 JASON, "An Analysis of Data and Hypotheses Related to the Embassy Incidents," 6.
47 David Relman and Julie A. Pavlin, eds., *An Assessment of Illness in U.S. Government Employees and Their Families at Overseas Embassies* (Washington, DC: National Academies of Sciences, 2020), 48.
48 Relman and Pavlin, eds., *An Assessment of Illness in U.S. Government Employees and Their Families at Overseas Embassies*, 8.
49 Relman and Pavlin, eds., *An Assessment of Illness in U.S. Government Employees and Their Families at Overseas Embassies*, XI.
50 Relman and Pavlin, eds., *An Assessment of Illness in U.S. Government Employees and Their Families at Overseas Embassies*, 15.
51 Relman and Pavlin, eds., *An Assessment of Illness in U.S. Government Employees and Their Families at Overseas Embassies*, 15.
52 Relman and Pavlin, eds., *An Assessment of Illness in U.S. Government Employees and Their Families at Overseas Embassies*, 21–2.
53 Relman and Pavlin, eds., *An Assessment of Illness in U.S. Government Employees and Their Families at Overseas Embassies*, 23.
54 Relman and Pavlin, eds., *An Assessment of Illness in U.S. Government Employees and Their Families at Overseas Embassies*, 24.
55 Relman and Pavlin, eds., *An Assessment of Illness in U.S. Government Employees and Their Families at Overseas Embassies*, 26.
56 Relman and Pavlin, eds., *An Assessment of Illness in U.S. Government Employees and Their Families at Overseas Embassies*, 27.
57 Relman and Pavlin, eds., *An Assessment of Illness in U.S. Government Employees and Their Families at Overseas Embassies*, 18.
58 Relman and Pavlin, eds., *An Assessment of Illness in U.S. Government Employees and Their Families at Overseas Embassies*, 20.
59 Relman and Pavlin, eds., *An Assessment of Illness in U.S. Government Employees and Their Families at Overseas Embassies*, XI, 1.
60 Robert E. Bartholomew and Robert W. Baloh, "'Havana Syndrome': A Post-Mortem," *International Journal of Social Psychiatry* 70, no. 2 (2024): 403.
61 US Office of the Director of National Intelligence, "Anomalous Health Incidents: Analysis of Potential Mechanisms," *IC Experts Panel*, September 2022, V.

62 US Office of the Director of National Intelligence, "Anomalous Health Incidents," IX.
63 US Office of the Director of National Intelligence, "Anomalous Health Incidents," V.
64 US Office of the Director of National Intelligence, "Anomalous Health Incidents," V.
65 US Office of the Director of National Intelligence, "Anomalous Health Incidents," 1.
66 US Office of the Director of National Intelligence, "Anomalous Health Incidents," 1.
67 US Office of the Director of National Intelligence, "Anomalous Health Incidents," 5.
68 US Office of the Director of National Intelligence, "Anomalous Health Incidents," 7.
69 US Office of the Director of National Intelligence, "Anomalous Health Incidents," 7.
70 US Office of the Director of National Intelligence, "Anomalous Health Incidents," 9.
71 US Office of the Director of National Intelligence, "Anomalous Health Incidents," VI.
72 US Office of the Director of National Intelligence, "Anomalous Health Incidents," 24.
73 US Office of the Director of National Intelligence, "Anomalous Health Incidents," 25.
74 US Office of the Director of National Intelligence, "Anomalous Health Incidents," 27.
75 US Office of the Director of National Intelligence, "Anomalous Health Incidents," 28.
76 Julian E. Barnes, "Most 'Havana Syndrome' Cases Unlikely Caused by a Foreign Power," *New York Times*, January 20, 2024; US Office of the Director of National Intelligence, "Updated Assessment of Anomalous Health Incidents," *National Intelligence Council*, March 1, 2023, 1.
77 Barnes, "Most 'Havana Syndrome' Cases Unlikely Caused by a Foreign Power."
78 US Office of the Director of National Intelligence, "Updated Assessment of Anomalous Health Incidents," 1.
79 US Office of the Director of National Intelligence, "Updated Assessment of Anomalous Health Incidents," 1.
80 National Review Editors, "A Havana Syndrome Cover-Up?," *National Review*, April 2, 2024, available at: https://www.nationalreview.com/2024/04/a-havana-syndrome-cover-up/.
81 Calder McHugh, "The 'Havana Syndrome' Report Has Not Convinced Everyone," *Politico*, March 1, 2023, available at: https://www.politico.com/newsletters/politico-nightly/2023/03/01/the-havana-syndrome-report-hasnt-convinced-everyone-00085112.
82 Olivier Knox and Caroline Anders, "Is 'Havana Syndrome' Settled Now? White House Won't Say: The New Intelligence Report Seems to Land with a Thud at 1600 Penn," *Washington Post*, March 2, 2023.
83 Kylie Atwood and Jennifer Hansler, "US Intelligence Community Cannot Link 'Havana Syndrome' Cases to Foreign Adversary," *CNN*, March 2, 2023, available at: https://www.cnn.com/2023/03/01/politics/us-intel-community-havana-syndrome/index.html.
84 Atwood and Hansler, "US Intelligence Community Cannot Link 'Havana Syndrome' Cases to Foreign Adversary."

85 Shane Harris and John Hudson, "'Havana Syndrome' Not Caused by Energy Weapon or Foreign Adversary, Intelligence Review Finds," *Washington Post*, March 1, 2023.
86 Peter Weber, "Havana Syndrome Not Caused by Foreign Adversaries, Energy Weapons, or Aliens, U.S. Intelligence Assesses," *Newsweek*, March 2, 2023, available at: https://theweek.com/health-and-science/1021446/havana-syndrome-not-caused-by-foreign-adversaries-energy-weapons-or.
87 Glenn Hastedt, "The Politics of Intelligence and the Politicization of Intelligence: The American Experience," *Intelligence and National Security* 28, no. 1 (2013): 6.
88 Hastedt, "The Politics of Intelligence and the Politicization of Intelligence," 14–29.
89 J. Michael Waller, *Big Intel: How the CIA and FBI Went from Cold War Heroes to Deep State Villains* (Washington, DC: Regnery Publishing, 2024), 270.
90 US Department of State, "Fact Sheet: Activity at the Wuhan Institute of Virology," *Office of the Spokesperson*, January 15, 2021, available at: https://2017-2021.state.gov/fact-sheet-activity-at-the-wuhan-institute-of-virology/.
91 US Office of the Director of National Intelligence, "Updated Assessment of COVID-19 Origins," *National Intelligence Council*, October 29, 2021, available at: https://www.dni.gov/files/ODNI/documents/assessments/Declassified-Assessment-on-COVID-19-Origins.pdf.
92 John Ratcliffe and Cliff Sims, "The CIA Politicizes Intelligence on China and COVID; A Whistleblower Says That Analysts Who Favored the Lab-Leak Theory Were Paid to Change Positions," *Wall Street Journal*, September 18, 2023.
93 Robert F. Kennedy Jr., *The Wuhan Cover-Up and the Terrifying Bioweapons Arms Race* (New York: Skyhorse Publishing, 2023), 232.
94 Kennedy Jr., *The Wuhan Cover-Up and the Terrifying Bioweapons Arms Race*, 233.
95 Kennedy Jr., *The Wuhan Cover-Up and the Terrifying Bioweapons Arms Race*, 237, 243.
96 Kennedy Jr., *The Wuhan Cover-Up and the Terrifying Bioweapons Arms Race*, 237.
97 David Ignatius, "Dealing with 'Havana Syndrome' Is a Policymaker's Nightmare," *Washington Post*, October 28, 2021.
98 Julian Borger, "Microwave Weapons that Could Cause Havana Syndrome, Experts Say," *The Guardian*, June 2, 2021, available at: https://www.theguardian.com/science/2021/jun/02/microwave-weapons-havana-syndrome-experts.
99 Matthew Phelan, "New NIH Study Sheds Light on Mysterious 'Havana Syndrome': Victims' Symptoms Are 'Real' and 'Quite Profound'—But Injuries Don't Show Up on MRI Much Like 'Mini Stroke', One Pentagon Medical Consultant Told DailyMail.com," *Daily Mail*, March 18, 2024, available at: https://www.dailymail.co.uk/sciencetech/article-13210727/NIH-study-Havana-Syndrome-Victims-symptoms-energy-weapons-microwave-acoustic-mystery.html.

100 Nicky Woolf, "Havana Syndrome Might Be Real and It Is Scary as Hell," *The Daily Beast*, February 2, 2023, available at: https://www.thedailybeast.com/havana-syndrome-might-be-real-and-its-scary-as-hell?ref=scroll.

101 Nicky Woolf, "The Sound: Mystery of the Havana Syndrome—A Conversation with Nicky Woolf," University of Boston, November 1, 2023, available at: https://www.youtube.com/watch?v=kVZyDRBil8U.

102 Joyeux Noel Womac, "Marked as Dangerous: An Investigative Analysis of No-Touch Torture on Targeted Individuals" (Master Thesis, University of Purdue, 2022).

103 David Guyatt, "Anti-Personnel 'Soft Kill' Weaponry," *World Affairs* 9, no. 2 (2005): 50.

104 Edl Schamiloglu, "Experts Suggest US Embassies Were Hit with High-Power Microwaves—Here's How the Weapons Work," *The Conversation*, December 10, 2020, available at: https://theconversation.com/experts-suggest-us-embassies-were-hit-with-high-power-microwaves-heres-how-the-weapons-work-151730.

105 US Congress, "Silent Weapons: Examining Foreign Anomalous Health Incidents Targeting Americans in the Homeland," Homeland Security Committee, May 8, 2024, testimony of Christo Grozev.

106 See for example, Beatrice Alexandra Golomb, "Diplomats' Mystery Illness and Pulsed Radiofrequency/ Microwave Radiation," *Neural Computing* 30, no. 11 (2018): 2882–985; Vladimir Binhi and Andrei B. Rubin, "Theoretical Concepts in Magnetobiology after 40 Years of Research," *Cells* 11, no. 2 (2022): 1–15.

7

What Might Be the Intent behind the Covert Attacks?

The public debate on Havana Syndrome has largely focused on the question as to whether Havana Syndrome is a deliberate attack, while less attention has been given to the question as to what could be the strategic intent, assuming that the AHIs were caused by deliberate covert attacks. Former National Security Advisor John Bolton suggested in an interview on *60 Minutes Australia* that "our adversaries are looking for ways, using directed energy or perhaps other techniques, to be able to disable senior officials or large military formations through this new technology in ways that we don't have adequate defenses and we just don't have enough evidence yet to make a judgment one way or the other."[1] Bolton did not identify any particular adversary he thought was responsible for Havana Syndrome or why exactly the AHIs occurred at the locations or times that they did. This chapter seeks to make some educated guesses about the possible perpetrators and their motivations and to put these likely covert attacks in the larger context of what NATO analysts have called cognitive warfare. It is argued that most of the available circumstantial evidence points toward Russia but also allows for the possibility that other actors may be responsible for some of the reported AHIs. The cognitive warfare concept discussed in the final chapter suggests that the AHIs may be only part of a much broader and much more dangerous attack on US national security.

The Impact of the Havana Syndrome

It is undeniable that Havana Syndrome has had a substantial impact on the US government and on US diplomatic relations with Cuba and other countries. A significant number of US officials have been injured and this has hurt morale within the US Department of State and other US agencies. It is difficult to estimate the overall damage, but it is apparent that Havana Syndrome cannot and should not be ignored as there is a potential for further escalation and much more damage if the aggressor is not exposed and punished, and if no effective countermeasures are taken, since this would invite further aggressions. The slow pace at which the US government has responded to the initial attacks in Cuba may have encouraged further attacks against US personnel in many other locations around the world that mainly occurred in 2018 and 2021. There is no reason to believe that Havana Syndrome would simply go away by ignoring the issue.

Effect on Diplomatic Relations

AHIs have impacted US diplomatic relations with different countries, mostly in the locations where the AHIs did occur. The diplomatic relations with Cuba were disrupted as the US embassy reopened in Havana in 2015 was temporarily closed and as US Cuba sanctions were reimposed. The US embassy in Cuba is currently operating at a much lower staff level than before.[2] Havana Syndrome has affected the travel for senior US officials, whose staff members had been targeted. A CIA officer, who was travelling with CIA Director William Burns to India, suffered a mysterious health condition consistent with the Havana Syndrome.[3] A diplomatic visit of Vice President Kamala Harris to Vietnam was delayed for several hours due to the occurrence of a potential covert attack on two US personnel at the Hanoi embassy, who had to be medevacked.[4] Different agencies have advised against officials travelling overseas because of these and other incidents.[5] If the AHIs continue and expand to more locations, it could become more difficult for the United States to maintain strong relations with key allies and to have a sufficient diplomatic presence in certain countries that are neutral or adversarial. The consequence of this could be a less effective US foreign policy and, with it, a decline of US influence in the world.

Morale of US Government Personnel

Mark Zaid stated in his Congressional testimony on May 8, 2024, that "AHIs are having a very profound and adverse impact on morale and dissuading officers from accepting overseas assignments. Some officers have even quit specifically because of AHI concerns. The relevant workforce, which is comprised of many of our best and brightest, do not believe they are being provided with sufficient information or protection."[6] The more US government personnel are harmed, the more difficult it becomes to find qualified personnel to fill positions in certain locations, especially if it becomes more widely known that there is a high risk of harmful exposure of some kind. The US Department of State had to offer diplomats the highest rate for hardship and cut staff from fifty-four to eighteen at the US embassy in Cuba, and the CIA shut down their station in Havana completely in 2017.[7] The Havana Syndrome allegedly "'dramatically hurt' morale in the diplomatic service and affected recruitment" for the foreign service.[8] The consequence is that the best and the brightest will no longer find it attractive to work in government jobs that require them to be in certain overseas locations if that comes with a risk of severe damage to their health and the health of their family members. It is even more damaging to morale for the US government not to honestly acknowledge the risks and not to provide adequate care to those who have been harmed. Many of the US government employees who have suffered from an AHI still struggle to receive adequate financial support and healthcare.

Adversarial Activity Not Motivated by Causing Harm

There is the possibility that adversarial activity is responsible for health damage to US personnel, but that the motivation is not actually to deliberately harm people. It has been suggested in the case of the Moscow Signal and in the case of US diplomats in Cuba that the intent for using directed energy was electronic surveillance. An adversary may use eavesdropping devices that emit some kind of electromagnetic or acoustic signal that inadvertently produces negative health effects to those who get exposed to these signals. As mentioned before, the leading theory for the Moscow Signal is that the Soviets used RF imposition, where a radiofrequency signal sent toward a target captures voice-induced vibrations that are reflected back.[9] The Soviets may have primarily wanted to listen to the conversations in the Moscow embassy when they beamed microwaves at them and may not have cared whether that exposure was harmful. An alternative explanation is that the Soviets may have used RF/microwave signals to interfere with the electronic eavesdropping equipment based in the US embassy.[10] A third possibility is that there was an inadvertent exposure of US embassy personnel by electronic surveillance equipment inside the embassy. All of these possibilities should also be considered in relation to Havana Syndrome.

In 2017, James Lewis, a former State Department official with expertise in surveillance technology, argued that an acoustic device used by Cuban intelligence designed to pick up the vibrations of speech could have been incorrectly configured, resulting in harmful emissions. He stated: "We know with 100% certainly that the embassies are under surveillance, and the technology being used could just be crude and over-powered."[11] In other words, Cuban intelligence officers may have used poorly designed equipment or may not have known how to use the equipment correctly, resulting in unintended harm to the people under their surveillance.

While this more benign explanation has some merit, there are several reasons why it is overall not plausible. First, most of the AHIs occurred in residencies rather than in embassies or offices, which suggests that there would be less benefit for aggressive surveillance since sensitive matters would not be discussed by diplomats or intelligence officers at home when family members are present. Secondly, an adversarial intelligence service would have figured out, at least after complaints made by the US government to a host government, that harm to US personnel had occurred. A responsible host government would then have stopped the harmful surveillance activities unless there was an intention to do harm. If harmful exposures continue to occur over many years, it is hard not to conclude that the harm was deliberate. Finally, the nature of the injuries suffered by some AHI patients seems to indicate that this was caused by a sophisticated weapon and not by some electronic surveillance device. This concerns specifically the sudden onset of symptoms, including the loud high-pitched sound, strong headaches, vertigo, and the traumatic brain injury, all of which are not normally observed in cases of strong electromagnetic or acoustic wave exposure.

Potential Perpetrators

The list of likely perpetrators is quite short since the technology used in the Havana Syndrome can be assumed to be very advanced and hence only within reach of a few major nations and perhaps a few select nonstate actors. Unfortunately, no weapon that could cause Havana Syndrome and no perpetrator for any of the incidents has ever been captured. There is only circumstantial evidence subject to interpretation and with a high possibility of deception. This leaves quite a bit of speculation as to who is responsible and what their motives are. This section will discuss the most likely perpetrators in terms of their possible motives, opportunity, and means.

Cuba

The Trump administration and Senator Marco Rubio were quick to blame Cuba for the AHIs when they became public in summer 2017. President Trump said at a press conference in early October 2017: "I do believe Cuba's responsible. I do believe that. . . . And it's a very unusual attack, as you know. But I do believe Cuba is responsible."[12] The State Department did not call out Cuba as the responsible party but noted that it was Cuba's responsibility under international law to protect American diplomats on their soil. The White House chief of staff, John Kelly stated that "[w]e believe that the Cuban government could stop the attacks on our diplomats," which means that at a minimum they allowed the attacks to happen.[13] During the January 2018 Western Hemisphere Subcommittee hearing chaired by Senator Marco Rubio, Senator Menendez claimed that "it is unfathomable that the Castro regime, and the intelligence services specifically, were not aware of these attacks. If senior Cuban officials did not directly order these attacks, they must have been aware or given tacit approval to foreign agents to operate in Cuba. The scope of the attacks is too specific."[14] It is unavoidable to conclude that the Cuban intelligence services were involved in some shape or form in the early AHIs in Cuba, although they may have acted on behalf of another power.

Motive

Although relations between the United States and Cuba were improving from 2015, it appears that at least a subgroup within the Cuban national security apparatus was opposed to the presence of US diplomats and intelligence officers in Cuba that resulted from the diplomatic initiatives of the Obama administration. It is uncontroversial that Cuban intelligence engaged in various forms of harassment against US personnel in Cuba from 2016.[15] This makes it likely that they would not have cared to damage the health of US personnel, if this could have been accomplished covertly and with reduced odds of attribution because of the secret technology used. It may even be the case that the Cuban government was highly suspicious of the American overtures for the normalization of relations.[16] The Cuban government was perhaps looking for a way to instead improve relations with Russia or China, which do not criticize the Cuban government for human rights violations and democracy deficits and which may have made better offers to the regime. The Obama administration had secretly funded the social messaging platform ZunZuneo, which was meant to bypass Cuban government censorship and was sending subversive messages to Cubans, which was revealed in 2014.[17] In short, the Cuban government had reasons not to trust the US government.

Opportunity

Almost all the known AHIs of late 2016 and 2017 occurred in Cuba. Cuban intelligence did conduct electronic and physical surveillance of US personnel, enabling them to track American diplomats and to covertly attack them when there was an opportunity to do so. Senator Rubio claimed that "Cuba, by all accounts, is by far the most heavily monitored and surveilled country in the Western Hemisphere."[18] Cuban intelligence services are modeled after the KGB, which trained them, and are widely known to be extremely proficient in counterintelligence. Brian Latell, a former CIA analyst and expert on Latin American intelligence services, claimed that Cuba has "the best damn intelligence service in the world."[19] The US diplomats who came to Cuba after the resumption of diplomatic relations in 2015 believed that they were under constant physical and electronic surveillance by the Cubans.[20] Cuban intelligence had access to the homes of the diplomats and could track them at any time in Cuba. However, it seems far less likely that Cuban intelligence services would have covertly attacked US personnel outside of Cuba and especially outside of the Western hemisphere. Cuban intelligence operations seem to be directed primarily against the United States and are focused on Latin America.

Means

It is plausible that the Cuban government would have DEW technology necessary for covert attacks on personnel. They could have received the technology from China or from Russia, or they could have developed the technology themselves. It is not unreasonable to suggest that electromagnetic antipersonnel weapons may have already proliferated across the world and that some Latin American states have access to it. According to Cuban defector Julio Antonio de Marmol, the Castro government received a "Pulsing Radiowave Frequency machine" from China in the early 1960s. De Marmol suggested that "[t]he microwave radiation focused on an ultrasonic wavelength" could read brainwaves and turn them into readable text through computerized analysis.[21] "This machine, decades later, was classified as a tool that caused Havana Syndrome," according to de Marmol.[22] In 2009 the ousted Honduran president Manuel Zelaya complained that he was attacked by an "electron bombardment with microwaves" that caused "headache and organic destabilisation" while he was sheltering in the Brazilian embassy after the coup.[23] When interviewed by Amy Goodman on *Democracy Now!* Zelaya made the following remarks: "There are two kinds of unconventional weapons that have been used against us by the regime. There's a high-frequency pitch that has been used against protesters. And another weapon that has been used against us is an electronic device that issues microwaves, which is very harmful for your health. It causes headaches." When asked whether he knew whether the Honduran military had these weapons in their arsenal, he said: "Yes, of course."[24] If a small country like Honduras would have access to secret electromagnetic weaponry, it would follow that Cuba would also have it. Cuban intelligence is known to operate quite successfully inside the United States, which makes it plausible that some of the US incidents could be connected to them as well.

Russia

The great majority of analysts and commentators, who believe that AHIs are caused by some kind of weapon and amount to deliberate attacks, strongly suggest that the responsible party is Russia. Although the "smoking gun" evidence is missing to clearly implicate Russia, it is frequently pointed out that many of the supposed attacks and victims have a Russia connection, that Russia likely has the technology for a DEW that could produce these effects, and that Russia has a motive for covertly attacking US personnel in overseas locations.[25] Former senior CIA officer Marc Polymeropoulos stated on *60 Minutes Australia*: "I'm convinced that Russia has the motive, the mandate, the capability and the presence, and I believe Russia is behind at least some of the attacks of Havana syndrome incidents."[26] Similarly, Greg Edgreen told the Homeland Security Committee that in all the AHI cases "consistently there was a Russia nexus."[27]

Motive

The Russian government had several plausible motives for targeting US diplomats and intelligence officers in Cuba and a few other countries. First, Russia had an interest in spoiling the improved relations between the United States and Cuba as this could have made it more difficult for Russian intelligence and the Russian military to use Cuba as a base of operations against the United States. The Soviet Union established a SIGINT base at Lourdes, Cuba, in 1962, which provided them with the ability to collect US telephone, microwave, and satellite communications. In 2001, it was announced that Russia would close the base, but by 2008, Russian politicians declared that Cuba was of geostrategic importance to Russia and Russian–Cuban relations should be restored. Head of the Russian Security Council, Nikolai Patrushev visited Cuba in the same year to improve cooperation in all areas, including military cooperation.[28] In July 2014, there were rumors about Russia planning to reopen the SIGINT base.[29] In the same month, Russia wrote off $32 billion in Cold War era Cuban debt.[30] The Obama administration's effort to normalize relations with Havana, announced in December 2014, would have been an obstacle to a reopened Russian spy base on the island. If it was a Russian plan to reorient Cuba again toward Russia as their main partner by covertly attacking US diplomats in Cuba, it succeeded brilliantly. The Trump administration reintroduced sanctions against Cuba, which reversed some of the normalization measures of the previous administration and allowed lawsuits by Cubans who fled the island in the 1960s to reclaim confiscated property they had left behind.[31] This has forced the Cuban government to again strengthen their economic ties with Russia. In June 2024, a small Russian flotilla arrived in Havana before sailing for Venezuela, signaling that Russia wants to maintain a permanent military presence in the Western hemisphere.[32] The targeting of Canadian diplomats in Cuba was no accident either. According to Don Munton, "[d]iplomats at the Canadian embassy in Havana collected human intelligence, especially of a political and military nature, through covert as well as overt means," on behalf of the CIA from the 1960s to the early 1970s.[33] Canada is also a member of the Five Eyes SIGINT alliance and hence, the Canadians in Cuba may have been considered by Russia as US partners in intelligence operations against Cuba. It also appears that the worldwide campaign to target US intelligence officers and diplomats may have started in 2014 when the United States and Europe were imposing heavy sanctions on Russia over Ukraine.[34] The Russian attacks on US personnel may have been motivated by the desire to disrupt US foreign policy, signal Russian determination, and punish the United States for their meddling in Ukraine during the Euromaidan revolution and the subsequent support to the new pro-Western Ukrainian government. According to *The Insider* report, at least three CIA officers who had served at Kyiv station from 2015 had later suffered Havana Syndrome in other locations, which could suggest that they were specifically targeted for working with the Ukrainians.[35]

Opportunity

Mark Lowenthal pointed out that "Cuban intelligence has had a longtime deep association with Soviet and now Russian intelligence, and observers assume that this continues."[36] The KGB worked with the Cuban intelligence service DGI on both intelligence and covert operations directed against the United States. For example, the DGI trained and armed the Nicaraguan Sandinista guerrillas in Cuba in collaboration with the KGB in the 1970s, which eventually supported the success of the Sandinista revolution of 1979.[37] There is some speculation that Cuba may have traded secrets with Russia it obtained through their successful intelligence operations directed against the United States (e.g., Ana Belen Montes, Kendall Myers, and Manuel Rocha among others) for political favors and goods.[38] The relations between Russia and Cuba were a lot better in 2016 than the improved relations between Cuba and the United States. It is very likely that either Cuban intelligence acted on behalf of Russian intelligence to attack the United States and Canadian diplomats in Havana, or that they would not have interfered with Russian intelligence officers carrying out such attacks. The other major locations in which AHIs were reported also seem to be either former or current Russian client states, or well-known hotspots for Russian intelligence operations, namely Russia, China, Uzbekistan, Vietnam, Austria, and Germany. There was clearly an opportunity to attack Polymeropoulos in Moscow as he was meeting officially with representatives of Russian intelligence. Russia and China may not be perfect allies, but they are military partners with increasingly close military cooperation, who both consider the United States as their main adversary. In short, China may have allowed Russian operatives to carry out the attack on the Guangzhou consulate staffers. The Soviet Union and later Russia maintained a naval base in Cam Ranh Bay from 1979 to 2002, but in 2016 it was announced that Russia wanted to reopen a base in Vietnam. In 2019 a new Russian military logistics facility was established in Vietnam, indicating some Russian military presence in that country.[39] Vienna has been known for decades to be a hotspot for Russian intelligence and a location where Russian intelligence and the Russian mafia were laundering money.[40] Needless to say, Russian intelligence has a record for infiltrating the German government in Berlin, although these intelligence operations suffered a massive setback after 600 Russian diplomats were expelled from European countries in 2022.[41] However, this happened after the alleged Havana Syndrome case in Berlin of late summer 2021.

Means

Considering the long history of Soviet/Russian DEW research and the persistent rumors of Russian psychotronic weapons that can disrupt brains and the central nervous system, Russia is the most obvious country that would have and would use such weapons. The *60 Minutes* investigation of 2024 made the case that members of the Russian military intelligence (GU) Unit 29155 were the likely perpetrators. The unit is known for its role in assassinations and sabotage operations.[42] The unit was formed in the aftermath of the 2008 Georgia War and was commanded (as of 2020) by Major General Andrey Averyanov. According to Christo Grozev, Unit 29155 can be linked strongly to one AHI that occurred in Tbilisi, Georgia, in September 2021 when the wife of a US diplomat was seemingly attacked with a sonic weapon through her window. One individual who was standing near her home when it happened was later identified as the son of Major General Averyanov, Albert Averyanov, who is a member of Unit 29155.[43] Several other members of Unit 29155 were spotted near locations where AHIs occurred during the time they occurred, which includes Frankfurt in 2014 and possibly China in 2018. *The Insider* report claimed that the deputy commander of Unit 29155, Colonel Ivan Terentiev, is an engineer who had researched nonlethal acoustic weapons and that he had been rapidly promoted to a Kremlin position following a potential breakthrough in technological development.[44] This research was possibly based on a much older Soviet research program called *Reduktor* that began in 1984 and that investigated "electromagnetic radiation to influence the behavior and reactions of biological objects, [including] people."[45] A newer program, perhaps initiated in 2010, focused on the "development of basic technologies for the creation of a new generation of sonar and acoustic weapons systems."[46] During the May 2024 Homeland Security Committee meeting, Grozev testified that he had personally seen a 1991 version of the Russian DEW that could cause Havana Syndrome. Grozev said:

> [I]t looks like a satellite dish with the with a unit this size attached to it and of course over the years miniaturization has been possible. Obviously, there is a limitation to how miniaturized it can be because of the antenna size which can always is always related to the wave but still it is something that can be well contained in a in the trunk of a car or even a large backpack.[47]

China

Although China is rarely considered a potential perpetrator for the AHIs, there are also good reasons to look seriously into a China connection to the Havana Syndrome. First, China has invested even more money and effort into the development of DEW than either Russia or the United States.[48] There is a good amount of literature on Chinese biowarfare and neuroweapons research, which they have been conducting for many decades. If Russia would have the capability to conduct covert DE attacks on personnel, it is a safe bet that China would also have this capability. Several AHIs occurred in China, which is one of the most surveilled countries in the world.[49] It would follow that the Chinese government was at a minimum complicit in the incidents that occurred inside China as they failed to protect US diplomats. Furthermore, China has a global presence and the Chinese government has become increasingly hostile toward the United States, which has resulted in some analysts suggesting that China is already in a "stealth war" with the United States and that open war may be inevitable.[50] China has used gray zone tactics to keep the US Navy out of the South China Sea and is engaged in cyber warfare directed against the United States, Taiwan, and a long list of other countries. At least some of the AHIs could have been conceivably caused by Chinese operatives.

Motive

China has an interest in expanding its influence in Cuba and in undermining Cuban relations with the United States for a similar reason that Russia does. In 2014, Chinese president Xi Jinping visited Cuba to meet with Raoul and Fidel Castro, and in 2016 Chinese prime minister Li Keqiang came to Cuba to sign over twenty cooperation agreements between China and Cuba, which seemed to have included Cuba granting the Chinese military permission to construct a SIGINT base on the island for collecting signals from the United States. All of this Chinese diplomatic activity occurred when US–Cuban relations were supposedly improving. In 2016, a new radome was spotted near Bejucal, possibly related to Chinese SIGINT operations.[51] In 2023, the Biden administration acknowledged that China had in fact established a SIGINT base in Cuba, just 100 miles from Florida.[52] The Guangzhou AHIs also occurred at a curious time frame in late 2017 and spring 2018. At the beginning of his presidency, Donald Trump was undecided about China, but toward late 2017 he was swayed by the China hawks in his administration. On December 18, 2017, the Trump White House released a new National Security Strategy, which identified China as an adversary and blatantly accused them of stealing hundreds of billions of dollars of intellectual property per year.[53] This set the tone for US Trade Representative Robert Lightizer's report, published in late March 2018, which identified 1,333 Chinese companies producing per year over $50 billion worth of goods that violated US intellectual property. This justified President Trump's China sanctions and kicked off the US–China trade war.[54] It is notable that two Department of Commerce employees suffered an AHI in China (Catherine Werner and Robyn Garfield) in the late 2017 to mid-2018 time period, which indicates that this was some kind of Chinese retaliation for the US–China trade dispute. A third incident that looks like it could be connected to China is the series of AHIs in Hanoi in August 2021, which delayed Vice President Kamala Harris' visit to Vietnam for 3 hours. Several members of her advance team fell sick. Harris came to Vietnam to offer Covid vaccines and discuss Chinese expansionism in the South China Sea.[55] When her arrival was delayed, the Chinese ambassador to Vietnam requested an urgent meeting with Vietnamese prime minister Pham Minh Chinh, in which he offered them 2 million doses of the Chinese Covid vaccine.[56]

Opportunity

China has the largest intelligence apparatus in the world. The Chinese government has an estimated 600,000 people working in intelligence and security, both within China and outside China, which is more than any other country.[57] Chinese HUMINT benefits from a large Chinese global diaspora with many Chinese living outside China to be willing to support China when called upon. China has even established overseas police stations in several countries to exercise control over Chinese communities outside China.[58] Although there is only a small Chinese population in Cuba, Chinese warships visit the island regularly, and China seems to operate a listening post there since 2016, which means that they likely had military/intelligence personnel on the island when the first AHIs happened. There was clearly an opportunity for the Chinese government to attack US personnel in Guangzhou and Shanghai in late 2017 and 2018. Furthermore, Vietnam is in China's backyard, which means that their intelligence services would naturally have a presence in this country. Even some of the incidents inside the United States could have been carried out by Chinese intelligence, considering the sheer scale of Chinese intelligence operations in the United States. In 2021, the FBI had over 2,000 active counterintelligence investigations related to China, more than for any other country.[59]

Means

China is known to have developed "new concept weapons" that include novel types of DEWs and are part of China's "assassin's mace" strategy. In short, China has been looking for revolutionary niche technologies that can offset conventional

American military strength. Timothy Thomas has pointed out that the Chinese new concept weapons include "infrasound weapons, lasers, microwave and particle beam weapons and incoherent light sources."[60] Thomas quoted a Chinese military journal that claimed infrasound waves could cause "cardiac, respiratory, digestive and central nervous system malfunction, disorientation and emotional disorders" and that such weapons are being developed and tested in China. One of the weapons under development would use super-high frequency capable of interfering with the central nervous system and causing "unbearable noise and whistling sounds."[61] There is a direct quote in Thomas' article from the Chinese journal, which suggests that microwave weaponry that interferes with the central nervous system was already widely utilized and that medical protection against microwaves was already being developed.[62] A more recent report from the think tank *CCP Biothreats Initiative* claims that "the Chinese Communist Party (CCP) and its People's Liberation Army (PLA) have established themselves as world leaders in the development of NeuroStrike weapons. These platforms directly attack, or even control, mammalian brains (including humans) with microwave/directed energy weapons via standalone platforms (i.e., handheld gun) or the broader electromagnetic spectrum."[63] The US government seems to be aware of Chinese research in this area as the Department of Commerce imposed sanctions on select Chinese entities in December 2021 for using "biotechnology processes to support Chinese military end-uses and end-users, to include purported brain-control weaponry."[64] China tested a new HPM weapon for planned use on PLA Navy ships that can generate a magnetic field 68,000 times stronger than the earth's magnetic field, consumes a fifth of the energy of other systems, operates continuously for 4 hours, and is compact enough to be fitted into a truck.[65] The picture that emerges is that China has very clearly the technology to carry out covert attacks with acoustic or electromagnetic weaponry.

Nonstate Actors

At this point, even nonstate actors, either acting on their own initiative or as proxies for a foreign power, cannot be ruled out as perpetrators, which greatly complicates the issue. Relevant nonstate actors would include transnational criminal organizations, terrorist organizations, and private security/military companies (PSCs/PMCs). Yes, the weaponry capable of inducing Havana Syndrome can be assumed to be technologically advanced since the effects are more immediate and more severe than those of known nonlethal DEWs, and since the equipment would need to be miniaturized. Unfortunately, nonstate have been able to acquire other advanced weaponry in the past, and there is no reason to assume that they would not be able to acquire secret acoustic or electromagnetic weapons with or without the help of state actors.

Motive

A nonstate actor may carry out covert attacks on US government personnel on behalf of a state actor that sponsors them. Many analysts have pointed out that Russian intelligence uses Russian organized crime for their intelligence collection and covert operations. Mark Galeotti claimed that "[w]hile some of these murders appear to be the handiwork of government assassins, others seem to have been subcontracted to RBOC [Russian-based Organized Crime], especially groups from the North Caucasus themselves or with links to Chechnya."[66] The Russian government may pay ethnic Russian criminal groups to carry out covert attacks on Americans for reasons of operational security and plausible deniability—individuals connected to Russian organized crime may not face the same surveillance as Russian diplomats and intelligence/military operatives abroad, and if one of the criminals gets caught, it would be easier for the Russian government to deny responsibility for the attacks. Alternatively, a terrorist organization might target American government employees with DEWs for the purpose of revenge or retaliation. A potential suspect could be Hezbollah, which often acts as an overseas covert action arm of the Islamic Republic of Iran. Hezbollah has used drones, dazzling lasers, anti-tank missiles, and anti-aircraft missiles with great effect. They may have even received electromagnetic weapons or HPMs from Iran to disable electronics, as was reported by a Kuwaiti newspaper.[67] PSCs/PMCs, especially the bigger and leading firms, are often staffed by individuals with intelligence and military backgrounds, which means that they would be familiar with some of the highly classified surveillance and weapons technology. Some of the PSCs/PMCs are effectively fronts for government intelligence agencies. An obvious example is the Russian Wagner Group, which was established by Russian military intelligence in 2010.[68] There has been speculation that some of these PSCs/PMCs may have access to very advanced surveillance technology and electromagnetic weaponry, which they could employ on behalf of their clients, that could be governments, corporations, or NGOs, against unsuspecting targets. The use of nonstate proxies for governments or other actors creates a huge analytical challenge as proxies will sometimes act on their own initiative and sometimes act as directed by their sponsors. This makes it very hard to understand who is actually responsible for actions and what the intent is behind these actions.

Opportunity

Nonstate actors are generally considered to have far lesser capabilities compared to state actors, which makes them considerably less dangerous. However, it is also easier for nonstate actors to stay below the radar of government surveillance and security measures that are more capable of detecting threats associated with nation-states. Some nonstate actors can operate globally. For example, the Russian mafia has a presence in numerous countries around the world, including Europe, North America, and Asia. Globalization has made it easier for nonstate actors to travel around the world because of cheap communication and transportation. Although it has gotten harder to utilize forged passports because of biometrics, many Western countries now have poorly protected borders that allow people to enter without ID papers or going through the normal visa process. Terrorists could illegally enter the EU or the United States by illegally crossing a land border or by sea, mixing with thousands of ordinary migrants. For example, over the last few years, DHS detained over 294 individuals on the terror watchlist, with an unknown number of terrorists who may have slipped through.[69] Once they are in a target location, they could put together a primitive DEW, using off-the-shelf components.[70] Getting away would be also easier for individuals illegally in a country and not associated in any way with an adversarial government. The FBI or CIA may be looking primarily for Russian or Chinese intelligence operatives but may have a blind spot when it comes to clandestinely operating nonstate actors with less obvious motives and capabilities.

Means

There are two potential ways for nonstate actors to acquire DEWs that could induce Havana Syndrome: either they received the technology from a nation-state that has developed it by way of theft, corruption, or gifting, or they developed such a weapon themselves, using readily available parts that one could find in a consumer electronics store. When the Cold War ended rather suddenly in December 1991, the former Soviet Republics were sitting on the largest arsenal of weapons and weapons technology ever amassed in human history. The economic hardship, out-of-control corruption, rampant organized crime, and the general chaos in Russia and other former Soviet states at the time meant that pretty much every weapon was for sale on black markets with the exception of nuclear weapons.[71] Various terror and criminal groups made attempts in the early 1990s to buy various weapons systems, biological agents, and nuclear materials. It is hence conceivable that Soviet psychotronic weapons technology may have ended up in the hands of transnational criminal organizations.[72] As it concerns DIY electromagnetic weapons, the cost and technological barrier for building a primitive one is not high. One can find instructions on the internet on how to convert a microwave oven into a High-Energy Radiofrequency (HERF) device that can be used to destroy electronics or harm people (from a close distance). Journalist Nicky Woolf claimed that he was able to build a primitive HERF device by using an old microwave oven and some additional parts and he was able to measure the energy it emitted at a distance.[73] It is definitely not outside of the realm of possibility that US government personnel and also random civilians could be covertly attacked by terrorists or criminals with hard-to-detect and self-made DEWs.

Conclusion

The likely perpetrators for the AHIs are Cuba, Russia, and China, which may cooperate with nonstate actors such as criminal or terror groups, or PSCs/PMCs. The Cuban government is a primary suspect with respect to the AHIs that occurred on the island in 2016 and 2017. They may have decided to seek better military and intelligence relations with Russia and China, making the US diplomatic initiative to normalize relations an obstacle to their shift in policy. Many of the AHIs around the world, especially the ones that occurred in Europe, Russia, and the United States, have been connected to Russia, which has the motive, the global presence, and the technological capability for these covert attacks. It is notable that the attacks seemed to have started in 2014, the year in which Russia's diplomatic relations with the West were breaking down over Ukraine. China should not be neglected as a prime suspect for several of the AHIs, namely the ones that occurred in China in 2017 and 2018 and the one that occurred in Vietnam in 2021. US–Chinese relations took a turn toward openly adversarial with the shift in policy by the Trump administration that occurred at that exact time. China has been developing DEWs and, in particular, HPMs that could be used for covert attacks. It therefore appears that the AHIs may involve several different foreign powers and possibly also nonstate actors, pursuing different objectives. This would explain that different types of DEWs were used in different incidents, some of which appear to be caused by acoustic weapons and some appear to have been caused by electromagnetic weapons.

Notes

1 60 Minutes Australia, "Havana Syndrome: Is Russia Behind the Mysterious Illness?," *60 Minutes Australia*, April 28, 2024, available at: https://www.youtube.com/watch?v=aq7dTOPMViI.
2 Carol Morello, "U.S. Declares Reduced Staffing Levels 'Permanent' at Embassy in Havana: The State Department Also Extended an Advisory Urging Americans to Reconsider Travel to Cuba for Months After 24 U.S. Diplomats Suffered Unexplained Injuries," *Washington Post*, March 2, 2018.
3 Barnes, "C.I.A. Officer Suffer Havana Syndrome Symptoms," *New York Times*, September 20, 2021.
4 Michele Kelemen and Deepa Shivaram, "VP Harris' Flight Delayed After Possible 'Havana Syndrome' Incident in Hanoi," *NPR*, August 24, 2021, available at: https://www.npr.org/2021/08/24/1030663913/kamala-harris-havana-syndrome-vietnam-delay-embassy.
5 Barnes, "C.I.A. Officer Suffer Havana Syndrome Symptoms."
6 Mark Zaid, "Testimony of Mark S. Zaid Esq.," Homeland Security Committee, May 8, 2024, 9, available at: https://homeland.house.gov/wp-content/uploads/2024/05/2024-05-08-CTI-HRG-Testimony.pdf.
7 Jamey Essex and Joshua Bowman, "From the Green Zone to the Havana Syndrome: Making Geographic Sense of Rotationality and Hardship in Diplomacy," *Diplomatica* 4, no. 1 (2022): 94; Adam Entous, "Are U.S. Officials Under Silent Attack?," The New Yorker (May 24, 2021), available at: https://cs.brown.edu/people/jsavage/sources/2021_05_24_NewYorker_AreUSOfficialsUnderSilentAttack.pdf.
8 Julian Borger, "Havana Syndrome has 'Dramatically Hurt' Morale, US Diplomats Say," *The Guardian*, February 10, 2022, available at: https://www.theguardian.com/us-news/2022/feb/10/havana-syndrome-cuba-us-diplomats-afsa.
9 Eric Haseltine, *The Spy in Moscow Station: A Counterspy's Hunt for a Deadly Cold War Threat* (New York: St. Martin's Griffin, 2019), 22.
10 New York Times Staff, "Soviet Halts Microwaves Aimed at U.S. Embassy," *New York Times*, May 30, 1979.
11 Julian Borger, "Botched Surveillance Job May Have Led to Strange Injuries at Embassy in Cuba," *The Guardian*, August 25, 2017, available at: https://www

.theguardian.com/world/2017/aug/25/botched-surveillance-job-may-have-led-to-strange-injuries-at-cuban-embassy.

12 The Guardian Staff, "Trump Says Cuba 'Responsible' for Alleged Sonic Attacks, but Offers No Evidence," *The Guardian*, October 16, 2017, available at: https://www.theguardian.com/world/2017/oct/16/trump-says-cuba-responsible-for-alleged-sonic-attacks-but-offers-no-evidence.

13 The Guardian Staff, "Trump Says Cuba 'Responsible' for Alleged Sonic Attacks, but Offers No Evidence."

14 US Congress, "Attacks on U.S. Diplomats in Cuba: Response and Oversight," Senate Subcommittee on Western Hemisphere, Transnational Crime, Civilian Security, Democracy, Human Rights, and Global Women's Issues, January 9, 2018, 3.

15 Frances Robles and Kirk Semple, "'Health Attacks' on U.S. Diplomats in Cuba Baffle Experts," *New York Times*, August 11, 2017.

16 Elise Labott, "John Kerry Reopens Embassy in Cube, But Tensions Remain," *CNN*, August 14, 2015, available at: https://www.cnn.com/2015/08/14/politics/cuba-embassy-opening-john-kerry-visit/index.html.

17 Desmond Butler, Jack Gillum, and Alberto Arce, "US Secretly Built 'Cuban Twitter' to Stir Unrest," *Associated Press*, April 3, 2014, available at: https://apnews.com/article/technology-cuba-united-states-government-904a9a6a1bcd46cebfc14bea2ee30fdf.

18 US Congress, "Attacks on U.S. Diplomats in Cuba," 29.

19 Brett Forrest and Warren P. Strobel, "How Cuba Recruits Spies to Penetrate Inner Circles of the U.S. Government," *Wall Street Journal*, March 16, 2024.

20 Joshua Partlow, "In Cuba, Harassment of U.S. Diplomats Even Extends to Their Pets. Will That Now Change?," *Washington Post Online*, January 1, 2015.

21 Julio Antonio del Marmol, *Black Tears: The Havana Syndrome* (Cuban Lightning Publications, 2022), 32.

22 Del Marmol, *Black Tears: The Havana Syndrome*, 242, note 8.

23 Fabiano Maisonnave, "Manuel Zelaya Undergoes Strange Siege Inside Brazilian Embassy," *The Guardian*, October 25, 2009, available at: https://www.theguardian.com/world/2009/oct/25/honduras-manuel-zelaya-embassy-siege.

24 Amy Goodman, "Ousted Honduran President Manuel Zelaya Speaks from Brazilian Embassy in Tegucigalpa," *Democracy Now!*, October 5, 2009, available at: https://www.democracynow.org/2009/10/5/ousted_honduran_president_manuel_zelaya_speaks.

25 Sean Power and Michael Miner, "Report—Havana Syndrome: American Officials Under Attack," *Belfer Center for Science and International Affairs*, Harvard University, November 4, 2021, available at: https://www.belfercenter.org/publication/report-havana-syndrome-american-officials-under-attack.

26 Dimitry Clancy, "Havana Syndrome: The Mysterious Illness Striking Down US Officials," *60 Minutes Australia*, April 2024, available at: https://9now.nine.com.au/60-minutes/havana-syndrome-the-mysterious-illness-striking-down-us-officials/27d3425c-274e-40a7-926f-ac33ff9e2d62.

27 US Congress, "Silent Weapons: Examining Foreign Anomalous Health Incidents Targeting Americans in Homeland," Homeland Security Committee, May 8, 2024, 4, https://homeland.house.gov/wp-content/uploads/2024/05/2024-05-08-CTI-HRG-Testimony.pdf.

28 Xinhua Staff, "Russia Resumes Military Presence on Cuba: Russian Lawmaker," *Xinhua News Agency*, August 3, 2008.

29 Mark Lowenthal, *Intelligence: From Secrets to Policy* (Thousand Oaks: Sage, 2020), 473.

30 Audrey Ostroukh, "Russia Writes Off Cuba Debt," *Dow Jones Institutional News*, July 11, 2014.

31 Karen DeYoung, "Trump Administration Announces New Measures Against Cuba," *Washington Post*, April 17, 2019.

32 Patrick Oppmann, AnneClaire Stapleton, Natasha Bertrand, Haley Britzky, Sergey Gudkov, and Sophie Tanno, "Russian Ships Arrive in Cuba as Cold War Allies Strengthen Their Ties," *CNN*, June 12, 2024, available at: https://www.cnn.com/2024/06/12/americas/russian-navy-cuba-intl/index.html.

33 Don Munton, "Our Men in Havana: Canadian Foreign Intelligence Operations in Castro's Cuba," *International Journal* 70, no. 1 (2015): 24.

34 Roman Dobrokhotov, Christo Grozev, and Michael Weiss, "Unraveling Havana Syndrome: New Evidence Links the GRU's Assassination Unit 29155 to Mysterious Attacks on U.S. Officials and Their Families," *The Insider*, March 31, 2024, available at: https://theins.ru/en/politics/270425.

35 Dobrokhotov, Grozev, and Weiss, "Unraveling Havana Syndrome: New Evidence Links the GRU's Assassination Unit 29155 to Mysterious Attacks on U.S. Officials and Their Families."

36 Lowenthal, *Intelligence*, 491.

37 Christopher Andrew and Vasili Mitrokhin, *The Mithrokin Archive: The KGB in Europe and the West* (London: Penguin, 1999), 503–5.

38 Stéphane Lefebvre, "Cuban Intelligence Activities Directed at the United States, 1959-2007," *International Journal of Intelligence and Counterintelligence* 22, no. 3 (2009): 464.

39 Prashanth Parameswaran, "What's in Russia's New Military Facility in Vietnam?," *The Diplomat*, April 30, 2019, available at: https://thediplomat.com/2019/04/whats-in-russias-new-military-facility-in-vietnam/.

40 Bojan Pancevski, "A Den of Spies: Vienna Emerges as a Hub for Russian Espionage," *Wall Street Journal*, June 27, 2024.
41 Thomas Escritt and Sarah Marsh, "Russia Buying Spies to Make Up for Expelled Diplomats, Germany Agency Says," *Reuters*, June 18, 2024, available at: https://www.reuters.com/world/europe/russia-buying-spies-make-up-expelled-diplomats-german-agency-says-2024-06-18/.
42 John Haltiwanger, "The Shadowy Russian Intel Unit That Allegedly Paid Afghan Militants to Kill US Troops Is the Same One Running Assassinations in Europe," *Business Insider*, June 29, 2020, available at: https://www.businessinsider.com/unit-29155-russian-intel-branch-allegedly-behind-bounties-us-troops-2020-6.
43 Dobrokhotov, Grozev, and Weiss, "Unraveling Havana Syndrome: New Evidence Links the GRU's Assassination Unit 29155 to Mysterious Attacks on U.S. Officials and Their Families."
44 Dobrokhotov, Grozev, and Weiss, "Unraveling Havana Syndrome: New Evidence Links the GRU's Assassination Unit 29155 to Mysterious Attacks on U.S. Officials and Their Families."
45 Dobrokhotov, Grozev, and Weiss, "Unraveling Havana Syndrome: New Evidence Links the GRU's Assassination Unit 29155 to Mysterious Attacks on U.S. Officials and Their Families."
46 Quoted from Dobrokhotov, Grozev, and Weiss, "Unraveling Havana Syndrome: New Evidence Links the GRU's Assassination Unit 29155 to Mysterious Attacks on U.S. Officials and Their Families."
47 US Congress, "Silent Weapons: Examining Foreign Anomalous Health Incidents Targeting Americans in Homeland," Homeland Security Committee, May 8, 2024, available at: https://www.youtube.com/watch?v=LCYH_K850Lw&t=3930s.
48 Edl Schamiloglu, "Experts Suggest US Embassies Were Hit with High-Power Microwaves—Here's How the Weapons Work," *The Conversation*, December 10, 2020, available at: https://theconversation.com/experts-suggest-us-embassies-were-hit-with-high-power-microwaves-heres-how-the-weapons-work-151730.
49 Josh Chin and Liza Lin, *Surveillance State: Inside China's Quest to Launch a New Era of Social Control Quest to Launch a New Era of Social Control* (New York: St. Martin's Press, 2022), 7.
50 Robert Spalding, *Stealth War: How China Took Over While America's Elite Slept* (New York: Penguin, 2019); Hal Brands and Michael Beckley, *Danger Zone: The Coming Conflict with China* (New York: W.W. Norton & Co., 2019).
51 Victor Robert Lee, "Satellite Images: A (Worrying) Cuban Mystery," *The Diplomat*, June 8, 2018, available at: https://thediplomat.com/2018/06/satellite-images-a-worrying-cuban-mystery/.

52 Warren P. Strobel and Gordon Lubold, "Cuba to Host Secret Chinese Spy Base Focusing on US," *Wall Street Journal*, June 8, 2023.
53 US White House, National Security Strategy of the United States, December 2017, 21.
54 Josh Rogin, *Chaos Under Heaven: Trump, Xi, and the Battle for the 21st Century* (Boston: Hougton Mifflin Harcourt, 2021), 136.
55 RFA Vietnamese, "Report: US Officials Had Sudden Symptoms Before Harris' Hanoi Visit," *Radio Free Asia*, April 3, 2024, available at: https://www.rfa.org/english/news/vietnam/hanoi-havana-syndrome-report-04032024152734.html.
56 James Pearson and Nandita Bose, "U.S. VP Harris Forges on with Vietnam Trip Despite Mystery 'Health Incident,'" *BBC News*, August 24, 2021, available at: https://www.reuters.com/world/asia-pacific/eve-harris-trip-vietnam-tells-china-it-does-not-pick-sides-2021-08-24/.
57 Gordon Corera, "China's Spy Threat Is Growing, But the West Has Struggled to Keep Up," *BBC News*, May 15, 2024, available at: https://www.bbc.com/news/articles/cmm33rm32veo.
58 Emile Dirks and Diana Fu, "China's Overseas Police Stations: An Imminent Security Threat," *Brookings*, February 16, 2024, available at: https://www.brookings.edu/articles/chinas-overseas-police-stations-an-imminent-security-threat/.
59 Mike Conte, "FBI Opens a New Investigation Into China 'Every 10 Hours,' Bureau Director Says," *CNN*, April 14, 2021, available at: https://www.cnn.com/2021/04/14/politics/fbi-director-china-investigations-intl-hnk/index.html.
60 Timothy Thomas, "Human Network Attacks," *Military Review* 79, (September/October 1999): 28.
61 Thomas, "Human Network Attacks," 28–9.
62 Thomas, "Human Network Attacks," 29.
63 Ryan Clarke, Xiaoxu Sean Lin, and L. J. Eads, "Enumerating, Targeting and Collapsing the Chinese Communist Party's NeuroStrike Program: Aggregating Intelligence Fragments and the Power of Network Graphs," *The CCP's Biothreats Initiative Research Report*, June 2023, 2, available at: https://www.ccpbiothreats.com/initiatives/project-one-ephnc-23hjt-xkgdj.
64 Quoted from: Bill Gertz, "China Crafts Weapons to Alter Brain Function; Report Says Tech Meant to Influence Government Leaders," *Washington Times*, July 6, 2023, available at: https://www.washingtontimes.com/news/2023/jul/6/chinas-military-leading-world-brain-neurostrike-we/.
65 Stephen Chen, "Chinese Scientists Build Powerful Microwave Weapon That Can Fire From a Moving Truck, Using Stirling Engine to Cool Technology," *South China Morning Post*, February 8, 2024, available at: https://www.scmp.com/news/china/

science/article/3251381/chinese-scientists-build-powerful-stirling-engine-based-microwave-weapon-can-fire-moving-truck.

66 Mark Galeotti, "CRIMINTERN: How the Kremlin Uses Russia's Criminal Networks in Europe," *European Council on Foreign Relations*, April 2017, 7, available at: https://ecfr.eu/wp-content/uploads/ECFR208_-_CRIMINTERM_-_HOW_RUSSIAN_ORGANISED_CRIME_OPERATES_IN_EUROPE02.pdf.

67 Matan Wasserman, "'Even Cockroaches Won't Survive': Expert Discusses Hezbollah's New EMP Weapon," *The Jerusalem Post*, July 28, 2024, available at: https://www.jpost.com/middle-east/article-812168.

68 Kimberley Marten, "Russia's Use of Semi-State Security Forces: The Case of the Wagner Group," *Post-Soviet Affairs* 35, no. 3 (2019): 187.

69 US Congress, "Border Sector Chiefs Confirm Operational Impacts of Border Chaos: Increased Gotaways, Closed Checkpoints, and Empowered Cartels," Homeland Security Committee, December 20, 2023, available at: https://homeland.house.gov/2023/12/20/border-sector-chiefs-confirm-operational-impacts-of-border-chaos-increased-gotaways-closed-checkpoints-and-empowered-cartels/.

70 US Congress, "Silent Weapons: Examining Foreign Anomalous Health Incidents Targeting Americans in Homeland."

71 Ian Anthony, ed., *Russia and the Arms Trade* (Oxford: Oxford University Press, 1998), 217–18.

72 Tom Bearden claimed that the Japanese Yakuza could lease a Soviet scalar interferometer to influence weather and affect behavior in the United States. Thomas Bearden, *Oblivion: America at the Brink* (Cheniere Press, 2005), 2–3.

73 Nicky Woolf, "The Sound: Mystery of the Havana Syndrome—A Conversation with Nicky Woolf," University of Boston, November 1, 2023, available at: https://www.youtube.com/watch?v=kVZyDRBil8U.

8

Cognitive Warfare

The possible motivations for a foreign power targeting a few US government personnel around the world remain unclear when just looking at each incident in isolation. It is, therefore, necessary to put the AHIs into a much broader theoretical context of what has been called "unrestricted warfare," "hybrid warfare," "psychological warfare," "gray zone conflict," "fifth generation warfare," "non-kinetic threats," and most recently "cognitive warfare." Here is not the place to go into the different nuances of these concepts and theories or to discuss their respective merits. However, it is worthwhile to review some of the key ideas in the general debate on conflict short of war that started in the early 1990s.[1] The underlying assumption in this debate is that adversaries, both state and nonstate actors, may engage in hostile activities that are covert or ambiguous to avoid an escalation to an open war that they most likely would lose. Instead, they weaken their enemies in a manner that is not apparent or difficult to attribute and hence deniable. Obviously, there is no major strategic advantage to be gained by a foreign power to injure relatively few US diplomats and intelligence officers unless this was part of a bigger effort or unless this was merely a testing phase before much more serious attacks would be carried out on a much larger scale.

Cognitive Warfare Defined

The debate on cognitive warfare within NATO began in late 2020, and there is continuing interest in and an expansion of the general concept. NATO analysts have defined cognitive warfare in the following way:

> Cognitive Warfare includes activities conducted in synchronization with other Instruments of Power, to affect attitudes and behaviours, by influencing, protecting, or disrupting individual, group, or population level cognition, to gain an advantage over an adversary. Designed to modify perceptions of reality,

> whole-of-society manipulation has become a new norm, with human cognition shaping to be a critical realm of warfare.[2]

The underlying idea of cognitive warfare is that "the human mind becomes the battlefield" and that "[t]he aim is to change not only what people think, but how they think and act."[3] In addition to the use of propaganda and disinformation, cognitive warfare also includes "neuro-weapons. . . . Its field of action is global and aimed to seize control of human beings (civilian as well as military), organisations, nations, but also of ideas, psychology, especially behavioural, thoughts as well as the environment."[4] Francois du Cluzel defined cognitive warfare as "the art of using technologies to alter the cognition of human targets, most often without their knowledge and consent."[5] Furthermore, "[c]ognitive warfare is the art of using technological tools to alter the cognition of human targets, who are often unaware of any such attempt—as are those entrusted with countering, minimizing, or managing its consequences, whose institutional and bureaucratic reactions are too slow or inadequate."[6] In short, cognitive warfare is a more sophisticated version of psychological warfare in the sense that it utilizes a broader range of instruments and benefits from knowledge gained from neuroscientific research, combined with adjacent technology areas, including neurotechnology, biotechnology, nanotechnology, information technology, and artificial intelligence, to ultimately understand, influence, and control human behavior individually and on a macroscale.

Havana Syndrome relates to cognitive warfare in the sense that it is very likely caused by what can be called a neuroweapon, designed to injure the brain, interfere with the brain, and possibly remotely monitor the brain. These attacks have, up to now, targeted individuals and small groups of individuals (e.g., families), but there is a possibility that the technology will advance to the point that larger groups of people, if not entire nations, could be targeted to damage or otherwise interfere with their brains and cognitive processes.

Attack on Leadership

Attacks on enemy leadership are nothing new in warfare and political conflicts. Many governments have used political assassinations as a means to overthrow regimes, alter the domestic politics of another country, or impose punishment on an adversarial government. However, political assassination is fraught with obvious problems that have made the practice often ineffective: political leaders tend to be well-protected, making it less likely that an assassination attempt would succeed; assassination attempts that can be traced back to a sponsoring government could result in a serious diplomatic crisis, if not war; a leader who survives an assassination attempt may double down on policies that prompted the assassination attempt in the first place; and a successful assassination attempt may result in a successor worse than the one who was eliminated. Bruce Berkowitz has claimed that because of these reasons, "*every* U.S. effort to kill a high-ranking official since World War II outside a full-scale war has failed. This record is so poor that it would be hard to find an instrument of national policy that has been less successful in achieving its objectives than assassination."[7]

Nonlethal cognitive attacks on leaders seem to be a better option. One objective in cognitive warfare is to undermine the ability of enemy decision-makers to make good decisions, which could mean manipulating their perceptions, degrading their mental or cognitive capacity for good decision-making, or to more directly influencing their thinking and behavior without the leaders realizing that they had been attacked.[8] Decision-makers could be pushed into taking rash and sweeping actions when not acting or acting carefully would be best or into not acting when swift action was absolutely essential.[9] There are, in principle, many possibilities to accomplish this, using tailored information or disinformation, provocations aimed at causing a predetermined desirable response by the adversary ("reflexive control"), biological or chemical agents that affect mental states and capacity, acoustic or electromagnetic waves that affect mental states or capacity, and incoherent light sources that can disorient and paralyze ("bucha effect").

Attacking leaders in a nonlethal way that leaves them in place but degrades their cognitive abilities or distorts their perception could prove to be much more effective than outright assassination. First, assassination is difficult to disguise as anything other than what it is, which makes the use of this tactic politically risky, while conditions caused by covert cognitive attacks may not be discovered at all as deliberate attacks, making this an almost risk-free approach for the attacker. As Robert McCreight stated, "[s]ymptoms of its victims cannot be readily evaluated by physicians as no case definition or peer reviewed research exists to verify its authenticity."[10] Secondly, it could be more difficult to protect officials against covert non-kinetic attacks than to protect them against bullets and poisons, especially if the threat is inadequately understood. Currently, the US government does not seem to have an effective approach as to how to protect their officials against DEWs that have invisible beams that go through walls and windows. Thirdly, targeted leaders or officials may be even reluctant to report potential covert attacks on their mental capacity as this could result in their removal from a leadership position because of a permanent disability they may have incurred.[11] This natural reluctance of officials to self-report potentially career-ending health incidents means that these officials remain longer in office than they should due to their mental impairment, which can affect the organization in which they hold a leadership position. It also makes the overall detection and response to attacks a lot more difficult. Fourthly, if a cognitively impaired leader remains in place and makes a series of poor decisions, an organization must contend not only with the direct consequences of these poor decisions but also with the delegitimization of their leadership as a whole, which can be organizationally and politically destabilizing as general trust in the leadership evaporates. In cognitive warfare, "[t]rust . . . is a targeted vulnerability," which means that cognitive attacks often seek to actively undermine trust in leadership.[12] Finally, if a whole leadership class or professional class with a rare set of experience and skills were to be targeted, it could be extremely difficult to replace such high-value individuals, as pointed out by Joshua D. Gramm and Brian A. Branagan:

> The United States cannot mass produce CIA officers with almost three decades of experience and losing someone of his caliber ultimately hurts national security. If this is continued in a targeted, deliberate, systematic fashion, serious damages to national security will accumulate as key people in senior leadership positions are no longer willing and/or able to do their jobs.[13]

Without skilled professionals with sufficient experience and knowledge, or in other words human capital, an organization cannot be successful. Hence, it makes sense to systematically target talented and experienced individuals in an adversarial organization to cause long-term damage to the organization.

Political and Societal Destabilization

Cognitive warfare can also be directed toward an entire society with the aim of political or social destabilization. A NATO paper suggests the following: "The first fundamental goal of cognitive warfare is to destabilize target populations. Destabilization is done by disrupting the organization and unity of a population's systems and people."[14] Cognitive warfare "seeks to sow doubt, to introduce conflicting narratives, to polarise opinion, to radicalise groups, and to motivate them to acts that can disrupt or fragment an otherwise cohesive society."[15] This may be enabled by divisive narratives, propaganda, and disinformation, but may also include more nefarious and sophisticated means.

This process of societal destabilization can be further facilitated by way of attacking the mental capacity of a population more broadly. If one could lower the IQ of millions of people, it becomes easier to manipulate them as they lack the critical thinking ability to question supposed facts or narratives that simply do not make any sense. The declining average mental capacity within a society becomes, in many ways, a threat to national security as people are more likely to fall victim to enemy propaganda and lose their capacity and will to resist more direct and obvious aggression. In the long-term, a decline in average IQ is a disaster for any society as it will lose its ability to innovate and develop technology essential to a nation's defense. The United States depends on technological innovation for maintaining its current leading economic and military position, but unfortunately, China is in the process of overtaking the United States when it comes to scientific research publications and inventions.[16] In that case, the United States would have lost both its industrial manufacturing capability and also its ability to innovate to China.

A large-scale attack on mental capacity may already be happening in Western societies as IQs have been dropping significantly over the last few decades with no good explanation as to why.[17] According to one study, the average IQ has dropped an astonishing 13.35 points in Western nations between 1889 and 2004.[18] People are losing, on average, the ability to perform even the simplest calculations in their heads or to retain more complex new information longer than a few seconds. Since the early 2000s, the average attention span of Americans dropped from 2.5 minutes to currently 47 seconds, which is technically called attention deficit and hyperactivity disorder (ADHD).[19] The situation seems to have gotten much worse since the pandemic started in 2020. A *New England Journal of Medicine* study of 800,000 adults in England indicated that individuals who suffered from a Covid infection lost some IQ points, and those who suffered from long Covid lost up to 9 IQ points, which is massive. The researchers found that long Covid patients were likely to suffer from poor memory and from problems with concentrating and thinking ("brain fog").[20]

Interestingly, many Havana Syndrome patients have complained about poor memory and brain fog, which has sometimes ended their careers since they could no longer do intellectual work. Of course, Covid was a biological vector for inducing this condition while Havana Syndrome seems to be induced by some kind of acoustic or electromagnetic exposure, but there are certainly similarities in the effect. A Havana Syndrome weapon could be scalable to attack multiple individuals at a time, if not entire communities. Existing telecommunications and other technological infrastructure could be covertly repurposed in a nefarious way. For example, there are huge concerns about 5G technology and the ability of nefarious actors to weaponize it for taking control of all kinds of smart devices and infrastructure.[21] Even simple consumer electronics such as headphones or speakers could be turned into mind-scrambling neuroweapons by remotely hacking a computer and making it produce harmful sounds.[22]

Far less thought has been given to the possibility of taking over and using 5G infrastructure for attacking people and communities with harmful and possibly debilitating EMF exposures by just greatly increasing power outputs and using harmful frequencies and wave modulations. 5G can use the millimeter wave frequency, just like the ADS. There is only a difference in power output.[23] Covert attacks could aim not only causing a decline in mental capacity but could possibly induce psychotic behaviors in communities, something the proponents of psychochemical warfare in the Cold War had theorized could be done with hallucinogens added to the water or food, or sprayed in the air.[24]

Neuroweapons

Neuroweapons can be defined as weapons that target the brain to influence cognition and behavior.[25] This can include a wide range of biological, chemical, informational, acoustic, and electromagnetic means for altering brain function. Robert McCreight has proposed the term "NeuroStrike weapon" to describe novel types of weapons that can remotely degrade cognitive abilities and damage the brain. He defines a NeuroStrike weapon as a weapon that "entails a hand held, or platform mounted, mixture of an RF, directed energy pulse *or neurocognitive disrupter, combined with acoustic wave dynamics* which is designed to harm, disable or permanently damage a human brain."[26] The effect would be "debilitating, leaving its victims unable to perform brain functions for many years."[27]

Brain research or neuroscience has been "weaponized" since the 1950s or the beginning with the CIA MK ULTRA mind control research program. The initial focus of these efforts was the discovery or development of new drugs that had specific effects on the brain and behavior. At that time, a lot of research was conducted in relation to LSD and other hallucinogenic drugs, but from the early 1960s, research was conducted that examined the electrical stimulation of the brain.[28] The Havana Syndrome has led to growing concerns that directed energy could be used to stimulate and damage brains from a distance in a manner that remains, up to now, poorly understood. In any case, there are existing brain interventions and neurotechnologies that are typically developed in a health/therapeutic context but that could be conceivably used maliciously for remote attacks on brains.

Brain Stimulation

Dr. José Delgado was a leading brain researcher during the 1950s and 1960s, and he remains famous for having developed the "stimoceiver," which consisted of electrodes implanted into the brain and that could stimulate the brain to cause specific behavior. Delgado demonstrated this new technology by stopping a bull equipped with a stimoceiver that was charging at him by pressing a button.[29] Delgado also implanted monkeys and humans with electrodes to stimulate particular brain regions, and he was able to produce a consistent and predictable behavioral response when an electric stimulus was given.[30] The stimoceiver only weighed a few grams and enabled the remote stimulation of the brain and the simultaneous recording of brain waves.[31] There are good reasons to believe that individuals were unwittingly implanted with stimoceiver-like devices in the MK ULTRA era. The CIA was sued by veterans in 2010 for conducting mind control experiments on them, including implanting electrical devices in their brains to turn them into robots, which may have happened before 1975.[32] Delgado's early work with brain implants has led to a more recent DARPA SUBNETS program that includes Deep Brain Stimulation (DBS) for the purpose of treating PTSD, depression, and other neuropsychiatric illnesses with electrical impulses that are delivered directly to the brain by tiny implanted devices. DBS functions like a pacemaker for the brain that controls moods and suppresses brain disorders.[33]

DARPA hopes to eventually produce a brain chip that would allow commanders to remotely monitor the brains of their soldiers and relieve pain or anxiety by way of electrical impulses to improve combat effectiveness.[34] Other techniques for noninvasive brain stimulation that could manage the brain functions of soldiers via a helmet device include the application of weak electrical stimuli to the scalp (transcranial direct current stimulation), strong magnetic fields to the head (transcranial magnetic stimulation), and the use of ultrasound for stimulating the brain (transcranial ultrasound stimulation).[35] Brain stimulation is a key technology for the eventual development (or rather perfection) of a BCI.

Brain-Computer Interface

From the 1950s, neuroscientists believed that the brain was a biocomputer that used electrical signals to process information, which made it plausible that brains could be somehow connected to computers or computer networks to send or receive information.[36] This merely requires the ability to decode the brain by determining how the brain processes information. The development of a BCI was first proposed in 1973 by Jacques Vidal, who suggested that brain wave activity measured by an EEG could be interpreted by a computer and used for sending information from the brain directly to the computer, for example, for controlling machinery.[37] Neuroscientists have already succeeded in the development of cochlea implants and bionic eye implants that restore senses and allow people who are deaf to hear and people who are blind to regain some of their vision. Brain implants can allow quadriplegic patients to move a cursor on a screen or operate a phone with their minds and allow other patients with lost limbs to control robotic limbs.[38]

Currently, the technology requires drilling a hole in the skull to insert the brain implant, but soon it would be possible to use a far less risky noninvasive way of connecting brains to computers. The company *Neuralink* and DARPA are working on a noninvasive technology for BCIs that would make it possible to roll out BCIs to the masses as some kind of consumer technology or to healthy soldiers for controlling weapons systems with their minds and for silent (brain-to-brain) communication (also known as "synthetic telepathy").[39] According to a *Time* article from 2008,

> improvements in computing power and a better understanding of how the brain works have scientists busy hunting for the distinctive neural fingerprints that flash through a brain when a person is talking to himself. The Army's initial goal is to capture those brain waves with incredibly sophisticated software that then translates the waves into audible radio messages for other troops in the field.[40]

To make this a viable technology for the military (and consumers), it must be noninvasive, as few people would like to have permanent brain implants.

The main technology direction for a noninvasive BCI is the use of magnetic nanoparticles.[41]

Nanoparticles

Nanotechnology deals with the manipulation of matter at a molecular scale and was first proposed by physicist Richard Feynman in a lecture titled "There Is Plenty of Room at the Bottom" from 1959 and was first described by Eric Drexler in his 1986 book *Engines of Creation*. Drexler envisioned self-assembling nanomachines where molecular-size robots move atoms to the correct location.[42] Nanotechnology research was previously dominated by chemistry, physics, and material science, but it has become a key technology direction in the biosciences, pharmacology, and biotechnology. In general, nanotechnology deals with the manipulation of matter smaller than 100 nanometers.

Nanoparticles are so small that they can breach the blood-brain barrier and hence reach areas of the brain that normal drugs cannot.[43] This means that drugs could be delivered with precision to particular areas of the brain or other parts of the body, reducing some of the risks of side effects of drugs. Another application is the use of magnetic nanoparticles such as iron oxide to enhance the resolution of MRI neural imaging, providing a better diagnostic tool. The nanoparticles can be injected into the bloodstream and can thereby reach any part of the body, including the brain. Although some nanoparticles are known to have toxic and inflammatory effects, they remain insufficiently regulated and are likely to be ingested through drugs and foods.[44]

DARPA has funded a research project as part of their Next Generation Non-Surgical Neurotechnology (N3) program to develop a bidirectional BCI based on magnetoelectric nanoparticles, which could perform deep brain stimulation via a helmet-like device.[45] This technology could be weaponized by potentially spraying magnetic nanoparticles in the air to later degrade brain health and cognitive functions, perhaps in combination with electromagnetic fields applied to the head to achieve more specific effects on the brain and the mind. Another possibility for deployment is the surreptitious addition of nanoparticles to food, pharmaceuticals, and vaccines, which would, over time, enrich a population with harmful magnetic nanoparticles. The nanoparticles could be used for interfering with their brain processes and potentially for taking direct control over the behavior of people when used in combination with directed energy and manipulated with EMF emitted by devices such as smartphones. In the United States, metallic nanoparticles such as titanium oxide, zinc oxide, and graphene oxide are used as food additives, despite the health concerns that come with their ability to spread across the body and cross the blood-brain barrier.[46]

Neurodefense

Jonathan Moreno proposed the concepts of neurosecurity and neurodefense for countering the threats posed by advances in neuro S/T.[47] Moreno drew parallels to biosecurity and biological weapons development to explain the concept of neurosecurity. In 1972, the superpowers agreed to outlaw biological weapons in the Biological and Toxin Weapons Convention (BTWC), but the Soviet Union decided to violate the convention on a massive scale, hiding their biowarfare program within a biomedical research and pharmaceutical company called *Biopreparat*. *Biopreparat's* biowarfare activities were so secretive that the program lacked accountability and harmed the Soviet public, which was endangered by accidental releases and disease outbreaks.[48] The Soviets weaponized many existing disease agents and even produced new ones that were more transmissible and lethal than anything the world had seen before. They amassed tens of tons of anthrax, smallpox, and plague ready to be dispersed through special munitions, spraying mechanisms on ships and aircraft, and covert releases by human agents.[49] The Soviet biowarfare effort was so heavily compartmentalized that few senior Soviet officials were fully informed about it, which allowed *Biopreparat* to operate like an autonomous entity with little political oversight.[50] The lesson to be learned here is that it was possible for the Soviet Union to keep a large-scale biowarfare program and the bioweapons they produced secret from the world for over twenty years. As Moreno has argued, such a mistake should not be repeated in the area of future neuroweapons.

Prevention

The first objective for policymakers and national security officials should be the prevention of more covert attacks with neuroweapons against their own personnel, which requires a combination of measures that need to be taken.

Intelligence

The US IC needs to collect intelligence on research undertaken by foreign governments in the areas of DEWs, neuro S/T, and neuroweapons to be better able to assess threats and develop countermeasures. This would require a review of foreign publications, patents, conference papers, and gray literature (OSINT) to determine how advanced their research is and what kind of applications it could lead to. Since these areas of research tend to be highly secretive in all countries, it would be necessary to obtain critical information through human intelligence collection, which includes the recruitment of agents in foreign scientific communities and defectors with knowledge of neuroweapons programs, as well as the procurement of sensitive foreign neurotechnology and neuroweapons through capture or third parties. Unfortunately, the United States has scaled back HUMINT operations and is no longer very effective in this important intelligence collection discipline.[51] This means that HUMINT capabilities need to be strengthened and they may even benefit from neuro S/T in the form of improved ways of getting information from knowledgeable individuals through interviewing and interrogation, even if they are not cooperative.

Detection

It should be relatively straightforward to detect acoustic or electromagnetic signals emitted by DEWs. Existing sensors are sensitive enough to detect RF signals even with small power output from outer space. A new generation of geospatial intelligence satellites has the capability to geolocate RF signals up to 30 GHz with a power output as small as 5 W, which should be sufficient to detect and locate DEW usage that could cause Havana Syndrome.[52] Such sensors could be placed on buildings or could be located in public places. According to Mayor Eric Adams, New York City was developing a new sensor system for the subway against next-generation threats, to include electromagnetic weapons.[53] If they detect any unusual RF signals, they could automatically alert the authorities and trigger an investigation into the cause. RF sensors could be inside residences and sound an alarm just like a fire alarm, or they could be wearable. The British defense research company *Qinetiq* stated that the British Ministry of Defense was taking the threat posed by the Havana Syndrome incidents seriously and that *Qinetiq* is currently developing a wearable RF detection sensor "that will detect and document the exposure of personnel to injurious levels of RF energy."[54] The desired characteristics of such a system are: "[it] has an extremely small footprint in terms of space, weight and power (SWaP), is very low cost, has a very low false positive rate, and is easy to interpret."[55] If a DEW that causes Havana Syndrome exploited the Frey effect, then the most likely RF frequency range would be 0.4 GHz to 3 GHz.[56] In this case, fairly cheap and simple EMF meters could detect these signals when beamed at a target. Individuals could be able to detect attacks as they happen through EMF measurement. In any case, it would be important to make sensors that can detect DEW attacks commercially available so that the general public can benefit from them.

Hardening of Buildings

Most AHIs have occurred within buildings, which suggests two things: (1) this is a signal in the RF/microwave range that can penetrate walls and windows, and (2) most attacks could be prevented by hardening buildings, which would either be achieved through shielding or signal jamming. Electromagnetic shielding means reducing EMF in a specified area to render it harmless. It has been important in national security in relation to communications security as electromagnetic emanations could be picked up by others to reconstruct information that is created, stored, displayed, or transmitted on electronic devices.[57] Hence, particularly sensitive information must be stored, accessed, or received in facilities that are shielded against various forms of eavesdropping and that are known as "sensitive compartmented information facilities" or SCIFs. The electromagnetic shielding of a building is a complex task and it is not cheap as it requires special materials that need to cover all walls, windows, floors, and ceilings, grounding to dissipate EMF, and extensive measurement for any electromagnetic leakage. Apart from the high cost of shielding, a potential downside is that it would block external cell phone, Wi-Fi, and radio signals and would potentially amplify EMF levels from sources within a shielded building, which could lead to unhealthy EMF exposure.[58] Furthermore, the shielding would also block the natural Schumann resonances necessary for health and well-being.[59] The alternative option would be the jamming of signals that are malicious or harmful, which requires knowledge of the specific frequency and modulation of the signal to be jammed. The idea of electromagnetic jamming is to emit a signal that cancels out the unwanted or harmful signal or overpowers the enemy's signal.[60] Adversaries can defeat jamming activities by varying the signals that they use. There is also the obvious downside that people protected by way of electromagnetic jamming would now be constantly exposed to EMF emitted by the jamming devices, which is not ideal.

Protecting Key Personnel

There is already a growing industry that produces garments that promise to electromagnetically shield people who are electrosensitive against EMF. This includes shielded underwear, upper clothing, headgear, goggles, and gloves. Some of these garments are designed to look like ordinary pieces of clothing but are meant to substantially reduce EMF exposure to the human body. It is unclear whether EMF-shielded garments are effective in reducing EMF and in providing protection to the wearer, as there do not seem to be any scientific studies to back up the claims of the retailers. However, the general idea of EMF-shielded clothing to protect against covert DEW attacks may be sound. US Special Operations Command has been funding advanced uniforms and wearable equipment that can improve the survivability of soldiers against a range of threats that include protection against DEWs.[61] Wearable biosensors would monitor the biofunctions of soldiers, and a specially designed helmet with a head-up display would alert them of threats. The helmet would "counter blast forces and prevent traumatic brain injuries, as well as . . . erect an electromagnetic shield against directed energy weapons like those suspected to be behind Havana Syndrome."[62] Of course, EMF-shielded helmets may not be practical or fashionable for civilian officials.

Protecting the General Public

Some thought must be given to protecting the general public as, in principle, in this new non-kinetic type of conflict, everyone can be a target and a victim, regardless of whether they are connected to the government, just like in biological warfare and cyber warfare. The protection of the public begins with educating them about the threat, advising people to take reasonable steps to protect themselves, and to seek government assistance if there are indications that they are individually subjected to a covert DEW attack. It also means creating the knowledge and resources in the law enforcement community to investigate potential uses of neuroweapons.

Response

Up to now, the responses of the US government to the AHIs have been seemingly limited to scientific and intelligence investigations, to diplomatic initiatives such as expulsions of diplomats, and to providing medical support to affected government personnel and their dependents. There has not been any action to punish perpetrators or to deter future attacks of this kind, which makes it likely that future attacks will occur. Some clear and measured response is needed, or the problem is bound to get worse.

Ending Neuroweapons Secrecy

As argued in earlier chapters, there are many reasons to believe that governments of major countries (and perhaps of some smaller ones) have developed DEWs that can incapacitate and injure personnel, although the existence of such weapons or their capabilities tend to be obscured by excessive secrecy for reasons of national security. As Moreno has pointed out, "finding the balance between national security and democratic openness is easier said than done, but the right start seems to be to make transparency rather than opacity the default position."[63] If the US government could acknowledge that neuroweapons capable of causing Havana Syndrome exist, then it would be a lot easier to develop a public policy as to how to respond to AHIs. This could mean that a lot of the classified research into NLWs would have to be redone by academic researchers outside of classified programs in an ethical and accountable manner because of the need for human subject research.

Attribution of Attacks

The best option for attribution would be to catch an adversary in the act together with the weapon used in the AHIs, as this would amount to incontrovertible evidence that could be presented to the UN or another international body to expose the foreign power that was responsible and to seek international action against it.[64] Unfortunately, the attribution of attacks has been hampered by the fact that there is a delay of the effect on the target by the exposure and that it may only take an exposure of a few minutes to cause serious damage to the brain and central nervous system. This means that there is only a short time window for detecting an attack, determining the source of the attack, and catching the perpetrator(s). From the publicly known cases of AHIs, there does not seem to be a clear pattern for when and where attacks take place, which makes predicting future attacks difficult. There is simply a too large number of individuals an adversary could target in a location of their choosing. The second-best option is to collect circumstantial evidence after the fact, such as determining whether known operatives of an adversary were at the time in the location where an AHI occurred, or to match the injuries that our own personnel received to the fingerprint of a weapon that a particular adversary is known to possess.

Options for Responses

The problem of deterring covert attacks with neuroweapons seems to be similar to the problem of deterring cyberattacks. As in cyber warfare, attribution is difficult—if one cannot identify the aggressor, one cannot retaliate. In addition, as pointed out by Martin Libicki, a cyber-deterrence strategy must consider the following issues: "If retaliation does not deter, can it at least disarm? Will third parties join the fight? Does retaliation send the right message to our own side? Do we have a threshold response? Can we avoid escalation? What if the attacker has little worth hitting?"[65] In cognitive warfare, the last question could be replaced by: would a response in kind be ethical or morally justifiable? For reasons of effective deterrence, responses to AHIs should occur with little time delay and should be forceful enough to impose sufficiently high costs on the adversary to affect their future behavior without causing uncontrollable escalation. Ideally, responses should be based on public policy or a public declaration that threatens certain consequences, and they should also be carried out openly. There is a temptation for governments that have been at the receiving end of covert aggressions to respond in kind by using similar covert attacks against the aggressors since it accomplishes two things: they do not have to publicly admit the damage they had suffered in the covert aggression and they hope that a covert response in kind would make the management of escalation a lot easier. However, longer delays between an attack and a response and the use of covert measures (as opposed to overt action) aimed at imposing some cost on the adversary tend to weaken or obscure the message the response intended to send. The aggressor would be unsure about the determination and capability of the victim to respond to future aggressions and hence might believe that there would not be a serious consequence. The bottom line is that the best way of dealing with covert aggression and in the case of Havana Syndrome is to expose it and to take appropriate and effective overt actions to punish aggression to signal resolve.[66]

Prosecution of Perpetrators

In a domestic context, perpetrators who are caught using DEWs against others need to be arrested and prosecuted. This may require the creation of new laws that make it illegal for people to build, distribute, or use DEWs and other types of neuroweapons that cause permanent damage to the health of others. The prosecution of perpetrators has been hampered by the scarcity of technical and medical information on DEWs and other neuroweapons. Relevant information needs to be made available to legislators, law enforcement agencies, and the courts. There should be effective domestic enforcement, and this also means high penalties for perpetrators of these new types of human rights abuses.

Treatment

Public information suggests that many victims of AHIs have struggled to get treatment for managing or curing the conditions they have acquired. There are many reasons why this is the case: there is no universally accepted diagnosis for an AHI or Havana Syndrome, the medical profession is not familiar with the condition and how it is caused, there are no established treatments, and government bureaucracies have been slow in providing the needed medical and financial assistance to the victims.

Diagnosis

What has come out of the neuroscientific studies conducted on the AHI patients is that it has been exceedingly difficult to match the symptoms experienced by them to abnormalities in the brain or even to particular exposures that caused them. Neuroimaging has not been able to objectively prove that AHI patients have brain damage that was likely caused by a DEW or neuroweapon.[67] The best way forward would be to conduct public research on the effects of certain DEWs on the brain and central nervous system and make this research available to the medical profession so that it can help them develop better ways for diagnosing people who have been attacked with DEWs. It may also be necessary to develop specialized diagnostic tools and technologies that can detect abnormal brain changes caused by neuroweapons attacks.

Development of New Treatments

Since the condition of Havana Syndrome is fairly new and since the number of people diagnosed with it is quite small, there is no established or standard treatment available that could help victims. Data from 2024 suggest that over 300 individuals are currently being treated for Havana Syndrome.[68] There are experimental treatments, some of which show promise.[69] For example, transcranial magnetic stimulation (TMS) could relieve the symptoms in some of the AHI patients. It is a treatment that is being used for treating depression, PTSD, and traumatic brain injury. However, it is also a very expensive treatment that involves risk, as the magnetic fields applied to the brain are very strong and could cause seizures if overdosed.[70] The brain damage suffered by some AHI patients may be irreversible and may be a lifelong debilitating condition.[71] This means that some victims may require lifelong care. The US Army has recently announced the development of a "brain health strategy," partially in response to the AHIs, to improve all aspects of brain health for military personnel, including nutrition, exercise, and mitigating potential exposures.[72]

Support to Victims

The HAVANA Act has provided financial support to affected government employees and dependents and has improved their access to specialized treatments. Unfortunately, different agencies have different standards for determining eligibility, and it takes several weeks before there is any bureaucratic response. Although the lump sum provided through the HAVANA Act to victims is helpful, it is not nearly enough for those victims who suffered a permanent disability. Helping victims can restore some trust in the government and improve the morale of government employees, who may face a higher risk, such as diplomatic and intelligence personnel.

Governance of Neuroweapons

The challenges posed by advances in neuro S/T and DEWs need to be addressed internationally by way of establishing binding norms that restrict unethical uses of these technologies by governments and nonstate actors. The stakes are tremendously high since individual freedom is in jeopardy as it becomes technologically easier to not only damage brains remotely but also to read minds, externally manage mental states, inject thoughts and information directly into brains, and even coerce people to behave in a specific way.[73]

Neurorights

Neuroethics is a branch of bioethics that is concerned with the ethical dilemmas created by neuro S/T. Some neuroethicists have advocated for neurorights that include:

> (1) the right to identity, or the ability to control both one's physical and mental integrity; (2) the right to agency, or the freedom of thought and free will to choose one's own actions; (3) the right to mental privacy, or the ability to keep thoughts protected against disclosure; (4) the right to fair access to mental augmentation,

> or the ability to ensure that the benefits of improvements to sensory and mental capacity through neurotechnology are distributed justly in the population; and (5) the right to protection from algorithmic bias, or the ability to ensure that technologies do not insert prejudices.[74]

If governments were able to read the minds of citizens, to mentally coerce them, or to alter their personalities, it would result in the creation of a kind of totalitarian society that the world has never seen. Even in the Stalinist Soviet Union or Mao's China, people could keep at least their thoughts to themselves and retain some ability to resist tyranny. However, in a world where everyone's thoughts could be monitored in real time, combined with the ability to punish thought crimes and reform "deviants" through mandatory brain changes, there is no theoretical possibility for resistance to take place. Humanity may become enslaved forever by a tiny elite in control of the technology.[75] It becomes, therefore, critical that mental privacy, freedom of will, and a right to a self-determined identity are codified as human rights that shall not be infringed upon by governments, corporations, or other entities and individuals to preserve democratic government and freedom.

Arms Control

Neurorights afforded by governments to their citizens should be accompanied by new norms that govern armed conflict, both within states as well as between states. It is likely that governments want national security exceptions to neurorights, as it could be ethically justifiable to violate the mental privacy of a terrorist or the freedom of will of an enemy soldier in war.[76] It may still be ethically acceptable to allow the use of neuroweapons in these specific contexts, provided they do not violate existing international law, namely the prohibition of weapons that are indiscriminate or inhumane. This makes it even more important to create an ethical framework for the uses of neuro S/T in armed conflict, which would include restrictions on the use of neuroweapons. Currently, there are no specific rules, only a secretive competition for "neurosupremacy," which has, according to Nicholas Evans, the potential of triggering a "scientific arms race."[77] McCreight has labeled the current state of affairs "brain brinkmanship," as nations would hide their neurowarfare capabilities or may threaten others with neuroweapons, which could cause deterrence to fail.[78] More transparency in the area of neuroweapons technology could strengthen deterrence and thereby international stability.

Restrictions on Research

Neuroscience research is inherently dual-use, as knowledge derived from research can be used for the development of new therapeutics and the improvement of health/longevity or it can be used for national security, including predicting and shaping behaviors, human enhancement of soldiers, and the development of neuroweapons.[79] This makes the regulation of the underlying research tricky, as society would want to benefit from neuroscience research while avoiding applications that have a high potential for massive human rights abuses and for creating a politically more unstable and dangerous world. A huge concern relates to human subject research that involves the modification of the brain, the tampering with personality, and the ability of individuals to make self-determined decisions, which could be "stepping over some natural line and jeopardizing our essential nature or 'personhood.'"[80] Neuroscientists and medical professionals must be held to a strict ethical code in their research that protects individual autonomy and personhood and they should not participate in research that aims to develop neuroweapons that are inhumane in the sense of causing "superfluous injury and unnecessary suffering."[81] Professional organizations of neuroscientists can play a key role in the development of norms guiding neuroscience research, and they have also some ability to reinforce and police these norms in the profession through education, self-governance, and influence on national policymaking related to neuroscience.[82] Academic journals and grantmaking organizations can deny the publication or funding of unethical research or research that has a high potential for unethical applications. The downside to such an approach would be that it could drive certain research areas underground, which would hurt transparency. In short, key facts about neuroweapons still need to be part of the discussion without allowing or encouraging bad actors to develop them.

Accountability Mechanisms

Since the potential for abuses in military neuroscience research is very high, there must be some international mechanism to investigate these abuses and hold nation-states and internationally operating nonstate actors accountable in some form. At this time, the United Nations High Commissioner for Human Rights and other UN suborganizations remain the main international bodies to which individuals and groups who have been harmed by neuroethics abuses can turn. In 2008, UNESCO held a seminar on the potential of using electromagnetic radiation for terrorism, which is an allegation made by countless people around the world.[83]

Several victim groups turned to the UN Special Rapporteur on Torture and Other Cruel Inhumane Treatment or Punishment, Professor Nils Melzer, to bring attention to the phenomenon of "cyber torture," which is psychological torture using the internet and other electronic means.[84] Melzer argued in his report:

> In practice, cybertechnology already plays the role of an "enabler" in the perpetration of both physical and psychological forms of torture, most notably through the collection and transmission of surveillance information and instructions to interrogators, through the dissemination of audio or video recordings of torture or murder for the purposes of intimidation, or even live streaming of child sexual abuse "on demand" of voyeuristic clients (A/HRC/28/56, para. 71), and increasingly also through the remote control or manipulation of stun belts (A/72/178, para. 51), medical implants and, conceivably, nanotechnological or neurotechnological devices. Cybertechnology can also be used to inflict, or contribute to, severe mental suffering while avoiding the conduit of the physical body, most notably through intimidation, harassment, surveillance, public shaming and defamation, as well as appropriation, deletion or manipulation of information.[85]

There are governments that have reportedly conducted unethical human subject experiments for the purpose of developing neuroweapons and means of cyber torture in pursuit of cognitive warfare. These allegations need to be investigated by an international body, the evidence needs to be publicly presented, and there need to be some kind of consequences for the governments responsible for these abuses, which may include sanctions and the international prosecution for crimes against humanity of government officials implicated in these crimes. One can even imagine a future where Truth and Reconciliation Commissions, following the model of South Africa after Apartheid, could be established to investigate state-sanctioned crimes. The idea would be to encourage individuals who were guilty of past abuses that were part of a government research effort or covert action to testify before a Truth and Reconciliation Commission in exchange for indemnity, so that at least the truth can be known and future abuses can be prevented.[86]

Conclusion

The major powers of the world seem to be engaged in a new type of arms race for the development of neuroweapons and new approaches for cognitive warfare, which is designed to manipulate and internally collapse adversarial societies by way of non-kinetic destabilization that relies on covert or ambiguous measures. The current focus of NATO's cognitive warfare debate is on online propaganda and disinformation, but the larger context and future threat relate to neuroweapons that are designed to remotely monitor brains and other biofunctions, degrade mental capacity, manipulate perception and emotions, and even control thinking and behavior not only at an individual level but possibly at the level of a larger group. The relevant technologies have been under development since at least the 1960s, and the publicized Havana Syndrome incidents may only represent the tip of the iceberg as it concerns the current uses of neuroweapons. The first step in addressing these challenges to national and international security is to conduct research and investigations into the AHIs that are unclassified. There must be a serious public debate about the threat of neuroweapons and, with it, steps need to be taken to protect government officials and the public. More thorough investigations of possible attacks on individuals with covert technology by law enforcement and intelligence agencies should take place as the threat is real and growing. It is inevitable that a broader discussion of neuroethics must happen in view of a framework as to what could be acceptable military or national security applications and uses of neurotechnology. Havana Syndrome may be an opportunity to get this necessary and needed debate started and to spur action by governments and international organizations.

Notes

1 A notable research paper that explored the concept of conflict short of war in the 1990s was Steven Metz and James Kievit, "The Revolution in Military Affairs and Conflict Short of War," US Army War College, Strategic Studies Institute, July 25, 1994.

2 NATO, "Cognitive Warfare," Strategic Warfare Development Command Website, available at: https://www.act.nato.int/activities/cognitive-warfare/ (accessed August 10, 2024).

3 NATO, "Countering Cognitive Warfare: Awareness and Resilience," *NATO Review*, May 20, 2021, available at: https://www.nato.int/docu/review/articles/2021/05/20/countering-cognitive-warfare-awareness-and-resilience/index.html.

4 Francois du Cluzel, "Cognitive Warfare, a Battle for the Brain," NATO Science and Technology Organization, December 2023, 1.

5 Du Cluzel, "Cognitive Warfare, a Battle for the Brain," 2.

6 Bernard Claverie and Francois du Cluzel, "The Cognitive Warfare Concept," NATO Allied Command Transformation, December 2023, 2, available at: https://innovationhub-act.org/wp-content/uploads/2023/12/CW-article-Claverie-du-Cluzel-final_0.pdf.

7 Bruce Berkowitz, "Is Assassination an Option?," *Hoover Institution* website, January 30, 2002, available at: https://www.hoover.org/research/assassination-option.

8 Robert McCreight, "Non-Kinetic Threats and the Threshold Spectrum of Strategic Endgames," *Mad Scientist Laboratory blog*, May 11, 2023, available at: https://madsciblog.tradoc.army.mil/444-non-kinetic-threats-and-the-threshold-spectrum-of-strategic-endgame-warnings/.

9 Du Cluzel, "Cognitive Warfare, a Battle for the Brain," 2.

10 Robert McCreight, "Neuro-Cognitive Warfare: Inflicting Strategic Impact via Non-Kinetic Threat," *Small Wars Journal*, September 16, 2022, available at: https://smallwarsjournal.com/jrnl/art/neuro-cognitive-warfare-inflicting-strategic-impact-non-kinetic-threat.

11 Robert McCreight, "The Era of Cognitive Warfare: What Next??," Presentation given at East Carolina University on March 21, 2024.

12 August Cole and Hervé Guyader, "Cognitive: A 6th Domain of Operations?," NATO Innovation Hub, January 2023, 13, available at: https://www.projectcensored.org/wp-content/uploads/2023/01/Cognitive-a-6th-Domain-of-Operations.pdf.

13 Joshua D. Gramm and Brian A. Branagan, "Neurowar Is Here!" (Master's Thesis, Naval Postgraduate School, December 2021), 53, available at: https://apps.dtic.mil/sti/trecms/pdf/AD1164923.pdf.

14 Alonso Bernal, Cameron Carter, Ishpreet Singh, Kathy Cao, and Olivia Madreperla, "Cognitive Warfare: An Attack on Truth and Thought," NATO Allied Command Transformation, December 2020, 12, available at: https://innovationhub-act.org/wp-content/uploads/2023/12/Cognitive-Warfare.pdf.

15 Kathy Cao et al., "Cognitive Warfare: Awareness and Resilience," *NATO Review*, May 20, 2021, available at: https://www.nato.int/docu/review/articles/2021/05/20/countering-cognitive-warfare-awareness-and-resilience/index.html.

16 Ian Clay and Robert D. Atkinson, "Wake Up America, China Is Overtaking the United States in Innovation Capacity," *Information Technology & Innovation Foundation*, January 23, 2024, available at: https://itif.org/publications/2023/01/23/wake-up-america-china-is-overtaking-the-united-states-in-innovation-capacity/.

17 Evan Horowitz, "IQ Rates Are Dropping in Many Developed Countries and That Doesn't Bode Well for Humanity," *NBC News*, May 22, 2019, available at: https://www.nbcnews.com/think/opinion/iq-rates-are-dropping-many-developed-countries-doesn-t-bode-ncna1008576.

18 Michael A. Woodley, Jan de Nijenhuis, and Reagan Murphy, "Were the Victorians Cleverer Than Us? The Decline in General Intelligence Estimated from a Meta-Analysis of the Slowing of Simple Reaction Time," *Intelligence* 41, no. 6 (2013): 843–50.
19 Jamie Ducharme, "Why Everyone's Worried About Their Attention Span—and How to Improve Yours," *Time Magazine*, August 10, 2023, available at: https://time.com/6302294/why-you-cant-focus-anymore-and-what-to-do-about-it/.
20 Adam Hampshire, Adriana Azor, Christina Atchison, William Trender, Peter J. Hellyer, Valentina Giunchiglia, Masud Husein, and Paul Elliott, "Cognition and Memory after Covid-19 in a Large Community Sample," *The New England Journal of Medicine* 390, no. 9 (2024): 806–18.
21 Robert Spalding, *Stealth War: How China Took Over While America's Elite Slept* (New York: Penguin, 2019), 109–20.
22 Lily Hay Newman, "Hackers Can Turn Everyday Speakers Into Acoustic Cyberweapons," *Wired Magazine*, August 11, 2019, available at: https://www.wired.com/story/acoustic-cyberweapons-defcon/.
23 Anita O'Reilly, "An Australian Parliamentary Inquiry into the Deployment, Adoption, and Application of 5G in Australia," November 1, 2019, available at: https://www.aph.gov.au/DocumentStore.ashx?id=2de0d339-65e0-44d2-a576-31d22467e69c&subId=672968.
24 Raffi Katchadourian, "Operation Delirium," *The New Yorker*, December 9, 2012, available at: https://www.newyorker.com/magazine/2012/12/17/operation-delirium?currentPage=all&src=longreads&buffer_share=25d72.
25 Regan F. Lyon, Joshua Gramm, Brian Branagan, and Shannon C. Houck, "Implications of Neurological Directed Energy Weapons for Military Medicine," *Journal of Special Operations Medicine* 22, no. 3 (2022): 104.
26 McCreight, "Neuro-Cognitive Warfare: Inflicting Strategic Impact via Non-Kinetic Threat."
27 McCreight, "Non-Kinetic Threats and the Threshold Spectrum of Strategic Endgame Warnings."
28 Colin A. Ross, *The C.I.A. Doctors* (Richardson: Manitou Communications Inc., 2006), 88.
29 Jonathan Moreno, *Mind Wars: Brain Research and National Defense* (New York: Dana Press, 2006), 43.
30 These experiments were described in José Delgado, *The Physical Control of the Mind: Towards a Psychocivilized Society* (New York: Harper & Row, 1969).
31 Walter Bowart, *Operation Mind Control* (New York: Dell Publishing, 1978), 257.
32 Cheryl Welsh, "Cold War Nonconsensual Experiments: The Threat of Neuroweapons and the Danger It Will Happen Again," *Essex Human Rights Review* 9, no. 1 (2012): 9.

33 James Gorman, "Agency Initiative Will Focus on Deep Brain Stimulation," *New York Times*, October 25, 2013.

34 Annie Jacobsen, *The Pentagon's Brain: An Uncensored History of DARPA, America's Top Secret Military Research Agency* (New York: Little, Brown and Co., 2015), 424.

35 Clay Dillow, "DARPA Wants to Install Transcranial Ultrasonic Mind Control Devices in Soldier's Helmets," *Popular Science*, September 10, 2010, available at: https://www.popsci.com/technology/article/2010-09/darpa-wants-mind-control-keep-soldiers-sharp-smart-and-safe/.

36 The idea of the brain as a programmable biocomputer was proposed by neuroscientist John C. Lilly, who developed the theory in the 1950s.

37 Jacques J. Vidal, "Toward Direct Brain-Computer Communication," *Annual Review of Biophysics and Bioengineering* 2, no. 1 (1973): 157–80.

38 Jim Reed and Joe McFadden, "Neuralink: Can Musk's Brain Technology Change the World?," *BBC News*, February 3, 2024, available at: https://www.bbc.com/news/health-68169082.

39 Kyle Mizokami, "DARPA Wants Soldiers to Control Machines with Their Minds," *Popular Mechanics*, May 22, 2019, available at: https://www.popularmechanics.com/military/research/a27560088/darpa-soldier-machine/; Eric Bland, "Army Developing 'Synthetic Telepathy,'" *NBC News*, October 13, 2008, available at: https://www.nbcnews.com/id/wbna27162401.

40 Mark Thompson, "The Army's Totally Serious Mind Control Project," *Time*, September 14, 2008, available at: https://time.com/archive/6913384/the-armys-totally-serious-mind-control-project/.

41 Institute for Basic Science, South Korea, "New Technology to Control the Brain Using Magnetic Fields Developed," *EurekAlert!*, July 17, 2024, available at: https://www.eurekalert.org/news-releases/1051652.

42 K. Eric Drexler, *Engines of Creation: The Coming Era of Nanotechnology* (New York: Anchor Books, 1987), 58–9.

43 Sonia Contero, *Nano Comes to Life: How Nanotechnology Is Transforming Medicine and the Future of Biology* (Princeton: Princeton University Press, 2010), 116.

44 Vicki Stone, Elinor Johnston, and Martin J. D. Clift, "Air Pollution, Ultrafine and Nanoparticle Toxicology: Cellular and Molecular Interactions," *IEEE Transactions on Nanobioscience* 6, no. 4 (2007): 331–40.

45 Battelle, "Battelle-Led Team Wins DARPA Award to Develop Injectable, Bi-Directional Brain-Computer Interface," *Battelle Media Relations*, May 20, 2019, available at: https://www.battelle.org/insights/newsroom/press-release-details/battelle-led-team-wins-darpa-award-to-develop-injectable-bi-directional-brain-computer-interface.

46 Mićo Tatalović, "I Wash All My Food Like Crazy: Scientists Voice Concern Over Nanoparticles," *The Guardian*, May 29, 2019, available at: https://www.theguardian.com/us-news/2019/may/29/i-wash-all-my-food-like-crazy-researchers-voice-concern-about-nanoparticles.
47 Moreno, *Mind Wars*, 172–9.
48 Moreno, *Mind Wars*, 167.
49 Gregory D. Koblentz, *Living Weapons: Biological Warfare and National Security* (Ithaca: Cornell University Press, 2009), 37.
50 Koblentz, *Living Weapons*, 108–14.
51 Lewis A. Bradley, "The Death of Human Intelligence: How Human Intelligence Has Been Minimized Since the 1960s," *Military and Strategic Affairs* 8, no. 1 (2016): 75–90.
52 Victor Robert Lee, "Could Satellite Sensors Solve the Havana Syndrome Mystery? Recent Breakthroughs May Prove Forensically Useful," *The Diplomat*, August 30, 2021, available at: https://thediplomat.com/2021/08/could-satellite-sensors-solve-the-havana-syndrome-mystery/.
53 Joshua Philipp, "Next-Gen Weapons Detection Tech Being Deployed; 'Havana Syndrome' Confirmed by Pentagon Personnel as Real," *Epoch Times Crossroads*, April 4, 2024, available at: https://www.theepochtimes.com/epochtv/next-gen-weapons-detection-tech-being-deployed-5621381.
54 Qinetiq, "The U.S. Is Developing Wearable 'RF Weapon' Exposure Sensor," *Qinetiq* website, September 17, 2019, available at: https://www.qinetiq.com/en/blogs/wearable-rf-sensor.
55 Qinetiq, "The U.S. Is Developing Wearable 'RF Weapon' Exposure Sensor."
56 JASON, "An Analysis of Data and Hypotheses Related to the Embassy Incidents," *The MITRE Corporation*, October 2021, 65.
57 Derek Hawkins, Adrian Blanco, Perry Stein, and William Neff, "Inside the Fortified Rooms Securing U.S. Secrets," *Washington Post*, April 28, 2023.
58 Dimitris J. Panagopoulos and George P. Crousos, "Shielding Methods and Products Against Man-Made Electromagnetic Fields: Protection Versus Risk," *Science of the Total Environment* 667 (2019): 259.
59 Panagopoulos and Crousos, "Shielding Methods and Products Against Man-Made Electromagnetic Fields," 257.
60 Douglas Deason, *The E-Bomb: How America's New Directed Energy Weapons Will Change the Way Future Wars Will Be Fought* (Cambridge: Da Capo Press, 2005), 99–100.
61 Jeremy Bogaisky, "Helmets Like Iron Man's and a Smart T-Shirt that Calls for Help: The Pentagon's Wearable Tech Revolution," *Forbes*, October 28, 2022, available at: https://www.forbes.com/sites/jeremybogaisky/2022/10/28/helmet-iron-man-smart-shirt-pentagon-wearable-tech/.

62 Bogaisky, "Helmets Like Iron Man's and a Smart T-Shirt that Calls for Help."

63 Moreno, *Mind Wars*, 174.

64 US Congress, "Silent Weapons: Examining Foreign Anomalous Health Incidents Targeting Americans in Homeland," Homeland Security Committee, May 8, 2024, available at: https://homeland.house.gov/wp-content/uploads/2024/05/2024-05-08-CTI-HRG-Testimony.pdf.

65 Martin Libicki, *Cyberdeterrence and Cyberwar* (Santa Monica: RAND, 2009), 39.

66 Sean Power and Michael Miner, "Report—Havana Syndrome: American Officials Under Attack," *Belfer Center for Science and International Affairs*, Harvard University, November 4, 2021, available at: https://www.belfercenter.org/publication/report-havana-syndrome-american-officials-under-attack.

67 Matthew Phelan, "New NIH Study Sheds Light on Mysterious 'Havana Syndrome': Victims' Symptoms Are 'Real' and 'Quite Profound'—But Injuries Don't Show Up on MRI Much Like 'Mini Stroke,' One Pentagon Medical Consultant Told DailyMail.com," *Daily Mail*, March 18, 2024, available at: https://www.dailymail.co.uk/sciencetech/article-13210727/NIH-study-Havana-Syndrome-Victims-symptoms-energy-weapons-microwave-acoustic-mystery.html.

68 General Accounting Office Staff, "Havana Syndrome—Americans Affected by Mysterious Symptoms May Struggle to Get Care," *General Accounting Office*, July 29, 2024, available at: https://www.gao.gov/blog/havana-syndrome-americans-affected-mysterious-symptoms-may-struggle-get-care.

69 Marc Polymeropoulos mentioned in an interview that Walter Reed National Military Medical Center has turned to TMS to relieve Havana Syndrome symptoms and that in his case it has led to improvement. Shawn Ryan, "Marc Polymeropoulos—CIA Senior Intelligence Officer," *Shawn Ryan Show*, August 1, 2022, available at: https://www.youtube.com/watch?v=z2KDbESmZRk.

70 Mahdi Razafsha, Tracy A. Barbour, Amit Chopra, Michael D. Kritzer, and Theodore A. Stern, "Transcranial Magnetic Stimulation in Primary Care: Indications, Risks, and Outcomes," *The Psychiatrist.com*, March 12, 2024, available at: https://www.psychiatrist.com/pcc/transcranial-magnetic-stimulation-primary-care-indications-risks-and-outcomes/.

71 Julian E. Barnes, Edward Wong, and Eric Schmitt, "Mysterious Ailments Are Said to Be More Widespread Among U.S. Personnel," *New York Times*, May 13, 2021.

72 Brandi Vincent, "Army's New Brain Health Strategy to Address Anomalous Health Incidents, Havana Syndrome," *Defensescoop*, October 15, 2024, available at: https://defensescoop.com/2024/10/15/army-brain-health-strategy-address-anomalous-health-incidents-havana-syndrome/.

73 Adam Piore, "Building a Telepathic Army," *Discover Magazine*, November 11, 2019, available at: https://www.discovermagazine.com/mind/building-a-telepathic-army.

74 Rafael Yuste, Jared Genser, and Stephannie Hermann, "It's Time for Neuro-Rights: New Human Rights for the Age of Neurotechnology," *Horizons* 18 (2021): 161–2.
75 Bill Joy, "Why the Future Does Not Need Us," *Wired Magazine* 8.04 (April 2000), available at: https://www.wired.com/2000/04/joy-2/.
76 Moreno, *Mind Wars*, 176.
77 Nicholas G. Evans, *The Ethics of Neuroscience and National Security* (New York: Routledge, 2021), 133.
78 Robert McCreight, "Brain Brinkmanship: Devising Neuroweapons Looking at Battlespace, Doctrine, and Strategy," in *Neurotechnology in National Security and Defense: Practical Considerations, Neuroethical Concerns*, ed. James Giordano (Boca Raton: CRC Press, 2014), 115–32.
79 Moreno, *Mind Wars*, 57–8.
80 Moreno, *Mind Wars*, 19.
81 Michael L. Gross, "Medicalized Weapons & Modern War," *Hastings Center Report*, January–February 2010, 40.
82 Evans, *The Ethics of Neuroscience and National Security*, 153–4.
83 David Hambling, "UN Investigates Electromagnetic Terrorism," *Wired Magazine*, December 2, 2008, available at: https://www.wired.com/2008/12/un-investigates/.
84 Owen Bowcott, "UN Warns of Rise of 'Cybertorture' to Bypass Physical Ban," *The Guardian*, February 21, 2020, available at: https://www.theguardian.com/law/2020/feb/21/un-rapporteur-warns-of-rise-of-cybertorture-to-bypass-physical-ban.
85 Nils Melzer, "Torture and Other Cruel, Inhuman or Degrading Treatment or Punishment," United Nations Human Rights Council (A/HRC/43/49), March 20, 2020, available at: https://documents.un.org/doc/undoc/gen/g20/070/73/pdf/g2007073.pdf.
86 Bronwyn Lebow, *Judging State-Sponsored Violence, Imagining Political Change* (Cambridge: Cambridge University Press, 2011), 60–1.

Bibliography

Abbott, Daniel H., ed. *The Handbook of 5GW: A Fifth Generation of Warfare?* Ann Arbor: Nimble Books LLC, 2010.

Achenbach, Joel, and Shane Harris. "NIH Probe of 'Havana Syndrome' Finds No Sign of Brain Injuries." *Washington Post*, March 18, 2024.

Adams, Ronald M., and R. A. Williams. "Biological Effects of Electromagnetic Radiation (Radiowaves and Microwaves)—Eurasian Communist Countries." Defense Intelligence Agency, March 1976.

Aftergood, Steven. "Nonlethal Weapons." *Secrecy & Government Bulletin* 28 (1993): 1–2.

Aftergood, Steven. "The Soft-Kill Fallacy: The Idea of 'Non-Lethal Weapons' Is Politically Attractive and Purposefully Misleading." *The Bulletin of Atomic Scientists* 50, no. 5 (1994): 40–5.

Albarelli, H. P. *A Terrible Mistake: The Murder of Frank Olson and the CIA's Secret Cold War Experiments*. Walterville: TrineDay, 2009.

Alexander, John B. *Future War: Non-Lethal Weapons in Twenty-First-Century Warfare*. New York: St. Martin's Griffin, 1999.

Alexander, John B. "The New Mental Battlefield—Beam Me Up, Spock." *Military Review* 60, no. 12 (1980): 54–67.

Al Jazeera. "Pentagon Reveals Senior Official Reported Symptoms of 'Havana Syndrome.'" *Al Jazeera*, April 1, 2024, available at: https://www.aljazeera.com/news/2024/4/1/pentagon-reveals-senior-official-reported-symptoms-of-havana-syndrome.

Altmann, Jürgen. "Acoustic Weapons—A Prospective Assessment." *Science & Global Security* 9, no. 3 (1999): 165–234.

Altmann, Jürgen. "Non-Lethal Weapons Technologies—The Case for Independent Scientific Analysis." *Medicine, Conflict, & Survival* 17, no. 3 (2001): 234–47.

Ambinder, Marc, and D. B. Grady. *Deep State: Inside Government Secrecy*. Hoboken: Wiley & Sons, 2013.

Anderson, J. "'Brainwash' Attempt by Russians?" *Washington Post*, May 10, 1972, B15.

Anderssen, Erin. "Mad Gassers, Toxic Bussers, and the Havana Syndrome: What Society Still Gets Wrong About the Way Stress Can Make Us Sick." *The Globe and Mail*, May 22, 2019.

Andrew, Christopher, and Vasili Mithrokin. *The Mithrokin Archive: The KGB in Europe and the West*. London: Penguin, 1999.

Anthony, Ian, ed. *Russia and the Arms Trade*. Oxford: Oxford University Press, 1998.

Arquilla, John, and David Ronfeldt. *In Athena's Camp: Preparing for Conflict in the Information Age*. Santa Monica: RAND, 1997.

Atwood, Kylie. "Members of CIA Chief's Team Reported Havana Syndrome on Recent Trip to India." *CNN*, September 21, 2021, available at: https://www.cnn.com/2021/09/20/politics/cia-director-havana-syndrome-india-trip/index.html.

Atwood, Kylie, and Jennifer Hansler. "US Intelligence Community Cannot Link 'Havana Syndrome' Cases to Foreign Adversary." *CNN*, March 2, 2023, available at: https://www.cnn.com/2023/03/01/politics/us-intel-community-havana-syndrome/index.html.

Atwood, Kylie, Katie Bo Lillis, and Jennifer Hansler. "Biden Administration to Compensate Some 'Havana Syndrome' Victims Up to $187,000." *CNN*, June 24, 2022, available at: https://www.cnn.com/2022/06/23/politics/havana-syndrome-victims-compensation/index.html.

Axe, David. "Laser-Armed Trucks Are Coming to Shoot Drones Out of the Sky." *Daily Beast*, April 13, 2017, available at: https://www.thedailybeast.com/laser-armed-trucks-are-coming-to-shoot-drones-out-of-the-sky.

Backes, Oliver, and Andrew Swab. "Cognitive Warfare: The Russian Threat to Election Integrity in the Baltic States." *Belfer Center for Science and International Affairs*, Harvard University, November 2019.

Baier, Bret, and Amy Munneke. "Havana Syndrome: Foreign Adversaries' Microwave Weapons Capabilities Explained by Physicist." *Fox News*, April 18, 2023, available at: https://www.foxnews.com/politics/havana-syndrome-foreign-adversaries-microwave-weapons-capabilities-explained-physicist.

Baloh, Robert W. "Havana Syndrome Fits the Pattern of Psychosomatic Illness—But That Does Not Mean Symptoms Are Not Real." *The Conversation*, March 7, 2023, available at: https://theconversation.com/havana-syndrome-fits-the-pattern-of-psychosomatic-illness-but-that-doesnt-mean-symptoms-arent-real-167275.

Baloh, Robert W., and Robert E. Bartholomew. *Havana Syndrome: Mass Pyschogenic Illness and the Real Story Behind the Embassy Mystery and Hysteria*. Cham, Switzerland: Copernicus, 2020.

Bansal, Rajeev. "Microwave Surfing: Kaboom!" *IEEE Microwave Magazine* (May 2019): 12–13.

Barnes, Julian. "C.I.A. Begins Compensating Victims of Havana Syndrome." *New York Times*, August 25, 2022.

Barnes, Julian. "C.I.A. Officer Suffers Havana Symptoms." *New York Times*, September 20, 2021.

Barnes, Julian. "Foreign Power Not Seen by CIA as Cause of 'Havana Syndrome.'" *New York Times*, January 21, 2022.

Barnes, Julian. "New Studies Find No Evidence of Brain Injury in Havana Syndrome Cases." *New York Times*, March 18, 2024.

Barnes, Julian. "Panel Says Some Havana Syndrome Cases May Stem from Radio Energy." *New York Times*, February 2, 2022.

Barnes, Julian. "Report Criticizes C.I.A. Handling of Havana Syndrome Cases." *New York Times*, October 14, 2022.

Barnes, Julian. "U.S. Outlines Compensation Rules for Some Havana Syndrome Victims." *New York Times*, June 24, 2022.

Barnes, Julian E., and Adam Entous. "Foreign Adversaries 'Very Unlikely' to Blame for Havana Syndrome, Intelligence Review Finds." *New York Times*, March 1, 2023.

Barnes, Julian E., Edward Wong, and Eric Schmitt. "Mysterious Ailments Are Said to Be More Widespread Among U.S. Personnel." *New York Times*, May 13, 2021.

Bartholomew, Robert E. "60 Minutes Whips Up 'Havana Syndrome' Hysteria, Airs Sensational Segment on White House 'Attacks.'" *The Skeptic*, March 4, 2022, available at: https://www.skeptic.com/reading_room/60-minutes-whips-up-havana-syndrome-hysteria-airs-sensational-segment-on-white-house-attacks/ - note03.

Bartholomew, Robert E. "Newly Declassified Report on 'Havana Syndrome' Used the Wrong Criteria!" *Skeptic.com*, March 31, 2023, available at: https://www.skeptic.com/reading_room/newly-declassified-report-on-havana-syndrome-used-wrong-criteria/.

Bartholomew, Robert E., and Robert W. Baloh. "'Havana Syndrome': A Post-Mortem." *International Journal of Social Psychiatry* 70, no. 2 (2024): 402–5.

Bartholomew, Robert E., and Robert W. Baloh. "Challenging the Diagnosis of the 'Havana Syndrome' as Novel Clinical Entity." *The Journal of the Royal Society of Medicine* 113, no. 1 (2020): 7–11.

Bartholomew, Robert E., and Robert W. Baloh. "'Havana Syndrome': A Post Mortem." *International Journal of Social Psychology* (2023), https://doi.org/10.1177/00207640231208374.

Bartholomew, Robert E., and Chandra Sekaran Muniratnam. "How Should Mental Health Professionals Respond to Outbreaks of Mass Psychogenic Illness?" *Journal of Cognitive Psychotherapy* 25, no. 4 (2011): 235–9.

Battelle. "Battelle-Led Team Wins DARPA Award to Develop Injectable, Bi-Directional Brain-Computer Interface." *Battelle Media Relations*, May 20, 2019, available at: https://www.battelle.org/insights/newsroom/press-release-details/battelle-led-team-wins-darpa-award-to-develop-injectable-bi-directional-brain-computer-interface.

Bauer, Nicole. "Havana Syndrome Upsets so Many Americans Because of the Secrecy Involved." *Washington Post*, May 3, 2023.

Bazail-Eimil, Eric. "Havana Syndrome Won't Go Away." *Politico*, April 1, 2024, available at: https://www.politico.com/newsletters/national-security-daily/2024/04/01/havana-syndrome-wont-go-away-00149977.

BBC Staff. "World: Europe Dissidents Say Stasi Gave Them Cancer." *BBC*, May 25, 1999, available at: http://news.bbc.co.uk/2/hi/europe/352461.stm.

Bearden, Thomas. *Excalibur Briefing: Explaining Paranormal Phenomena*. San Francisco: Strawberry Hill Press, 1988.

Bearden, Thomas. *Oblivion: America at the Brink*. Cheniere Press, 2005.

Beasley, Deena. "No Evidence of Havana Syndrome Brain Injury, Study Finds." *Reuters*, March 18, 2024, available at: https://www.reuters.com/world/us/us-study-finds-no-evidence-havana-syndrome-brain-injury-2024-03-18/.

Beason, Doug. *The E-Bomb: How America's New Directed Energy Weapons Will Change Future Wars Will Be Fought*. Cambridge: Da Capo Press, 2005.

Becker, Robert O. *Cross Currents: The Perils of Electropollution, the Promise of Electromedicine*. New York: Penguin, 1990.

Becker, Robert O., and Gary Selden. *The Body Electric: Electromagnetism and the Foundation of Life*. New York: William Morrow, 1985.

Beeston, R. "Russian Micro-waves Plan 'to Drive U.S. Envoys Mad.'" *London Daily Telegraph*, May 11, 1972.

Belpomme, Dominique, Lennart Hardell, Igor Belyaev, Ernesto Burgio, and David O. Carpenter. "Thermal and Non-Thermal Health Effects of Low-Intensity Non-Ionizing Radiation: An International Perspective." *Environmental Pollution* 242 (2018): 643–58.

Belpomme, Dominique, and Philippe Irigaray. "Electrohypersensitivity as a Newly Identified and Characterized Neurologic and Pathologic Disorder: How to Diagnose, Treat, and Prevent It." *International Journal of Molecular Sciences* 21, no. 1915 (2020): 1–20, https://doi.org/10.3390/ijms21061915.

Berezow, Alex. "Havana Syndrome: Were Our Diplomats Attacked with Microwave Weapons?" *American Council on Science and Health* website, October 23, 2020, available at: https://www.acsh.org/news/2020/10/23/havana-syndrome-were-our-diplomats-attacked-microwave-weapons-15107.

Berezow, Alex. "Sonic Attack: Cuba Playing Us for Fools." *American Council on Science and Health* website, October 23, 2020, available at: https://www.acsh.org/news/2017/12/06/sonic-attack-cuba-playing-us-fools-12245.

Berkowitz, Bruce. "Is Assassination an Option?" *Hoover Institution* website, January 30, 2002, available at: https://www.hoover.org/research/assassination-option.

Bernal, Alonso, Cameron Carter, Ishpreet Singh, Kathy Cao, and Olivia Madreperla. "Cognitive Warfare: An Attack on Truth and Thought." NATO Allied Command Transformation, December 2020, available at: https://innovationhub-act.org/wp-content/uploads/2023/12/Cognitive-Warfare.pdf.

Betz, Bradford. "Florida Car Chase in 2020 May Be Linked to Havana Syndrome: Report." *New York Post*, April 1, 2024, available at: https://nypost.com/2024/04/01/us-news/florida-car-chase-in-2020-may-be-linked-to-mysterious-havana-syndrome/.

Binhi, Vladimir, and Andrei B. Rubin. "Theoretical Concepts in Magnetobiology after 40 Years of Research." *Cells* 11, no. 2 (2022): 1–15.

Bland, Eric. "Army Developing 'Synthetic Telepathy.'" *NBC News*, October 13, 2008, available at: https://www.nbcnews.com/id/wbna27162401.

Blank, Stephen. "Russian Information Warfare as Domestic Counterinsurgency." *The Journal of the National Committee on American Foreign Policy* 35, no. 1 (2013): 31–4.

Bogaisky, Jeremy. "Helmets Like Iron Man's and a Smart T-Shirt that Calls for Help: The Pentagon's Wearable Tech Revolution." *Forbes*, October 28, 2022, available at: https://www.forbes.com/sites/jeremybogaisky/2022/10/28/helmet-iron-man-smart-shirt-pentagon-wearable-tech/.

Bokat-Lindell, Spencer. "Is 'Havana Syndrome' an 'Act of War' or 'Mass Hysteria?'" *New York Times*, October 26, 2021.

Bolton, Alexander. "Rubio Rejects Intelligence Finding That 'Havana Syndrome' Not Linked to Foreign Adversary." *The Hill*, March 2, 2023, available at: https://thehill.com/homenews/senate/3880776-rubio-rejects-intelligence-finding-that-havana-syndrome-not-linked-to-foreign-adversary/.

Borger, Julian. "Botched Surveillance Job May Have Led to Strange Injuries at Embassy in Cuba." *The Guardian*, August 25, 2017, available at: https://www.theguardian.com/world/2017/aug/25/botched-surveillance-job-may-have-led-to-strange-injuries-at-cuban-embassy.

Borger, Julian. "Havana Syndrome: NSA Officer's Case Hints at Microwave Attacks Since 90s." *The Guardian*, May 2, 2021, available at: https://www.theguardian.com/world/2021/may/02/havana-syndrome-nsa-officer-microwave-attacks-since-90s.

Borger, Julian. "Havana Syndrome Could Be Caused by Pulsed Energy Devices—US Export Report." *The Guardian*, February 3, 2022.

Borger, Julian. "Havana Syndrome has 'Dramatically Hurt' Morale, US Diplomats Say." *The Guardian*, February 10, 2022, available at: https://www.theguardian.com/us-news/2022/feb/10/havana-syndrome-cuba-us-diplomats-afsa.

Borger, Julian. "Microwave Weapons That Could Cause Havana Syndrome Exist, Experts Say; Russia and China Possibly Developed Technology Capable of Injuring Brain and a US Company Made a Prototype in 2004." *The Guardian*, June 2, 2021.

Borger, Julian. "US Officials Confirm 130 Incidents of Mysterious Havana Syndrome Brain Injury." *The Guardian*, May 14, 2021.

Bouchet, Nicolas. "Russia's 'Militarization' of Colour Revolutions." *Policy Perspectives* 4, no. 2 (2016): 2–3.

Bowart, Walter. *Operation Mind Control*. New York: Dell Publishing, 1978.

Bowcott, Owen. "UN Warns of Rise of 'Cybertorture' to Bypass Physical Ban." *The Guardian*, February 21, 2020, available at: https://www.theguardian.com/law/2020/feb/21/un-rapporteur-warns-of-rise-of-cybertorture-to-bypass-physical-ban.

Boyd-Barrett, Oliver, and Stephen Marmura. *Russiagate Revisited: The Aftermath of a Hoax*. Cham, Switzerland: Palgrave Macmillan, 2023.

Bradley, Lewis A. "The Death of Human Intelligence: How Human Intelligence Has Been Minimized Since the 1960s." *Military and Strategic Affairs* 8, no. 1 (2016): 75–90.

Brands, Hal, and Michael Beckley. *Danger Zone: The Coming Conflict with China*. New York: W.W. Norton & Co., 2019.

Broad, W. "Microwave Weapons Are Prime Suspect in Ills of U.S. Embassy Workers." *New York Times*, September 1, 2018.

Brodeur, Paul. *The Zapping of America: Microwaves, the Deadly Risk, and the Cover-Up*. New York: W.W. Norton & Co., 1977.

Bunker, Robert. "Unrestricted Warfare: Review Essay I." *Small Wars and Insurgencies* 11, no. 1 (2000): 115.

Burda, Robin. "Detection Tools for Cognitive Warfare: Leveraging the Cyber Domain." NATO Science and Technology Organization, 2023, available at: https://www.sto.nato.int/publications/STO%20Meeting%20Proceedings/STO-MP-SAS-OCS-ORA-2023/MP-SAS-OCS-ORA-2023-28.pdf.

Bures, Frank. "If a Weapon Didn't Cause Havana Syndrome, What Did?" *Slate*, February 1, 2022, available at: https://slate.com/technology/2022/02/havana-syndrome-health-weapon-functional-neurological-disorder.html.

Burleson, Nate, Catherine Herridge, and Gayle King. "Struggling with Havana Syndrome." *CBS Morning News*, March 31, 2022.

Burr, William, and Peter Kornbluh, eds. "The Moscow Signals Declassified: Irradiating Richard Nixon." *National Security Archive*, September 22, 2022, available at: https://nsarchive.gwu.edu/briefing-book/intelligence-nuclear-vault-russia-programs/2022-09-22/moscow-signals-declassified.

Butler, Desmond, Jack Gillum, and Alberto Arce. "US Secretly Built 'Cuban Twitter' to Stir Unrest." *Associated Press*, April 3, 2014, available at: https://apnews.com/article/technology-cuba-united-states-government-904a9a6a1bcd46cebfc14bea2ee30fdf.

Campion-Smith, Bruce. "Brain Injury Team to Study Havana Diplomats' Illness: Microwave Weapons Cited as Possible Cause of Canadians' Mysterious Health Problems." *Toronto Star*, October 1, 2018.

Cannarsa, Andrew. "CIA Official Who Traveled with Director to India Experienced Havana Syndrome: Report." *Washington Examiner*, September 21, 2021, available at: https://www.washingtonexaminer.com/news/102406/cia-official-who-traveled-with-director-to-india-experienced-havana-syndrome-symptoms-report/.

Cao, Kathy, Sean Glaister, Adriana Pena, Danbi Rhee, William Rong, Alexander Rovalino, Sam Bishop, Rohan Khanna, and Jatin Saini. "Countering Cognitive Warfare: Awareness and Resilience." *NATO Review*, May 20, 2021, available at: https://www.nato.int/docu/review/articles/2021/05/20/countering-cognitive-warfare-awareness-and-resilience/index.html.

Carpenter, David O. "Electromagnetic Fields and Cancer: The Cost of Doing Nothing." *Reviews on Environmental Health* 25, no. 1 (2009): 75–80.

Carter, Hana. "'Immaculate Concussion' Russians Use 'Secret Microwave Weapon' to Target American Spies Across the Globe . . . Including on US Soil, CIA Probe Claims." *The U.S. Sun*, October 21, 2020, available at: https://www.the-sun.com/news/1666632/russians-secret-microwave-weapon/.

CBS Staff. "After Several Childhood Cancer Cases at One School, Parents Question Radiation from Cell Tower." *CBS News*, April 4, 2019, available at: https://www

.cbsnews.com/news/cell-tower-shut-down-some-california-parents-link-to-several-cases-of-childhood-cancer/.

CBS Staff. "Havana Syndrome Symptoms Suggests Who May Be Responsible for Mysterious Brain Injuries." *60 Minutes*, March 31, 2024, available at: https://www.youtube.com/watch?v=JdPSD1SUYCY.

CDC. "Cuba Unexplained Events Investigation: Final Report." December 3, 2019, available at: https://nsarchive.gwu.edu/documents/cdc-report-havana-syndrome-medical-mystery-remains-unresolved/CDC%20%2320200983DOS255%20Final%20Report.pdf.

Celozzi, Salvatore, Rodolfo Araneo, Paolo Burghignoli, and Giampiero Lavat. *Electromagnetic Shielding: Theory and Applications*. Hoboken: Wiley, 2023.

Chavez, Nicole. "Using Sound to Attack: The Diverse World of Acoustic Devices." *CNN*, September 27, 2017, available at: https://www.cnn.com/2017/08/10/health/acoustic-weapons-explainer/index.html.

Chazan, Guy. "US Officials in Berlin Struck by 'Havana Syndrome' Symptoms." *Financial Times*, August 19, 2021.

Chekinov, S. G., and S. A. Bogdanov. "The Nature and Content of a New-Generation War." *Military Thought* 10 (2013).

Chen, Stephen. "Chinese Scientists Build Powerful Microwave Weapon That Can Fire From a Moving Truck, Using Stirling Engine to Cool Technology." *South China Morning Post*, February 8, 2024, available at: https://www.scmp.com/news/china/science/article/3251381/chinese-scientists-build-powerful-stirling-engine-based-microwave-weapon-can-fire-moving-truck.

Cheng, Amy. "Germany Investigates Possible 'Havana Syndrome' Sonic Attack on U.S. Embassy Staff." *Washington Post*, October 9, 2021.

Cheng, Amy. "U.S. Diplomat Said to Have 'Havana Syndrome' Sues State Dept. and Blinken, Alleging Discrimination." *Washington Post*, December 10, 2021.

Chin, Josh, and Liza Lin. *Surveillance State: Inside China's Quest to Launch a New Era of Social Control Quest to Launch a New Era of Social Control*. New York: St. Martin's Press, 2022.

Christensen, Jen. "NIH Cancels 'Havana Syndrome' Research, Citing Unethical Coercion of Participants." *CNN*, September 1, 2024, available at: https://www.cnn.com/2024/08/30/health/nih-havana-syndrome-study/index.html.

Clancy, Dimitry. "Havana Syndrome: The Mysterious Illness Striking Down US Officials." *60 Minutes Australia*, April 2024, available at: https://9now.nine.com.au/60-minutes/havana-syndrome-the-mysterious-illness-striking-down-us-officials/27d3425c-274e-40a7-926f-ac33ff9e2d62.

Clarke, Ryan, Xiaxou Sean Lin, and J. J. Eads. "Enumerating, Targeting and Collapsing the Communist Chinese Communist Party's NeuroStrike Program: Aggregating Intelligence Fragments and the Power of Network Graphs." *The CCP Biohazard Initiative*, Research Report, June 2023.

Claverie, Bernard, and Francois du Cluzel. “The Cognitive Warfare Concept.” NATO Allied Command Transformation, December 2023, available at: https://innovationhub-act.org/wp-content/uploads/2023/12/CW-article-Claverie-du-Cluzel-final_0.pdf.

Claverie, Bernard, B. Prébot, N. Buchler, and Francois Du Cluzel, eds. *Cognitive Warfare: The Future of Cognitive Dominance*. Neuilly, France: NATO, 2022, available at: https://innovationhub-act.org/wp-content/uploads/2023/12/210601-Cognition-Workshop-Report-v3.pdf.

Clay, Ian, and Robert D. Atkinson. “Wake Up America, China Is Overtaking the United States in Innovation Capacity.” *Information Technology & Innovation Foundation*, January 23, 2024, available at: https://itif.org/publications/2023/01/23/wake-up-america-china-is-overtaking-the-united-states-in-innovation-capacity/.

CNN. “Ex-CIA Operative Calls for New Election.” *CNN*, December 10, 2016, available at: https://www.youtube.com/watch?v=erRf6CONfco.

Coates, J. *Nonlethal and Non-Destructive Combat in Cities*. Washington, DC: Institute for Defense Analysis, 1970.

Cochrane, Emily. “Health Drove US Envoys Out of Cuba.” *New York Times*, August 11, 2017.

Cohen, Eliot. “The Mystique of U.S. Airpower.” *Foreign Affairs* 73, no. 1 (1994): 109–24.

Cole, August, and Hervé Guyader. “Cognitive: A 6th Domain of Operations?” NATO Innovation Hub, January 2023, available at: https://www.projectcensored.org/wp-content/uploads/2023/01/Cognitive-a-6th-Domain-of-Operations.pdf.

Conolly, Amanda. “Canadian Officials Warned Staff Bound for Cuba to Stay Silent on ‘Havana Syndrome.’” *Global News*, October 25, 2020, available at: https://globalnews.ca/news/7365888/havana-syndrome-canadian-diplomats-cuba/.

Conte, Mike. “FBI Opens a New Investigation Into China ‘Every 10 Hours’. Bureau Director Says.” *CNN*, April 14, 2021, available at: https://www.cnn.com/2021/04/14/politics/fbi-director-china-investigations-intl-hnk/index.html.

Contero, Sonia. *Nano Comes to Life: How Nanotechnology Is Transforming Medicine and the Future of Biology*. Princeton: Princeton University Press, 2010.

Copp, Tara. “U.S. Defense Department Official Had ‘Havana Syndrome’ Symptoms During a 2023 NATO Summit, the Pentagon Confirms.” *PBS News Hour*, April 1, 2024, available at: https://www.pbs.org/newshour/politics/u-s-defense-official-had-havana-syndrome-symptoms-during-a-2023-nato-summit-the-pentagon-confirms.

Corera, Gordon. “China’s Spy Threat Is Growing, But the West Has Struggled to Keep Up.” *BBC News*, May 15, 2024, available at: https://www.bbc.com/news/articles/cmm33rm32veo.

Corera, Gordon. “Havana Syndrome—Most Cases Not Caused by Foreign Power—CIA.” *BBC News*, January 20, 2022, available at: https://www.bbc.com/news/world-us-canada-60068483.

Corera, Gordon. "'Havana Syndrome' and the Mystery of Microwaves." *BBC News*, September 8, 2021, available at: https://www.bbc.com/news/world-58396698.

Crane, Emily. "FBI Acknowledges Agents May Have Had 'Havana Syndrome' Symptoms." *New York Post*, November 24, 2021, available at: https://nypost.com/2021/11/24/fbi-acknowledges-agents-may-have-had-havana-syndrome-symptoms/.

Croxton, Will. "5-Year Havana Syndrome Investigation Finds Evidence Who Might Be Responsible." *CBS News*, July 7, 2024, available at: https://www.cbsnews.com/news/5-year-havana-syndrome-investigation-finds-new-evidence-of-who-might-be-responsible-60-minutes/.

Cuiller, David. "Overclassification Overkill: The US Government Is Drowning in a Sea of Secrets." *The Conversation*, March 2, 2023, available at: https://theconversation.com/overclassification-overkill-the-us-government-is-drowning-in-a-sea-of-secrets-198917.

Cunliffe, Kyle S. "Hard Target Espionage in the Information Era: New Challenges for the Second-Oldest Profession." *Intelligence and National Security* 36, no. 7 (2021): 1018–34.

Dando, Malcolm. *The Chemical and Biological Nonproliferation Regime after the Covid-19 Pandemic: Dealing with the Scientific Revolution in the Life Sciences*. New York: Palgrave Macmillan, 2023.

Davison, Neil. "The Early History of 'Non-Lethal' Weapons." Bradford Non-Lethal Weapons Research Project, Occasional Paper No. 1, 2006.

Davison, Neil. *Non-Lethal Weapons*. London: Macmillan, 2009.

The Daily Beast. "Havana Syndrome Might Be Real and It's Scary as Hell." *TDB*, February 2, 2023, available at: https://www.thedailybeast.com/havana-syndrome-might-be-real-and-its-scary-as-hell?ref=scroll.

De Caro, Chuck. "Weapons of War: Is There an RF Gap?" *CNN Special Assignment*, November 1985, available at: https://rumble.com/v2fw85s-electromagnetic-frequency-weapons-1985-cnn-special-reports.html.

De Caro, Chuck. "The Zap Gap: The Soviets May Be Ahead of US in the Development of Radio-Frequency Weapons." *The Atlantic*, March 1987.

Delgado, Jose. *The Physical Control of the Mind: Towards a Psychocivilized Society*. New York: Harper & Row, 1969.

Della Sala, Sergio, and Roberto Cubelli. "Alleged 'Sonic Attack' Supported by Poor Neuropsychology." *Cortex* 103 (2018): 387–8.

Del Marmol, Julio Antonio. *Black Tears: The Havana Syndrome*. Cuban Lightning Publications, 2022.

Del Monte, Louis A. *Nanoweapons: A Growing Threat to Humanity*. Lincoln: Potomac Books, 2017.

Del Monte, Louis A. *War at the Speed of Light: Directed Energy Weapons and the Future of Twenty-First Century Warfare*. Lincoln: Potomac Books, 2022.

Der Spiegel. "Berliner Landeskriminalamt ermittelt wegen Havana Syndrom." *Der Spiegel*, October 10, 2021, available at: https://www.spiegel.de/politik/deutschland/berliner-landeskriminalamt-ermittelt-wegen-havanna-syndrom-a-637fbcd2-8229-447e-956b-350e34b4174c.

Deruelle, Fabien. "The Different Sources of Electromagnetic Fields: Dangers Are Not Limited to Physical Health." *Electromagnetic Biology and Medicine* 29, no. 2 (2020): 166–75.

Desiderio, Andrew. "Lawmakers Skewer Interim CIA Report on Havana Syndrome." *Politico*, January 20, 2022, available at: https://www.politico.com/news/2022/01/20/havana-syndrome-cia-congress-527527.

DeYoung, Karen. "Trump Administration Announces New Measures Against Cuba." *Washington Post*, April 17, 2019.

Dilanian, Ken. "FBI Acknowledges Some Agents May Have Havana Syndrome Symptoms." *NBC News*, November 24, 2021, available at: https://www.nbcnews.com/health/health-news/fbi-acknowledges-agents-may-havana-syndrome-symptoms-rcna6504.

Dilanian, Ken. "'Havana Syndrome' Symptoms in Small Group Most Likely Caused by Directed Energy, Says U.S. Intel Panel of Experts." *NBC News*, February 2, 2022, available at: https://www.nbcnews.com/politics/national-security/havana-syndrome-symptoms-small-group-likely-caused-directed-energy-say-rcna14584.

Dilanian, Ken, Andrea Mitchell, and Brenda Breslauer. "CIA Officer Suffered Crippling Symptoms in Moscow. What Is 'Havana Syndrome.'" *NBC News*, December 7, 2020, available at: https://www.nbcnews.com/news/world/cia-officer-suffered-crippling-symptoms-moscow-was-it-havana-syndrome-n1250177.

Dillow, Clay. "DARPA Wants to Install Transcranial Ultrasonic Mind Control Devices in Soldier's Helmets." *Popular Science*, September 10, 2010, available at: https://www.popsci.com/technology/article/2010-09/darpa-wants-mind-control-keep-soldiers-sharp-smart-and-safe/.

Dirks, Emile, and Diana Fu. "China's Overseas Police Stations: An Imminent Security Threat." *Brookings*, February 16, 2024, available at: https://www.brookings.edu/articles/chinas-overseas-police-stations-an-imminent-security-threat/.

Dobrokhotov, Roman, Christo Grozev, and Michael Weiss. "Unraveling Havana Syndrome: New Evidence Links the GRU's Assassination Unit 29155 to Mysterious Attacks on U.S. Officials and Their Families." *The Insider*, March 31, 2024, available at: https://theins.ru/en/politics/270425.

Dommeyer, Frederick C. "Psychical Research at Stanford University." *The Journal of Parapsychology* 39, no. 3 (1975): 173–205.

Dorsey, Steve. "Pentagon Turns Focus to Cuba Health 'Attacks' Amid New Findings on American Victims." *CBS News*, September 12, 2018, available at: https://www.cbsnews.com/news/pentagon-turns-focus-to-cuba-attacks/.

Dorsey, Steve. "Uzbekistan Incident Raises Suspicions of Russian Involvement in Cuba Attacks." *CBS News*, November 28, 2017, available at: https://www.cbsnews.com/news/uzbekistan-incident-raises-suspicions-of-russian-involvement-in-cuba-attacks/.

Doswald-Beck, Louise, and Gerald C. Cauderey. "The Development of New Anti-Personnel Weapons." *International Review of the Red Cross* 30, no. 279 (1997): 565–77.

Drexler, K. Eric. *Engines of Creation: The Coming Era of Nanotechnology*. New York: Anchor Books, 1987.

Ducharme, Jamie. "Why Everyone's Worried About Their Attention Span—and How to Improve Yours." *Time Magazine*, August 10, 2023, available at: https://time.com/6302294/why-you-cant-focus-anymore-and-what-to-do-about-it/.

Du Cluzel, Francois. "Cognitive Warfare." NATO Innovation Hub, November 2020, available at: https://innovationhub-act.org/wp-content/uploads/2023/12/20210113_CW-Final-v2-.pdf.

Du Cluzel, Francois. "Cognitive Warfare, a Battle for the Brain." NATO Science and Technology Organization, December 2023.

Dutton, Jack. "Havana Syndrome Symptoms Have Been Reported in these Countries." *Newsweek*, September 21, 2021, available at: https://www.newsweek.com/havana-syndrome-china-austria-russia-1631102.

Dylan, Huw, and Thomas J. Maguire. "Secret Intelligence and Public Diplomacy in the Ukraine War." *Survival* 64, no. 4 (2022): 33–74.

Eads, L. J., Ryan Clarke, and Xiaoxu Sean Lin. "In the Shadows of Science: Unravelling China's Invisible Arsenal of Nanoweapons." *The CCP Biohazard Initiative*, August 2023, available at: https://static1.squarespace.com/static/6444894f2a886e74091c9e1b/t/64ea4f2e51a29b701d5c3456/1693077294703/In+the+Shadows+of+Science+-+Unravelling+Chinas+Invisible+Arsenals+of+Nanoweapons.pdf.

Eads, L. J., Ryan Clarke, Xiaoxu Sean Lin, and Robert McCreight. "Warfare in the Cognitive Age: NeuroStrike and the PLA's Advanced Psychological Weapons & Tactics." *The CCP Biohazard Initiative*, December 2023, available at: https://static1.squarespace.com/static/6444894f2a886e74091c9e1b/t/65824d9fd6d294583d8e859c/1703038367948/Warfare+in+the+Cognitive+Age+NeuroStrike+and+the+PLAs+Advanced+Psychological+Weapons+%26+Tactics.pdf.

Eberhart, Christopher. "CIA Evacuates Intelligence Officer from Serbia as 'Havana Syndrome' Attacks on American Spies and Diplomats Continue to Grow." *Daily Mail*, September 28, 2021, available at: https://www.dailymail.co.uk/news/article-10038159/CIA-evacuates-intelligence-officer-Serbia-result-Havana-Syndrome.html.

Ebon, Martin. *Psychic Warfare: Threat or Illusion*. New York: McGraw-Hill, 1983.

The Economist Staff. "Sung Tieu Unpacks 'Havana Syndrome' in Her Latest Work: Prisoners of Sound." *The Economist*, November 18, 2021.

Eggertson, Laura. "Military Claims Laser Dazzlers Have 'Negligible' Risk." *Canadian Medical Association Journal* 180, no. 11 (2009): 1099–100.

Eichar, Donnie. *Dead Mountain: The Untold True Story of the Dyatlov Pass Incident*. San Francisco: Chronicle Books, 2013.

Eichensehr, Kristen, ed. "Investigations Continue Into Mysterious Illness Affecting U.S. Officials in Havana and Elsewhere." *The American Journal of International Law* 115, no. 3 (2021): 527–35.

Elder, A., and C. K. Chou. "Auditory Response to Pulsed Radiofrequency Energy." *Bioelectromgnetics Supplement* 6 (2003): S.162–S.173, https://doi.org/10.1002/bem.10163.

Ellen, Francis. "Colombia Aware of 'Havana Syndrome' Reported at U.S. Embassy in Bogota." *Washington Post*, October 13, 2021.

Elwood, Mark J. "Microwaves in the Cold War: The Moscow Embassy Study and Its Interpretation. Review of a Retrospective Cohort Study." *Environmental Health* 11, no. 85 (2012): 1–10.

Entous, Adam. "Stealth Mode: How the Havana Syndrome Spread to the White House." *The New Yorker* 97, no. 14 (May 24, 2021).

Entous, Adam. "Vienna Is the New Havana Syndrome Hotspot." *The New Yorker*, July 16, 2021, available at: https://www.newyorker.com/news/news-desk/vienna-is-the-new-havana-syndrome-hotspot.

Entous, Adam, and John Lee Anderson. "Havana Syndrome." *The New Yorker*, November 19, 2018.

Erickson, Amanda. "All the Theories What's Happening to the Diplomats in Cuba: At Least 21 Americans Have Reported a Bizarre Rash of Symptoms." *Washington Post blogs*, September 30, 2017, available at: https://www.washingtonpost.com/news/worldviews/wp/2017/09/30/all-the-theories-about-whats-happening-to-the-diplomats-in-cuba/.

Erickson, Amanda. "Another Diplomat Was Diagnosed with 'Havana Syndrome'. Here Is What We Know." *Washington Post*, December 3, 2018.

Erickson, Dave. *Framing Flynn: The Scandalous Takedown of an American General*. New York: Post Hill Press, 2021.

Escritt, Thomas, and Sarah Marsh. "Russia Buying Spies to Make Up for Expelled Diplomats, Germany Agency Says." *Reuters*, June 18, 2024, available at: https://www.reuters.com/world/europe/russia-buying-spies-make-up-expelled-diplomats-german-agency-says-2024-06-18/.

Essex, Jamey, and Joshua Bowman. "From the Green Zone to the Havana Syndrome: Making Geographic Sense of Rotationality and Hardship in Diplomacy." *Diplomatica* 4, no. 1 (2022): 74–99.

Evans, Nicholas G. *The Ethics of Neuroscience and National Security*. New York: Routledge, 2021.

Evans, R., and R. Novak. "The Microwave Affair." *Washington Post*, March 8, 1976, A19.

Faherty, Anne. "Senior DoD Official Experienced 'Havana Syndrome' Symptoms at NATO Summit in July, Pentagon Says." *ABC News*, April 1, 2024, available at: https://abcnews.go.com/Politics/senior-dod-official-experienced-havana-syndrome-symptoms-nato/story?id=108714952.

Fields, Douglas R. "Why the Havana Syndrome Happened." *International Journal of Social Psychology* (2023), https://doi.org/10.1177/00207640231212865.

Finkbeiner, Ann. *The Jasons: The Secret History of Science's Postwar Elite*. New York: Viking, 2006.

Finnegan, Conor, and Cindy Smith. "CIA Says Foreign Actor May Be Behind Some Havana Syndrome Cases." *NBC News*, January 20, 2022, available at: https://abcnews.go.com/Politics/cia-foreign-actor-havana-syndrome-cases/story?id=82376545.

Forrest, Brett, and Warren P. Strobel. "How Cuba Recruits Spies to Penetrate Inner Circles of the U.S. Government." *Wall Street Journal*, March 16, 2024.

Foster, Kenneth R., David C. Garrett, and Marvin, C. Ziskin. "Can the Microwave Auditory Effect Be 'Weaponized?'" *Frontiers in Public Health* 9 (2021): 1–4.

Francis, Ellen. "Colombia Aware of 'Havana Syndrome' Cases Reported at U.S. Embassy in Bogotá." *Washington Post*, October 13, 2021.

Frey, A. H. "Human Auditory System Response to Modulated Electromagnetic Frequency." *Journal of Applied Physiology* 17, no. 4 (1962): 689–92.

Gaba, Arlen, and Sahil Munjal. "Havana Syndrome: Social Contagion or Mass Psychogenic Illness." *Psychiatrist.com*, March 7, 2024, available at: https://www.psychiatrist.com/pcc/havana-syndrome-social-contagion-mass-psychogenic-illness/.

Galeotti, Mark. "CRIMINTERN: How the Kremlin Uses Russia's Criminal Networks in Europe." *European Council on Foreign Relations*, April 2017, available at: https://ecfr.eu/wp-content/uploads/ECFR208_-_CRIMINTERM_-_HOW_RUSSIAN_ORGANISED_CRIME_OPERATES_IN_EUROPE02.pdf.

Galeotti, Mark. *The Weaponisation of Everything: A Field Guide to the New Way of War*. New Haven: Yale University Press, 2022.

Gamez Torres, Nora. "An FBI Agent Was Victim of a Havana Syndrome 'Attack' in Key West, Lawyer Tells Congress." *Miami Herald*, May 8, 2024, available at: https://www.miamiherald.com/news/nation-world/world/americas/cuba/article288423243.html.

Gardiner, H. "25th Person at U.S. Embassy Is Mysteriously Sickened." *New York Times*, June 21, 2018, available at: https://www.nytimes.com/2018/06/21/us/politics/us-diplomat-cuba-embassy-illness.html.

Gazis, Olivia. "State Department, CIA Establish Federal Payment Rules for 'Havana Syndrome' Victims." *CBS News*, June 24, 2022, available at: https://www.cbsnews.com/news/havana-syndrome-state-department-cia-establish-federal-payment-rules-for-victims/.

Gazis, Olivia. "U.S. Intensifies Efforts to Address 'Havana Syndrome', But Answers Remain Elusive." *CBS News*, July 27, 2021, available at: https://www.cbsnews.com/news/havana-syndrome-efforts-united-states/.

Gearan, Anne. "U.S. Expelled Two Cuban Diplomats After Embassy Employees Developed Ailments." *Washington Post*, August 9, 2017.

Geis, John P. "Directed Energy Weapons on the Battlefield: A New Vision for 2025." *Center for Strategy and Technology Air War College Occasional Paper* 32 (2003).

Genasys. "LRAD Overview & Product Guide," available at: https://genasys.com/wp-content/uploads/2024/03/LRAD-Product-Guide-2024.pdf.

General Accounting Office Staff. "Havana Syndrome—Americans Affected by Mysterious Symptoms May Struggle to Get Care." *General Accounting Office*, July 29, 2024, available at: https://www.gao.gov/blog/havana-syndrome-americans-affected-mysterious-symptoms-may-struggle-get-care.

Gertz, Bill. "China Crafts Weapons to Alter Brain Function; Report Says Tech Meant to Influence Government Leaders." *Washington Times*, July 6, 2023.

Gertz, Bill. "U.S. Military Facing Nonkinetic and 'NeuroStrike' Weapons." *The Washington Times*, May 26, 2023.

Giles, Keir. *Russia's War on Everybody and What It Means for You*. London: Bloomsbury Academic, 2022.

Giordano, James. "Intel Community's Havana Syndrome Report and Its Flawed Assumptions." *National Defense Magazine*, March 10, 2023, available at: https://www.nationaldefensemagazine.org/articles/2023/3/10/intel-communitys-havana-syndrome-report-and-its-flawed-assumptions.

Giordano, James. "Nation Must Come Together to Tackle Havana Syndrome." *National Defense*, October 15, 2021, available at: https://www.nationaldefensemagazine.org/articles/2021/10/15/nation-must-come-together-to-tackle-havana-syndrome.

Giordano, James. *Neurotechnology in National Security and Defense: Practical Considerations, Neuroethical Concerns*. Boca Raton: CRC Press, 2012.

Giordano, James. "Weaponizing the Brain: Neuroscience Advancements Spark Debate." *National Defense*, May 11, 2017, available at: https://www.nationaldefensemagazine.org/articles/2017/5/11/weaponizing-the-brain-neuroscience-advancements-spark-debate.

Giri, D. V. *High-Power Electromagnetic Radiators: Nonlethal Weapons and Other Applications*. Cambridge, MA: Harvard University Press, 2004.

Golden, Tim, and Sebastian Rotella. "The Strange Case of American Diplomats in Cuba: As the Mystery Deepens So Do Divisions in Washington." *ProPublica*, November 9, 2018, available at: https://www.propublica.org/article/the-strange-case-of-american-diplomats-in-cuba-as-the-mystery-deepens-so-do-divisions-in-washington.

Goldfeder, Jerry H., and Mitchell Lincoln. "A Donald Trump Coup If He Loses in 2020? With All the Norms He's Busted, Don't Rule It Out." *USA Today*, March 14, 2019.

Goldsmith, J. R. "Balancing the Interests of Patients, Science and Employees: Case Study of RF (Microwave) Exposure of US Embassy Staff in Eastern European Posts." *The Science of the Total Environment* 184 (1996): 83–9.

Golomb, Beatrice Alexandra. "Diplomats' Mystery Illness and Pulsed Radiofrequency/ Microwave Radiation." *Neural Computing* 30, no. 11 (2018): 2882–985.

Goodman, Amy. "Ousted Honduran President Manuel Zelaya Speaks from Brazilian Embassy in Tegucigalpa." *Democracy Now!*, October 5, 2009, available at: https://www.democracynow.org/2009/10/5/ousted_honduran_president_manuel_zelaya_speaks.

Gorman, James. "Agency Initiative Will Focus on Deep Brain Stimulation." *New York Times*, October 25, 2013.

Gramm, Joshua D., and Brian A. Branagan. "Neurowar Is Here!" Master's Thesis, Naval Postgraduate School, Monterrey, December 2021.

Griffin, Jennifer, and Liz Friden. "Havana Syndrome 'Patient Zero' Rejects Intelligence Community Findings that Foreign Adversary 'Very Unlikely.'" *Fox News*, March 2, 2023, available at: https://www.foxnews.com/politics/havana-syndrome-patient-zero-rejects-intelligence-community-findings-foreign-adversary-very-unlikely.

Gross, Michael L. "Medicalized Weapons & Modern War." *Hastings Center Report*, January–February 2010.

Gross, Michael L. "Military Medical Research in Britain and the USA: The Challenge of Informed Consent." *Journal of the Royal Army Medical Corps* 165 (2019): 298–302.

The Guardian Staff. "Havana Syndrome: FBI Warns Staff Amid Reports of Symptoms Among Agents." *The Guardian*, November 25, 2021, available at: https://www.theguardian.com/us-news/2021/nov/25/havana-syndrome-fbi-warns-staff-amid-reports-of-symptoms-among-agents.

The Guardian Staff. "Trump Says Cuba 'Responsible' for Alleged Sonic Attacks, but Offers No Evidence." *The Guardian*, October 16, 2017, available at: https://www.theguardian.com/world/2017/oct/16/trump-says-cuba-responsible-for-alleged-sonic-attacks-but-offers-no-evidence.

Gunzinger, Mark. "Changing the Game: The Promise of Directed Energy Weapons." Center for Strategic and Budgetary Assessments, 2012.

Guthrie, Savannah, and Andrea Mitchell. "U.S. Diplomats Speak Out on Mysterious Havana Syndrome." *Today*, October 14, 2021.

Guyatt, David. "Anti-Personnel 'Soft Kill' Weaponry." *World Affairs* 9, no. 2 (2005): 41–57.

Gwertzman, Bernard. "Moscow Rays Linked to U.S. Bugging." *New York Times*, February 26, 1976.

Gwertzman, Bernard. "U.S. Radio Spying in Soviet Suffers." *New York Times*, May 2, 1976.

Haas, Richard. "Cold War II." *Council on Foreign Relations*, February 23, 2018, available at: https://www.cfr.org/article/cold-war-ii.

Haley, Robert W., Gerald Kramer, Junhui Xiao, Jill A. Dever, and John F. Teiber. "Evaluation of a Gene Environment Interaction of P0N1 and Low-Level Nerve Agent Exposure with Gulf War Illness: A Prevalence Case-Control Study Drawn from the U.S. National Health Survey's National Population Sample." *Environmental Health Perspectives* 130, no. 5 (2022): 1–16.

Haltiwanger, John. "The Shadowy Russian Intel Unit That Allegedly Paid Afghan Militants to Kill US Troops Is the Same One Running Assassinations in Europe." *Business Insider*, June 29, 2020, available at: https://www.businessinsider.com/unit-29155-russian-intel-branch-allegedly-behind-bounties-us-troops-2020-6.

Hambling, David. "Pain Ray: The U.S. Military's Agony Beam Weapon." *New Scientist*, May 8, 2013, available at: https://www.newscientist.com/article/mg21829162-300-pain-ray-the-us-militarys-new-agony-beam-weapon/.

Hambling, David. "US Bioelectromagnetic Weapon Research." *Military.com*, November 26, 2006, available at: https://www.military.com/defensetech/2006/11/26/us-bioelectromagnetic-weapons-research.

Hambling, David. "UN Investigates Electromagnetic Terrorism." *Wired Magazine*, December 2, 2008, available at: https://www.wired.com/2008/12/un-investigates/.

Hammer, Alex. "US Diplomats Struck by 'Havana Syndrome' Share Agonizing Symptoms of the Condition Which Has Left Them BRAIN DAMAGED and Destroyed Their Careers, as They Tearfully Refute Claims Illness Doesn't Exist." *Daily Mail*, October 14, 2021, available at: https://www.dailymail.co.uk/news/article-10091839/Diplomats-struck-Havana-Syndrome-say-destroyed-careers.html.

Hammes, Thomas. *The Sling and the Stone: On War in the 21st Century*. St. Paul: Zenith Press, 2004.

Hammes, Thomas. "Fourth Generation Evolves, Fifth Emerges." *Military Review* (May–June 2007): 14–23.

Hammond, Andrew, Nicky Woolf, Marc Polymeropoulos, and Marc Ziad. "The Sound: Mystery of the Havana Syndrome." *International Spy Museum*, March 9, 2023, available at: https://www.youtube.com/watch?v=km3MvDZBTP4.

Hampshire, Adam, Adriana Azor, Christina Atchison, William Trender, Peter J. Hellyer, Valentina Giunchiglia, Masud Husein, and Paul Elliott. "Cognition and Memory after Covid-19 in a Large Community Sample." *The New England Journal of Medicine* 390, no. 9 (2024).

Harding, Luke. "The Hidden History of Trump's First Trip to Moscow." *Politico*, November 19, 2017, available at: https://www.politico.com/magazine/story/2017/11/19/trump-first-moscow-trip-215842/.

Harris, Shane. "CIA Officer Who Helped Find bin Laden Will Look for Cause of Mysterious 'Havana Syndrome.'" *Washington Post*, July 21, 2021.

Harris, Shane, and John Hudson. "'Havana Syndrome' Not Caused by Energy Weapon or Foreign Adversary, Intelligence Review Finds." *Washington Post*, March 1, 2023.

Haseltine, Eric. *The Spy in Moscow Station: A Counterspy's Hunt for a Deadly Cold War Threat*. New York: St. Martin's Griffin, 2019.

Hastedt, Glenn. "The Politics of Intelligence and the Politicization of Intelligence: The American Experience." *Intelligence and National Security* 28, no. 1 (2013): 5–31.

Hawkins, Derek, Adrian Blanco, Perry Stein, and William Neff. "Inside the Fortified Rooms Securing U.S. Secrets." *Washington Post*, April 28, 2023.

Hayes, Chris, Jon Lee Anderson, and Adam Entous. "Unpacking the 'Havana Syndrome' with Jon Lee Anderson and Adam Entous: Podcast and Transcript." *MSNBC*, February 22, 2023, available at: https://www.msnbc.com/msnbc-podcast/why-is-this-happening/unpacking-havana-syndrome-jon-lee-anderson-adam-entous-podcast-transcript-n1303083.

Herridge, Catherine. "'My Brain Is Broken': Former CIA Analyst Struggling with Havana Syndrome Says She Has Not Received Promised Care." *CBS News*, May 31, 2022, available at: https://www.cbsnews.com/news/havana-syndrome-cia-medical-care-financial-support/.

Hollings, Alex. "SR-91 Aurora: The U.S. Military's Secret Mach 5 Plane?" *The National Interest*, October 29, 2023, available at: https://nationalinterest.org/blog/buzz/sr-91-aurora-us-militarys-secret-mach-5-plane-207093.

Horowitz, Evan. "IQ Rates Are Dropping in Many Developed Countries and That Doesn't Bode Well for Humanity." *NBC News*, May 22, 2019, available at: https://www.nbcnews.com/think/opinion/iq-rates-are-dropping-many-developed-countries-doesn-t-bode-ncna1008576.

Hosenball, Mark. "FBI Calls Dealing with 'Havana Syndrome' a Top Priority." *Reuters*, November 24, 2021.

Hudson, John, and Shane Harris. "CIA Chief in Vienna Recalled Amid Criticism of Management and Handling of Mysterious 'Havana Syndrome' Incidents." *Washington Post*, September 24, 2021.

Ignatius, David. "Dealing with 'Havana Syndrome' Is a Policymaker's Nightmare." *Washington Post*, October 28, 2021.

Insel, Thomas R., Story C. Landis, and Francis S. Collins. "The NIH BRAIN Initiative." *Science* 340, no. 6133 (2013): 687–8.

The Insider Staff. "Undercover Chef: How the FBI Interrogator of a Russian Spy Arrested in Florida Later Came Down with Havana Syndrome." *The Insider*, April 1, 2024, available at: https://theins.ru/en/politics/270450.

Institute for Basic Science, South Korea. "New Technology to Control the Brain Using Magnetic Fields Developed." *EurekAlert!*, July 17, 2024, available at: https://www.eurekalert.org/news-releases/1051652.

Ioffe, Julia. "The Mystery of the Immaculate Concussion." *GQ Magazine*, October 20, 2020, available at: https://www.gq.com/story/cia-investigation-and-russian-microwave-attacks.

ITV. "High Tech Psychological Warfare Arrives in the Middle East." *ITV News*, March 23, 1991, available at: https://bibliotecapleyades.net/CIENCIA/ciencia_nonlethalweapons05.htm.

Jacobsen, Annie. *The Pentagon's Brain: An Uncensored History of DARPA, America's Top Secret Military Research Agency*. New York: Little, Brown and Co., 2015.

Jacobsen, Annie. *Phenomena: The Secret History of the U.S. Government's Investigation Into Extrasensory Perception and Psychokinesis*. New York: Little Brown and Company, 2017.

JASON. "Acoustic Signals and Physiological Effects on U.S. Diplomats on Cuba." *MITRE Corporation*, November 2018.

JASON. "An Analysis of Data and Hypotheses Related to the Embassy Incidents." *MITRE Corporation*, October 16, 2021.

Joy, Bill. "Why the Future Does Not Need Us." *Wired Magazine* 8.04 (April 2000), available at: https://www.wired.com/2000/04/joy-2/.

Justesen, Don R. "Microwaves and Behavior." *American Psychologist* (March 1975): 392–401.

Kaldor, Mary. *New and Old Wars: Organized Violence in a Global Era*. Cambridge: Polity, 2001.

Kania, Elsa B. "Minds at War: China's Pursuit of Military Advantage through Cognitive Science and Biotechnology." *Prism* 8, no. 3 (2019): 82–101.

Karem, Brian. "Exclusive: Declassified Report Suggests 'Havana Syndrome' Could Result from Directed Energy." *Salon*, March 29, 2023, available at: https://www.salon.com/2023/03/29/exclusive-declassified-report-suggests-havana-syndrome-could-result-from-energy-weapon/.

Katchadourian, Raffi. "Operation Delirium." *The New Yorker*, December 9, 2012, available at: https://www.newyorker.com/magazine/2012/12/17/operation-delirium?currentPage=all&src=longreads&buffer_share=25d72.

Kaurin, Pauline. "With Fear and Trembling: An Empirical Framework for Non-Lethal Weapons." *Journal of Military Ethics* 9, no. 1 (2010): 100–14.

Kelemen, Michele, and Deepa Shivaram. "VP Harris' Flight Delayed After Possible 'Havana Syndrome' Incident in Hanoi." *NPR*, August 24, 2021, available at: https://www.npr.org/2021/08/24/1030663913/kamala-harris-havana-syndrome-vietnam-delay-embassy.

Keller, John. "Air Force Deploys B-52 Missiles That Could Disable Enemy Military Electronics with High-Power Microwaves." *Military & Aerospace Electronics*, May 17, 2019, available at: https://www.militaryaerospace.com/rf-analog/article/14033453/air-force-deploys-b-52-missiles-that-could-disable-enemy-military-electronics-with-high-power-microwaves.

Kennedy Jr., Robert F. *The Wuhan Cover-Up and the Terrifying Bioweapons Arms Race*. New York: Skyhorse Publishing, 2023.

Kernbach, Serge. "Unconventional Research in USSR and Russia: Short Overview." June 14, 2022, available at: http://dx.doi.org/10.2139/ssrn.4136176.

Kirk, John M. "The Strange Case of the Havana 'Sonic Attacks.'" *International Journal of Cuban Studies* 11, no. 1 (2019): 24–42.

Klippenstein, Ken. "Pentagon Requests $36 Million for Havana Syndrome." *The Intercept*, April 20, 2023, available at: https://theintercept.com/2023/04/20/pentagon-budget-havana-syndrome/.

Knox, Olivier, and Caroline Anders. "Is 'Havana Syndrome' Settled Now? White House Won't Say: The New Intelligence Report Seems to Land with a Thud at 1600." *Washington Post*, March 2, 2023.

Koblentz, Gregory D. *Living Weapons: Biological Warfare and National Security*. Ithaca: Cornell University Press, 2009.

Koffler, Rebekah. *Putin's Playbook: Russia's Secret Plan to Defeat America*. Washington, DC: Regnery Gateway, 2021.

Kolbe, Paul, Marc Polymeropoulus, and John Sipher. "Havana and the Global Hunt for U.S. Officers." *The Cipher Brief*, October 24, 2021, available at: https://www.thecipherbrief.com/havana-syndrome.

Kols, Richards. "NATO Must Meet Russia's Hybrid Warfare Challenge." *Atlantic Council*, July 3, 2018, https://www.atlanticcouncil.org/blogs/new-atlanticist/nato-must-meet-russia-s-hybrid-warfare-challenge/.

Koplov, David A. *Non-Lethal Weapons: The Law and Policy of Revolutionary Technologies for the Military and Law Enforcement*. Cambridge: Cambridge University Press, 2006.

Koplov, David A. "Red-Teaming NLW: A Top Ten List of Criticisms About Non-Lethal Weapons." *Case Western Reserve Journal of International Law* 47 (Spring 2015): 229–38.

Kornbluh, Peter. "The Secrets of the So-Called 'Havana Syndrome.'" *The Nation*, November 17, 2021, available at: https://www.thenation.com/article/world/havana-syndrome-attacks-cia/.

Kotchetkov, Ivan S., Brian Y. Hwang, Geoffrey Appleboom, Christopher P. Kellner, and Sander Connolly. "Brain-Computer Interfaces: Military, Neurosurgical, and Ethical Perspective." *Neurosurgical Focus* 28, no. 5 (2010): 1–6.

Kress, Kenneth A. "Parapsychology in Intelligence: A Personal View and Conclusions." *Studies in Intelligence* 24, no. 4 (1977): 7–17.

Krishnan, Armin. *Military Neuroscience and the Coming Age of Neurowarfare*. New York: Routledge, 2017.

Kubis, Joseph F. "Saratoga Report." Institute for Defense Analysis, May 8, 1969.

Labott, Elise. "John Kerry Reopens Embassy in Cube, But Tensions Remain." *CNN*, August 14, 2015, available at: https://www.cnn.com/2015/08/14/politics/cuba-embassy-opening-john-kerry-visit/index.html.

Labott, Elise, and Patrick Oppman. "State Department Orders Nonessential Diplomats and Families Out of Cuba Following Mysterious Attacks." *CNN*, September 29, 2017, available at: https://www.cnn.com/2017/09/29/politics/us-cuba-sonic-attacks-pulls-out-diplomats/index.html.

LaMothe, John. "Controlled Offensive Behavior—USSR." Defense Intelligence Agency, January 31, 1972.

Leake, Christopher, and Will Stewart. "Putin Targets Foes with 'Zombie' Gun Which Attack Victims' Central Nervous System." *Daily Mail*, March 31, 2012, available at: https://www.dailymail.co.uk/news/article-2123415/Putin-targets-foes-zombie-gun-attack-victims-central-nervous-system.html.

Lebow, Bronwyn. *Judging State-Sponsored Violence, Imagining Political Change.* Cambridge: Cambridge University Press, 2011.

Lederman, Josh. "Canadian Diplomats Say Their Government Is Withholding Info on More 'Havana Syndrome' Brain Injury Cases." *NBC News*, April 28, 2021, available at: https://www.nbcnews.com/politics/national-security/canadian-diplomats-say-their-government-withholding-info-more-havana-syndrome-n1265702.

Lederman, Josh, and Brenda Breslauer. "Legal, Financial Fight Mounts as 'Havana Syndrome' Goes Unsolved." *NBC News*, December 22, 2021, available at: https://www.nbcnews.com/politics/national-security/legal-financial-fights-mount-havana-syndrome-goes-unsolved-n1286399.

Lederman, Josh, and Michael Weissenstein. "Dangerous Sound? What Americans Heard in Cuba Attacks." *Associated Press*, October 13, 2017, available at: https://apnews.com/article/88bb914f8b284088bce48e54f6736d84.

Lee, Matthew, and Michael Weissenstein. "Hearing Loss of U.S. Diplomats in Cuba Blamed on Covert Device." *Associated Press*, August 9, 2017, available at: https://apnews.com/article/51828908c6c84d78a29e833d0aae10aa.

Lee, Victor Robert. "Satellite Images: A (Worrying) Cuban Mystery." *The Diplomat*, June 8, 2018, available at: https://thediplomat.com/2018/06/satellite-images-a-worrying-cuban-mystery/.

Lefebvre, Stéphane. "Cuban Intelligence Activities Directed at the United States, 1959-2007." *International Journal of Intelligence and Counterintelligence* 22, no. 3 (2009): 452–69.

Leventhall, Geoff. "Big Noise in Baghdad." *Noise & Vibration Worldwide* 35, no. 6 (2004): 27–31.

Levgold, Robert. *Return to the Cold War*. Cambridge: Polity, 2016.

LeVine, Susan. "The Active Denial System: A Revolutionary, Non-Lethal Weapon for Today's Battlefield." Center for Technology and National Security Policy National Defense University, June 2009.

Lewer, Nick, and Steven Schofield. *Non-Lethal Weapons: A Fatal Attraction? Military Strategies and Technologies for the 21st Century*. London: Zed Books, 1997.

Lewis, Flora. "Émigré Tells of Research in Soviet Parapsychology for Military Use." *New York Times*, June 19, 1977.

Lexington Institute. “Directed-Energy Weapons: Technologies, Applications and Implications.” Directed-Energy Program, 2003.

Liang, Qiao, and Wang Xiansui. *Unrestricted Warfare*. Beijing: PLA Literature and Arts Publishing House, 1999.

Libicki, Martin. *Cyberdeterrence and Cyberwar*. Santa Monica: RAND, 2009.

Lilienfeld A. M., J. Tonascia, S. Tonascia, C. A. Libauer, and G. M. Cauthen. “Foreign Service Health Status Study. Evaluation of Health Status of Foreign Service and Other Employees from Selected Eastern European Posts.” U.S. Department of State, July 1978.

Lillis, Katie Bo. “CIA Doctor Hit by Havana Syndrome Says He Was in ‘Disbelief’ as He Suffered What He Was Investigating.” *CNN*, September 25, 2022, available at: https://www.cnn.com/2022/09/25/politics/havana-syndrome-cia-doctor-cnn-special/index.html.

Lillis, Katie Bo. “CIA Inspector General Dings Agency Care of Early Havana Syndrome Victims.” *CNN*, October 14, 2022.

Lillis, Katie Bo, and Jen Christensen. “Despite Symptoms, NIH Research Finds No Evidence of ‘Havana Syndrome’ in Brain Scans.” *CNN*, March 18, 2024, available at: https://www.cnn.com/2024/03/18/health/havana-syndrome-studies/index.html.

Lillis, Katie Bo, and Jen Christensen. “‘There Is So Much Anger’: Havana Syndrome Victims Frustrated CIA Isn’t Blaming Russia for Victims.” *CNN*, May 1, 2024, available at: https://www.cnn.com/2024/05/01/politics/havana-syndrome-victims-cia-russia/index.html.

Lillis, Katie Bo, Jeremy Herb, and Kylie Atwood. “Exclusive: Dozens of CIA Officers Accuse Intel Agency of Soft Peddling Its ‘Havana Syndrome’ Investigation.” *CNN*, October 5, 2022, available at: https://www.cnn.com/2022/10/05/politics/cia-investigation-havana-syndrome-mysterious-illness/index.html.

Lim, Dawn. “Real-Life Inception: Army Looks to ‘Counteract Nightmares’ with Digital Dreams.” *Wired*, October 21, 2011, available at: https://www.wired.com/2011/10/real-life-inception/.

Lin, James C. “Microwave Signal at the US Embassy in Moscow.” *IEEE Microwave Magazine* 3 (2018): 20–2.

Lin, James C. “Weaponizing the Microwave Auditory Effect and the Havana Syndrome.” *The Radio Science Bulletin* 376 (2021): 36–8.

Lind, William, Keith Nightingale, John Schmitt, Joseph Sutton, and Gary Wilson. “The Changing Face of War: Into the Fourth Generation.” *Marine Corps Gazette* (March 2016): 86–90.

Lockie, Alex. “Russia Threatens US with ‘Asymmetric’ and ‘Painful’ Retaliation If Sanctions Imposed.” *Business Insider*, October 19, 2016, available at: https://www.businessinsider.com/russia-threatens-us-sanctions-2016-10.

London, Douglas. "The 'Havana Syndrome' Mystery and It's Impacts Aren't Over." *The Hill*, March 8, 2023, available at: https://thehill.com/opinion/national-security/3884347-the-havana-syndrome-mystery-and-its-impact-arent-over/.

Los Angeles Times. "U.S. Dismantles Antenna at Embassy." *Los Angeles Times*, November 14, 1977.

Lowenthal, Mark. *Intelligence: From Secrets to Policy*. Thousand Oaks: Sage, 2020.

Lowery, Oliver. "Silent Subliminal Presentation System." Patent No. US5159703A.

Lucas, Edward. *The New Cold War: Putin's Russia and the Threat to the West*. New York: St. Martin's Press, 2009.

Lukasik, Stephen. "Review of Project Pandora Experiments." *RAND*, November 4, 1969.

Lyon, Regan F., Joshua Gramm, Brian Branagan, and Shannon, C. Houck. "Implications of Neurological Directed-Energy Weapons for Military Medicine." *Journal of Special Operations Medicine* 22, no. 3 (2022): 104–7.

Macleaod, Alan. "A CIA Officer Has a Headache. Media Blame Russia." *Fairness & Accuracy in Reporting*, December 16, 2020, available at: https://fair.org/home/a-cia-officer-has-a-headache-media-blame-russia/.

Magnuson, Stew. "Exclusive: Doctors Reveal Details of Neuro-Strike Attacks in Havana." *National Defense Magazine*, September 6, 2018, available at: https://www.nationaldefensemagazine.org/articles/2018/9/6/exclusive-doctors-reveal-details-of-neuroweapon-attacks-in-havana.

Mahncke, Hans. "New Russia Hoax: Report Blames Kremlin for 'Havana Syndrome', But Evidence Suggests Otherwise." *Epoch Times Truth Over News*, April 5, 2024, available at: https://www.theepochtimes.com/epochtv/new-russia-hoax-report-blames-kremlin-for-havana-syndrome-but-evidence-suggests-otherwise-truth-over-news-5622714.

Maire, Louis F., and John D. LaMothe. "Soviet and Czechoslovakian Parapsychology Research." Defense Intelligence Agency, September 1975.

Maisonnave, Fabiano. "Manuel Zelaya Undergoes Strange Siege Inside Brazilian Embassy." *The Guardian*, October 25, 2009, available at: https://www.theguardian.com/world/2009/oct/25/honduras-manuel-zelaya-embassy-siege.

Mandel, Robert. *Security, Strategy, and the Quest for Bloodless War*. Boulder: Lynne Rienner Publishers Inc., 2004.

Marcetic, Branko. "Havana Syndrome Is Fake. But Mainstream Media Couldn't Get Enough of It for Years." *The Jacobin*, March 4, 2023, available at: https://jacobin.com/2023/03/havana-syndrome-government-report-debunking-intelligence-establishment-media.

Margolis, Jonathan. *The Secret Life of Uri Geller: CIA Master Spy?* London: Watkins Publishing, 2013.

Marks, John. *The Search for the "Manchurian Candidate": The CIA and Mind Control*. New York: W.W. Norton & Co., 1979.

Marten, Kimberley. "Russia's Use of Semi-State Security Forces: The Case of the Wagner Group." *Post-Soviet Affairs* 35, no. 3 (2019): 181–204.

Martinez, Jose A. "The 'Moscow Signal' Epidemiological Study, 40 Years On." *Reviews on Environmental Health* 34, no. 1 (2019): 13–24.

May, Edwin C., Victor Rubel, Joseph McMoneagle, and Loyd Auerbach. *ESP Wars: East & West*. Hertford: Crossroad Press, 2015.

Mazarr, Michael J. *Mastering the Gray Zone: Understanding a Changing Era of Conflict*. Carlisle: U.S. Army War College Press, 2015.

McCaffrey, Michael. "The Curious Case of Mysterious Attacks, Microwave Weapons and Media Manipulation." *Counterpunch*, September 19, 2018, available at: https://www.counterpunch.org/2018/09/19/a-curious-case-of-mysterious-attacks-microwave-weapons-and-media-manipulation/.

McCammon, Sarah, Courtney Dorning, and Jonaka Mehta. "New Cases of 'Havana Syndrome' Grow as Cause Remains a Mystery." *NPR*, October 15, 2021, available at: https://www.npr.org/2021/10/15/1046519741/new-cases-of-havana-syndrome-grow-as-cause-remains-a-mystery.

McCandles Farmer, Brit, Michael Rey, and Oriana Zill De Granados. "The Youngest Victims of 'Havana Syndrome.'" *CBS News*, June 26, 2022, available at: https://www.cbsnews.com/news/havana-syndrome-children-60-minutes-2022-06-26/.

McCreight, Robert. "Analyzing & Refuting Various JAMA/ NIH Claims on Havana Syndrome." Statement from March 19, 2024.

McCreight, Robert. "Brain Brinkmanship: Devising Neuroweapons Looking at Battlespace, Doctrine, and Strategy." In *Neurotechnology in National Security and Defense: Practical Considerations, Neuroethical Concerns*, edited by James Giordano, 115–32. Boca Raton: CRC Press, 2014.

McCreight, Robert. "The Era of Cognitive Warfare: What Next??" Presentation given at East Carolina University on March 21, 2024.

McCreight, Robert. "Neuro-Cognitive Warfare: Inflicting Strategic Impact Via Non-Kinetic Effect." *Small Wars Journal*, September 16, 2022.

McCreight, Robert. "Non-Kinetic Threats and the Threshold Spectrum of Strategic Endgame Warnings." *Mad Scientist Laboratory blog*, May 11, 2023, available at: https://madsciblog.tradoc.army.mil/444-non-kinetic-threats-and-the-threshold-spectrum-of-strategic-endgame-warnings/.

McCreight, Robert. "The War Inside Your Mind: Unprotected Brain Battlefields and Neuro-Vulnerability." *Academia Biology*, February 6, 2024, https://doi.org/10.20935/AcadBiol6156.

McHugh, Calder. "The 'Havana Syndrome' Report Hasn't Convinced Everyone." *Politico*, March 1, 2023, available at: https://www.politico.com/newsletters/politico-nightly/2023/03/01/the-havana-syndrome-report-hasnt-convinced-everyone-00085112.

McKelvy, Dolan M. "Psychic Warfare: Exploring the Mind Frontier." Montgomery, Air War College, Research Report, 1988.

McMillan, Tim, and Tyler Rogoway. "Special Access Programs and the Pentagon's Ecosystem of Secrecy." *The Warzone*, December 1, 2019, available at: https://www.twz.com/29092/special-access-programs-and-the-pentagons-ecosystem-of-secrecy.

McRae, Ron. *Mind Wars: The True Story of Government Research into the Military Potential of Psychic Weapons*. New York: St. Martin's Press, 1984.

Melzer, Nils. "Torture and Other Cruel, Inhuman or Degrading Treatment or Punishment." United Nations Human Rights Council (A/HRC/43/49), March 20, 2020, available: https://documents.un.org/doc/undoc/gen/g20/070/73/pdf/g2007073.pdf.

Mendez, Antonio, and Joanna Mendez. *Moscow Rules: The Secret CIA Tactics that Helped America Win the Cold War*. New York: Public Affairs, 2019.

Metz, Steven, and James Kievit. "The Revolution in Military Affairs and Conflict Short of War." U.S. Army War College, Strategic Studies Institute, July 25, 1994.

Meyer, Josh, and Dan Morrison. "Havana Syndrome Attacks Linked to Russian Spy Unit, New 60 Minutes Report Reveals." *USA Today*, April 1, 2024, available at: https://www.usatoday.com/story/news/politics/2024/04/01/havana-syndrome-brain-injury-attacks-russia/73169833007/.

Meyers, S. L., and J. Perlez. "U.S. Diplomats Evacuated in China as Medical Mystery Grows." *New York Times*, June 6, 2018.

Michaelson, Sol M., Roderick A. E. Thomson, and Joe W. Howland. "Biologic Effects of Microwave Exposure." University of Rochester, September 1967.

Michel, Casey. "The Time Russians Really Did Target Americans with Microwaves." *Politico*, March 10, 2023, available at: https://www.politico.com/news/magazine/2023/03/10/russians-americans-microwaves-00086482.

Milner, Conan. "Tuning in to Microwave Sickness." *Epoch Times*, May 23, 2019.

Mitchell, Andrea, Ken Dilanian, and Brenda Breslauer. "'Seized by Some Invisible Hand': What It Feels Like to Have Havana Syndrome." *NBC News*, October 13, 2021, available at: https://www.nbcnews.com/politics/national-security/seized-some-invisible-hand-what-it-feels-have-havana-syndrome-n1281326.

Mizokami, Kyle. "DARPA Wants Soldiers to Control Machines with Their Minds." *Popular Mechanics*, May 22, 2019, available at: https://www.popularmechanics.com/military/research/a27560088/darpa-soldier-machine/.

Moon, Jin-Hwa. "Health Effects of Electromagnetic Fields on Children." *Clinical and Experimental Pediatrics* 63, no. 11 (2020): 422–8.

Morehouse, David. *Nonlethal Weapons: War Without Death*. Westport: Praeger, 1996.

Morehouse, David. *Psychic Warrior: The True Story of the CIA's Psychic Espionage Program*. London: Clairview Press, 2004.

Morello, Carol. "U.S. Declares Reduced Staffing Levels 'Permanent' at Embassy in Havana: The State Department Also Extended an Advisory Urging Americans to Reconsider Travel to Cuba for Months After 24 U.S. Diplomats Suffered Unexplained Injuries." *Washington Post*, March 2, 2018.

Moreno, Jonathan D. *Mind War: Brain Research and National Defense*. New York: Dana Press, 2006.

Morris, Dick, and Eileen McGann. *Rogue Spooks: The Intelligence War on Donald Trump*. New York: St. Martin's Press, 2017.

Mosbergen, Dominique. "Microwave Weapons Could Be the Culprit Behind the Mysterious U.S. Embassy Attacks." *Huffington Post*, September 2, 2018, available at: https://www.huffpost.com/entry/microwave-weapons-embassy-attack-cuba-china_n_5b8bdaf4e4b0cf7b00370cc8.

Mothershead, Jerry, Zygmunt F. Dembek, Todd A. Hann, Christopher G. Owens, and Aiguo Wu. "Havana Syndrome: Directed Attack or Crickets?" *Joint Force Quarterly* 108, no. 1 (2023): 16–20.

Mulraney, Frances. "'Havana Syndrome' Sickens 100 CIA Officers & Families with Mystery Illness that Sparks 'Brain Fog' & 'Screeching Noises.'" *The U.S. Sun*, July 23, 2021, available at: https://www.the-sun.com/news/3336655/havana-syndrome-cia-officers-fbi-cause-unknown/.

Mumford, Michael D., Andrew M. Rose, and David A. Goslin. "An Evaluation of Remote Viewing: Research and Applications." The American Institutes for Research, September 29, 1995.

Munton, Don. "Our Men in Havana: Canadian Foreign Intelligence Operations in Castro's Cuba." *International Journal* 70, no. 1 (2015): 23–39.

Myre, Greg. "Long Before Havana Syndrome, the U.S. Reported Microwaves Beamed at Embassy." *NPR*, October 21, 2021, available at: https://www.npr.org/2021/10/21/1047342593/long-before-havana-syndrome-u-s-reported-microwaves-beamed-at-an-embassy.

National Academy of Sciences. "New Report Assesses Illnesses Among U.S. Government Personnel and Their Families at Overseas Embassies." *News Release*, December 5, 2020, available at: https://www.nationalacademies.org/news/2020/12/new-report-assesses-illnesses-among-us-government-personnel-and-their-families-at-overseas-embassies.

National Review Editors. "A Havana Syndrome Cover-Up?" *National Review*, April 2, 2024, available at: https://www.nationalreview.com/2024/04/a-havana-syndrome-cover-up/.

NATO. "Cognitive Warfare." Strategic Warfare Development Command Website, available at: https://www.act.nato.int/activities/cognitive-warfare/ (accessed August 10, 2024).

NATO. "Countering Cognitive Warfare: Awareness and Resilience." *NATO Review*, May 20, 2021, available at: https://www.nato.int/docu/review/articles/2021/05/20/countering-cognitive-warfare-awareness-and-resilience/index.html.

NBC. "Fighting an Invisible Enemy: The Voices of Havana Syndrome." *NBC News*, December 22, 2021, available at: https://www.youtube.com/watch?v=-tmFJDpLuMI.

Nelson, Roxanne. "Havana Syndrome May Be Result of Energy Pulses." *The Lancet* 396 (2020): 1954.

Neukam, Stephen. "'Havana Syndrome' Could Be the Result of Electromagnetic Weapon: Declassified Report." *The Hill*, March 30, 2023, available at: https://thehill.com/policy/healthcare/3925810-havana-syndrome-could-be-the-result-of-electromagnetic-weapon-declassified-report/.

Neukam, Stephen. "Lawyer: 'Havana Syndrome' Victims Feel 'Betrayed.'" *The Hill*, March 2, 2023, available at: https://thehill.com/policy/international/3880772-lawyer-havana-syndrome-patients-feel-betrayed/.

Newman, Lily Hay. "Hackers Can Turn Everyday Speakers Into Acoustic Cyberweapons." *Wired Magazine*, August 11, 2019, available at: https://www.wired.com/story/acoustic-cyberweapons-defcon/.

New Space Economy Staff. "What Is Space-Based Radio Frequency (RF) Monitoring and Why Is It Important?" *New Space Economy*, September 5, 2023, available at: https://newspaceeconomy.ca/2023/09/05/what-are-radio-frequency-rf-monitoring-satellites/.

New York Times Staff. "Embassy Radiation Is Cut in Moscow." *New York Times*, April 26, 1976, 5.

New York Times Staff. "Soviet Halts Microwaves Aimed at U.S. Embassy." *New York Times*, May 30, 1979.

New York Times Staff. "U.S. Moscow Envoy Reported to Be Ill: Embassy Denies." *New York Times*, February 17, 1976.

NPR. "The Curious Case of 'Havana Syndrome.'" *NPR*, January 25, 2023, available at: https://www.npr.org/2023/01/25/1151421770/the-curious-case-of-havana-syndrome.

O'Grady, Mary Anastasia. "Havana Syndrome Revisited." *Wall Street Journal*, March 20, 2023.

Opal, Jason. "America Is on the Brink of Another Civil War, This One Fueled by Donald Trump." *The Conversation*, August 2, 2023, available at: https://theconversation.com/america-is-on-the-brink-of-another-civil-war-this-one-fuelled-by-donald-trump-210937.

Oppmann, Patrick, AnneClaire Stapleton, Natasha Bertrand, Haley Britzky, Sergey Gudkov, and Sophie Tanno. "Russian Ships Arrive in Cuba as Cold War Allies Strengthen Their Ties." *CNN*, June 12, 2024, available at: https://www.cnn.com/2024/06/12/americas/russian-navy-cuba-intl/index.html.

O'Reilly, Anita. "An Australian Parliamentary Inquiry into the Deployment, Adoption, and Application of 5G in Australia." November 1, 2019, available at: https://www.aph.gov.au/DocumentStore.ashx?id=2de0d339-65e0-44d2-a576-31d22467e69c&subId=672968.

Ostrander, Sheila, and Lynn Schroeder. *Psychic Discoveries*. New York: Marlow & Co., 1997.

Ostroukh, Audrey. "Russia Writes Off Cuba Debt." *Dow Jones Institutional News*, July 11, 2014.

Page, Lewis. "Boeing Announces 'Laser Gunship' Completion." *The Register*, December 11, 2007, available at: https://www.theregister.com/2007/12/11/boeing_atl_advanced_tactical_laser_fitted/.

Panagopoulos, Dimitris J., and George P. Crousos. "Shielding Methods and Products Against Man-Made Electromagnetic Fields: Protection Versus Risk." *Science of the Total Environment* 667 (2019): 255–62.

Pancevski, Bojan. "A Den of Spies: Vienna Emerges as a Hub for Russian Espionage." *Wall Street Journal*, June 27, 2024.

Pancevski, Bojan. "U.S. Officials in Germany Hit by Havana Syndrome." *Wall Street Journal*, August 18, 2021.

Panuszka, Ryszard, Zbigniew Damijan, Cezary Kasprzak, and James McGlothlin. "Infrasounds and Biorhythms of the Human Brain." *Acoustical Society of America Journal* 111, no. 5 (2002): 2335–6.

Parameswaran, Prashanth. "What's in Russia's New Military Facility in Vietnam?" *The Diplomat*, April 30, 2019, available at: https://thediplomat.com/2019/04/whats-in-russias-new-military-facility-in-vietnam/.

Paranormal TV. "KGB Psychic Weapons Research." November 15, 2007, available at: https://www.youtube.com/watch?v=jexw2TAliRc&t=126s.

Partlow, Joshua. "In Cuba, Harassment of U.S. Diplomats Even Extends to Their Pets. Will That Now Change?" *Washington Post Online*, January 1, 2015.

Pasternak, Douglas. "Wonder Weapons: The Pentagon's Quest for Nonlethal Weapons Is Amazing. But Is It Smart?" *U.S. News & World Report* 123, no. 1 (1997): 38–44.

Payne, Elizabeth. "The Havana Syndrome: Why Canadian Diplomats Have Accused Their Government of Abandoning Them." *Ottawa Citizen*, February 25, 2019, available at: https://ottawacitizen.com/news/national/our-men-women-and-children-in-havana-how-a-dream-posting-became-a-nightmare.

Payne, Elizabeth. "Havana Syndrome Part 2: How a Dog's Brain May Help Solve the Mystery of Canadian Diplomats' Cuban Nightmare." *Ottawa Citizen*, February 27, 2019, available at: https://ottawacitizen.com/news/local-news/havana-syndrome-part-2-how-a-dogs-brain-may-help-solve-the-mystery-of-canadian-diplomats-cuban-nightmare.

Pearson, James, and Nandita Bose. "U.S. VP Harris Forges on with Vietnam Trip Despite Mystery 'Health Incident.'" *BBC News*, August 24, 2021, available at: https://www.reuters.com/world/asia-pacific/eve-harris-trip-vietnam-tells-china-it-does-not-pick-sides-2021-08-24/.

Peck, Michael. "Pentagon Fears that Microwave Weapons Are Undetectable." *Forbes*, March 2, 2021, available at: https://www.forbes.com/sites/michaelpeck/2021/03/02/the-pentagon-fears-that-deadly-microwave-weapons-are-undetectable/?sh=50d6ed72cc3f.

Pedrozo, Raul Pete. "The International Legal Implications of 'Havana Syndrome.'" *Lawfare blog*, December 23. 2020, available at: https://www.lawfareblog.com/international-legal-implications-havana-syndrome.

Pelley, Scott. "Havana Syndrome: High-Level National Security Official Stricken with Unexplained Illness on White House Grounds." *CBS News*, June 26, 2022, available at: https://www.cbsnews.com/news/havana-syndrome-white-house-cabinet-60-minutes-2022-06-26/.

Pelley, Scott. "'Havana Syndrome' Stumps Investigators as U.S. Officials Report Injuries on White House Grounds." *60 Minutes*, February 20, 2022, available at: https://www.youtube.com/watch?v=1meGH0Dts9M.

Pengelly, Martin. "John Bolton Chose Not to Brief Trump on Russia Havana Syndrome Suspicion." *The Guardian*, March 13, 2023, available at: https://www.theguardian.com/us-news/2023/mar/13/john-bolton-donald-trump-russia-havana-syndrome.

PETA Staff. "Victory! Army Ends Brain-Damage Testing on Ferrets at Wayne State Following PETA Pressure." *PETA Press Release*, November 16, 2023, available at: https://www.peta.org/media/news-releases/victory-army-ends-brain-damage-testing-on-ferrets-at-wayne-state-following-pressure-from-peta/.

Phelan, Matthew. "New NIH Study Sheds Light on Mysterious 'Havana Syndrome' Victims: Victims' Symptoms Are 'Real' and 'Quite Profound'—But Injuries Do Not Show Up on MRI Much Like a 'Mini-Stroke', One Pentagon Medical Consultant Tells DailyMail.com." *Daily Mail*, March 18, 2024, available at: https://www.dailymail.co.uk/sciencetech/article-13210727/NIH-study-Havana-Syndrome-Victims-symptoms-energy-weapons-microwave-acoustic-mystery.html.

Philipp, Joshua. "Next-Gen Weapons Detection Tech Being Deployed; 'Havana Syndrome' Confirmed by Pentagon Personnel as Real." *Epoch Times Crossroads*, April 4, 2024, available at: https://www.theepochtimes.com/epochtv/next-gen-weapons-detection-tech-being-deployed-5621381.

PHR and INCLO. "Lethal in Disguise: The Health Consequences of Crowd Control Weapons." Physicians for Human Rights/International Network of Civil Liberties Organizations, April 2014, available at: https://www.aclu.org/wp-content/uploads/publications/lethal_in_disguise_inclo_single_page.pdf.

Pichtel, John. *Terrorism and WMD: Awareness and Response*. Boca Raton: CRC Press, 2011.

Pierpaoli, Carlo, Amritha Nayak, Rabikul Hafiz et al. "Neuroimaging Findings in US Government Personnel and Their Family Members Involved in Anomalous Health Incidents." *JAMA* 331, no. 13 (2024): 1122–34.

Pilkington, Mark. "The Remote Viewers." *The Guardian*, June 4, 2005, available at: https://www.theguardian.com/science/2003/jun/05/research.science1.

Piore, Adam. "Building a Telepathic Army." *Discover Magazine*, November 11, 2019, available at: https://www.discovermagazine.com/mind/building-a-telepathic-army.

Platt, Brian. "In Court Filing, Canadian Government Argues Diplomats Exaggerated 'Havana Syndrome' Claims Behind $28 Million Lawsuit." *National Post*, November 26, 2019, available at: https://nationalpost.com/news/politics/in-court-filings-canadian-government-argues-havana-syndrome-claims-are-exaggerated-by-diplomats.

Poindexter, Lauren. "ARDEC Engineers Develop Solid State Active Denial Technology for Nonlethal Crowd Control." *U.S. Army* website, October 16, 2016, available at: https://www.army.mil/article/176579/ardec_engineers_develop_solid_state_active_denial_technology_for_non_lethal_crowd_control.

Pollack, H. "Epidemiologic Data on American Personnel in the Moscow Embassy." *Symposium on Health Aspects of Non-Ionizing Radiation*, New York, April 9–10, 1979.

Polymeropoulos, Marc. "'All I Wanted Was to See a Doctor': Ex-CIA Officer Tells All About His Battle with Havana Syndrome—and His Former Agency." *The Insider*, March 31, 2024, available at: https://theins.ru/en/opinion/marc-polymeropoulos/270427.

Pompeo, Michael. "Establishment of the Health Incidents Response Task Force." *U.S. Department of State Press Statement*, June 5, 2018, available at: https://2017-2021.state.gov/establishment-of-the-health-incidents-response-task-force/.

Power, Sean, and Michael Miner. "Report—Havana Syndrome: American Officials Under Attack." *Belfer Center for Science and International Affairs*, Harvard University, November 4, 2021, available at: https://www.belfercenter.org/publication/report-havana-syndrome-american-officials-under-attack.

Pradhan, S. D. "Chinese Neurostrike Programme: Pushing Cognitive Warfare to a New Level." *The Times of India*, July 8, 2023, available at: https://timesofindia.indiatimes.com/blogs/ChanakyaCode/chinese-neuro-strike-programme-pushing-cognitive-warfare-to-a-new-level/.

Pradhan, S. D. "NeuroStrike: A New Weapon of Warfare Requiring Prophylactic Steps." *The Times of India*, October 10, 2023, available at: https://timesofindia.indiatimes.com/blogs/ChanakyaCode/neurosrtike-a-new-weapon-of-warfare-requiring-urgent-prophylactic-steps/.

Pugh, Jonathan, Laurie Pycroft, Anders Sandberg, Tipu Aziz, and Julian Savulescu. "Brainjacking in Deep Brain Stimulation and Autonomy." *Ethics and Information Technology* 20, no. 3 (2018): 219–32.

Purvis, Vaughan. "The Nautilus Affair." 1997, available at: https://www.transformation.dk/www.raven1.net/mcf/hambone/nauti.html.

Qinetiq. "The U.S. Is Developing Wearable 'RF Weapon' Exposure Sensor." *Qinetiq* website, September 17, 2019, available at: https://www.qinetiq.com/en/blogs/wearable-rf-sensor.

Ratcliffe, John, and Cliff Sims. "The CIA Politicizes Intelligence on China and COVID; A Whistleblower Says That Analysts Who Favored the Lab-Leak Theory Were Paid to Change Positions." *Wall Street Journal*, September 18, 2023.

Razafsha, Mahdi, Tracy A. Barbour, Amit Chopra, Michael D. Kritzer, and Theodore A. Stern. "Transcranial Magnetic Stimulation in Primary Care: Indications, Risks, and Outcomes." *The Psychiatrist.com*, March 12, 2024, available at: https://www.psychiatrist.com/pcc/transcranial-magnetic-stimulation-primary-care-indications-risks-and-outcomes/.

Reed, Jim, and Joe McFadden. "Neuralink: Can Musk's Brain Technology Change the World?" *BBC News*, February 3, 2024, available at: https://www.bbc.com/news/health-68169082.

Regenstein, Lewis. "The Havana Syndrome: The History Behind the Mystery." *Foreign Policy Research Institute*, April 1, 2024, available at: https://www.fpri.org/article/2024/04/havana-syndrome-the-history-behind-the-mystery/.

Relman, David A., and Julie A. Pavlin, eds. *An Assessment of Illness in U.S. Government Employees and Their Families in Overseas Embassies*. Washington, DC: National Academies Press, 2020.

Reppert, B. "Zapping an Embassy: 35 Years Later, the Mystery Lingers." *Times Daily*, May 22, 1988, 6D.

Research Advisory Committee on Gulf War Veterans' Illness. *Gulf War Illness and the Health of Gulf War Veterans: Scientific Findings and Recommendations*. Washington, DC: U.S. Government Printing Office, 2008.

Reston, Richard. "Soviet 'Bugs' Find in U.S. Embassy Walls." *Los Angeles Times*, May 20, 1964.

Reuters. "'Havana Syndrome' U.S. Diplomats Get Benefits in Spending Bill." *Reuters*, December 16, 2019, available at: https://www.reuters.com/article/us-usa-budget-congress-diplomats/havana-syndrome-u-s-diplomats-get-benefits-in-spending-bill-idUSKBN1YK24Z.

RFA Vietnamese. "Report: US Officials Had Sudden Symptoms Before Harris' Hanoi Visit." *Radio Free Asia*, April 3, 2024, available at: https://www.rfa.org/english/news/vietnam/hanoi-havana-syndrome-report-04032024152734.html.

Richelson, Jeffrey. *The Wizards of Langley: Inside The CIA's Directorate of Science and Technology*. Boulder: Westview Press, 2001.

Robles, Frances. "U.S. Diplomats with Mysterious Illness in Cuba Had Inner-Ear Damage, Doctors Say." *New York Times*, December 12, 2018.

Robles, Frances, and Kirk Semple. "U.S. and Cuba Baffled by 'Health Attacks' on American Envoys in Havana." *New York Times*, August 12, 2017, A6.

Rodriguez Poleo, Germania. "Ex-National Security Advisor John Bolton Warns Russia 'Very Likely' Behind Havana Syndrome Amid Fears It's Being Used as Energy Weapon—as He Claims 'It Isn't Being Taken Seriously.'" *Daily Mail*, April 1, 2024, available at: https://www.dailymail.co.uk/news/article-13260299/john-bolton-russia-havana-syndrome.html.

Rofer, Cheryl. "Claims of Attacks with Microwaves Are Scientifically Implausible." *Foreign Policy*, May 10, 2021, available at: https://foreignpolicy.com/2021/05/10/microwave-attacks-havana-syndrome-scientifically-implausible/.

Rogin, Josh. *Chaos Under Heaven: Trump, Xi, and the Battle for the 21st Century*. Boston: Hougton Mifflin Harcourt, 2021.

Rogin, Josh. "Russia Is Harassing U.S. Diplomats All Over Europe." *Washington Post*, June 27, 2016.

Romo, Vanessa. "Canadian Diplomats Suing Government for $28 Million Over Mysterious Illness." *NPR*, February 7, 2019, available at: https://www.npr.org/2019/02/07/692548213/canadian-diplomats-suing-government-for-28-million-over-mysterious-illness.

Rosenberg, Yuval. "Trump Administration Asks for $81.1 Billion 'Black Budget', the Largest Ever." *Fiscal Times*, February 28, 2018, available at: https://www.thefiscaltimes.com/2018/02/28/Trump-Administration-Asks-811-Billion-Black-Budget-Largest-Ever.

Ross, Colin A. *The C.I.A. Doctors*. Richardson: Manitou Communications Inc., 2006.

Rubin, Rita. "More Questions Raised by Concussion-like Symptoms Found in US Diplomats Who Served in Havana." *JAMA* 319, no. 11 (2018): 1079–80.

Ryan, Shawn. "Marc Polymeropoulos—CIA Senior Intelligence Officer." *Shawn Ryan Show*, August 1, 2022, available at: https://www.youtube.com/watch?v=z2KDbESmZRk.

Safire, William. "Ockham's Razor's Close Shave." *New York Times*, January 31, 1999.

Sakelaris, Nicholas. "Diplomats Sue Canada Over 'Havana Syndrome' from Sonic Attacks." *UPI*, February 7, 2019, available at: https://www.upi.com/Top_News/World-News/2019/02/07/Diplomats-sue-Canada-over-Havana-Syndrome-from-sonic-attacks/1541549537662/.

Salama, Vivian. "U.S. Diplomats in Geneva, Paris Struck with Suspected 'Havana Syndrome'; Mysterious Neurological Ailment Has Afflicted as Many as 200 U.S. Officials in Diplomatic Posts Worldwide." *Wall Street Journal*, January 13, 2022.

Savitz, Scott, and Krista Romita Grocholski. "Revealing the Impact of Non-Lethal Weapons." *RAND Commentary*, July 15, 2022, available at: https://www.rand.org/pubs/commentary/2022/06/revealing-the-impact-of-non-lethal-weapons.html.

Scarf, Maggie. "Brain Researcher José Delgado Asks—'What Kind of Humans Would You Like to Construct?'" *New York Times*, November 15, 1970.

Schamiloglu, Edl. "Experts Believe US Embassies Were Hit with High-Power Microwaves—Here's How the Weapons Work." *SciTechDaily*, February 12, 2022, available at: https://scitechdaily.com/experts-believe-us-embassies-were-hit-with-high-power-microwaves-heres-how-the-weapons-work/.

Schamiloglu, Edl. "Microwave Weapon Behind Havana Syndrome: Report." *Asia Times*, February 7, 2022, available at: https://asiatimes.com/2022/02/microwave-weapon-behind-havana-syndrome-report/.

Schindler, John. "How Many American Spies Have to Die Before We Do Something Here?" *Top Secret Umbra*, April 30, 2021, available at: https://topsecretumbra.substack.com/p/how-many-american-spies-have-to-die.

Schnabel, Jim. *Remote Viewers: The Secret History of America's Psychic Spies*. New York: Dell Publishing, 1997.

Schumaker, James. "Before Havana Syndrome, There Was Moscow Signal." *Foreign Service Journal*, January/February 2022, available at: https://afsa.org/havana-syndrome-there-was-moscow-signal.

Schuster, Evylene. "Fifty Years Later: The Significance of the Nuremberg Code." *The New England Journal of Medicine* 337, no. 20 (1997): 1436–40.

Schuster, Steve. "Alleged CIA Developed Havana Syndrome Directed Energy Weapon, Attorney Says One Possible Theory for Coverup." *Wisconsin Law Journal*, April 10, 2024, available at: https://wislawjournal.com/2024/04/10/cia-developed-havana-syndrome-energy-weapon-attorney-says-possible-reason-for-coverup-2/.

Sciolino, Elaine. "The Bugged Embassy Case: What Went Wrong." *New York Times*, November 15, 1988.

Seldin, Jeff. "Energy Weapon Only 'Plausible' Explanation for Some Cases of Havana Syndrome." *Voice of America News*, February 2, 2022.

Seldin, Jeff. "'Havana Syndrome': Scans Show Differences in Affected Diplomat's Brain." *Voice of America News*, July 23, 2019.

Seldin, Jeff. "US Still Looking for 'Havana Syndrome' Answers." *Voice of America News*, January 21, 2022.

Seligman, Lara. "The Pentagon Is Funding Experiments on Animals to 'Recreate Havana Syndrome.'" *Politico*, March 9, 2023.

Seligman, Lara, and Erin Banco. "Pentagon Still Probing Would Caused 'Havana Syndrome', Even After Spy Agencies Found No Smoking Gun." *Politico*, March 6, 2023, available at: https://www.politico.com/news/2023/03/06/havana-syndrome-pentagon-research-00085686.

Seligman, Lara, and Andrew Desiderio. "'It Is an Act of War': Trump Acting Pentagon Chief Urges Biden to Tackle Directed Energy Attacks." *Politico*, March 5, 2021, available at: https://www.politico.com/news/2021/05/03/acting-pentagon-chief-miller-attacks-485236.

Seligman, Lara, Andrew Desiderio, and Betsy Woodruff Swann. "U.S. Troops Increasingly Vulnerable to Directed-Energy Attacks, Pentagon Tells Lawmakers." *Politico*, April 22, 2021, available at: https://www.politico.com/news/2021/04/22/troops-directed-energy-attacks-484246.

Shamlian, Janet. "New Study Finds Alarming Rise in Cancer Rates Among People Under 60." *CBS Evening News*, September 6, 2023, available at: https://www.cbsnews.com/news/study-alarming-rise-cancer-people-under-50/.

Shapira, Ian. "Was a Spy's Parkinson's Disease Caused by a Secret Microwave Weapon Attack?" *Washington Post*, December 5, 2017.

Sherman, Jason. "Boeing's Phantom Works Tapped to Design Airborne Laser in New MDA Tech Effort." *Inside the Pentagon's Inside Missile Defense* 23, no. 25 (2017), https://www.proquest.com/trade-journals/boeings-phantom-works-tapped-design-airborne/docview/1978600660/se-2.

Shorter, Edward. "'Havana Syndrome' Symptoms of Diplomats in Cuba Are Not Mass Hysteria." *The Conversation*, July 3, 2019, https://theconversation.com/havana-syndrome-symptoms-of-diplomats-in-cuba-are-not-mass-hysteria-118678.

Shukman, David. *Tomorrow's War: The Threat of Technology Weapons*. New York: Harcourt Brace & Co., 1995.

Singh, Ajay. "Non-Lethal Warfare." *Strategic Analysis* 22, no. 1 (1998): 5–15.

Spalding, Robert. *War Without Rules: China's Playbook for Global Domination*. New York: Sentinel, 2022.

Spetalnick, Matt. "U.S. Expels Cuba's UN Diplomats, Citing 'Influence Operations.'" *Reuters*, September 19, 2019, available at: https://www.reuters.com/article/idUSKBN1W42W1/.

Sputnik International Staff. "Russia Eyes Development of Futuristic Weaponry." *Sputnik International*, March 23, 2012, available at: https://sputnikglobe.com/20120322/172332421.html.

Starr, Barbara, Katie Bo Williams, and Jeremy Herb. "Pentagon Considering Telling Troops to Report 'Havana Syndrome' Incidents." *CNN*, May 26, 2021.

Steneck, Nicholas H. *The Microwave Debate*. Boston: MIT Press, 1984.

Stone, Vicki, Elinor Johnston, and Martin J. D. Clift. "Air Pollution, Ultrafine and Nanoparticle Toxicology: Cellular and Molecular Interactions." *IEEE Transactions on Nanobioscience* 6, no. 4 (2007): 331–40.

Strobel, Warren P. "Havana Syndrome Attacks Widen with CIA Officer's Evacuation from Serbia." *Wall Street Journal*, September 28, 2021.

Strobel, Warren P., and Gordon Lubold. "Cuba to Host Secret Chinese Spy Base Focusing on US." *Wall Street Journal*, June 8, 2023.

Stubbs, Alexander, and Fernando Montealegre-Zapata. "Recordings of 'Sonic Attacks' on U.S. Diplomats in Cuba Spectrally Matches the Echoing Call of a Caribbean Cricket." bioRxiv, January 2019.

Swanson, Ana, and Edward Wong. "Report Points to Microwave 'Attack' as Likely Source of Mystery Illnesses That Hit Diplomats and Spies." *New York Times*, December 5, 2020.

Swanson, Ana, Edward Wong, and Julian E. Barnes. "U.S. Diplomats and Spies Battle Trump Administration Over Suspected Attacks." *New York Times*, October 19, 2020.

Swanson, Randal L., Stephen Hampton, Judith Green-McKenzie, Ramon Diaz-Arrastia, Sean Grady, Ragini Verma, Rosette Biester, Diana Duda, Ronald L. Wolf, and Douglas H. Smith. "Neurological Manifestations Among US Government Personnel Reporting Directional Audible and Sensory Phenomena in Havana, Cuba." *JAMA* 319, no. 11 (2019): 1125–33.

Tadjdeh, Yasmin. "Innovation Hub Connects Industry, Academia and NATO." *National Defense* 102, no. 768 (2017): 28–9.

Tapscott, Mark. "DOD, Intel Agencies Look at Russian Mind Control Technology, Claims." *Defense Electronics*, July 1993.

Targ, Russell, and Harold Puthoff. "Information Transmission Under Conditions of Electromagnetic Shielding." Nature 251, no. 5476 (1974): 602–7.

Tatalović, Mićo. "I Wash All My Food Like Crazy: Scientists Voice Concern Over Nanoparticles." *The Guardian*, May 29, 2019, available at: https://www.theguardian.com/us-news/2019/may/29/i-wash-all-my-food-like-crazy-researchers-voice-concern-about-nanoparticles.

Thomas, Timothy. "Human Network Attacks." *Military Review* (September/October 1999): 23–33.

Thomas, Timothy. "Information Weapons: Russia's Nonnuclear Strategic Choice." *The Cyber Defense Review* (Summer 2020): 125–41.

Thomas, Timothy. "The Mind Has No Firewall." *Parameters* (Spring 1998): 84–92.

Thomas, Timothy. "The Russian View of Information War." In *The Russian Armed Forces at the Dawn of the Millenium*, edited by Michael C. Crutcher, 335–60. Carlisle: U.S. Army War College, December 2000.

Thomas, William. "Microwaving Iraq: 'Pacifying' Rays Pose New Hazards to Iraqi." January 25, 2005, available at: https://rense.com/general62/mciro.htm.

Thompson, Dennis. "No Brain Injuries Seen Among 'Havana Syndrome' Patients." *U.S. News*, March 19, 2024, available at: https://www.usnews.com/news/health-news/articles/2024-03-19/no-brain-injuries-seen-among-havana-syndrome-patients.

Thompson, Mark. "The Army's Totally Serious Mind Control Project." *Time*, September 14, 2008, available at: https://time.com/archive/6913384/the-armys-totally-serious-mind-control-project/.

United Nations. "The Convention on Prohibitions or Restrictions on the Use of Certain Conventional Weapons Which May Be Deemed to Be Excessively Injurious or to Have Indiscriminate Effects." October 10, 1980, available at: https://disarmament.unoda.org/the-convention-on-certain-conventional-weapons/.

UPI. "Report: N. Korea Fired Laser at Troops." *UPI.com*, May 13, 2003, available at: https://www.upi.com/Odd_News/2003/05/13/Report-N-Korea-fired-laser-at-troops/31591052808827/.

U.S. Advanced Research Projects Agency. "Justification Memorandum for Project Pandora." October 15, 1965, available at: https://nsarchive.gwu.edu/document/28787-document-3-arpa-richard-s-cesaro-memorandum-justification-memorandum-project-pandora.

U.S. Advanced Research Projects Agency. "Memorandum for Director, Defense Research & Engineering." Memorandum, September 27, 1967.

U.S. Advanced Research Projects Agency. "Minutes of Pandora Meetings." August 12 and 13, 1969.

U.S. Advanced Research Projects Agency. "PANDORA-BIZARRE Test Results." Memorandum, December 15, 1966.

U.S. Air Force. "Personnel Hatling and Stimulation Response (PHaSR) Fact Sheet." *Air Force Research Laboratory*, April 2006.

U.S. Centers for Disease Control. "Cuba Unexplained Events Investigation—Final Report." December 3, 2019.

U.S. Congress. "Attacks on U.S. Diplomats in Cuba: Response and Oversight." Senate Hearing 115-783, January 9, 2018.

U.S. Congress. "Border Sector Chiefs Confirm Operational Impacts of Border Chaos: Increased Gotaways, Closed Checkpoints, and Empowered Cartels." Homeland Security Committee, December 20, 2023, available at: https://homeland.house.gov/2023/12/20/border-sector-chiefs-confirm-operational-impacts-of-border-chaos-increased-gotaways-closed-checkpoints-and-empowered-cartels/.

U.S. Congress. "Chairman Pfluger Opens 'Havana Syndrome' Hearing: 'It Is Paramount That We Acknowledge the Gravity of the Situation.'" House Homeland Security Committee, May 8, 2024, available at: https://homeland.house.gov/2024/05/08/chairman-pfluger-opens-havana-syndrome-hearing-it-is-paramount-that-we-acknowledge-the-gravity-of-the-situation/.

U.S. Congress. "House Homeland Security Committee Holds Hearing on Foreign Anomalous Health Incidents." *Forbes Breaking News*, May 8, 2024, available at: https://www.youtube.com/watch?v=bwlCmtLCM2U.

U.S. Congress. H.R.4914 passed on August 3, 2021, available at: https://www.congress.gov/117/bills/hr4914/BILLS-117hr4914ih.pdf, Section 2 (13).

U.S. Congress. "Silent Weapons: Examining Foreign Anomalous Health Incidents Targeting Americans in the Homeland and Abroad: Written Testimonies." House Homeland Security Subcommittee on Counterterrorism, Law Enforcement, and Intelligence, May 8, 2024, available at: https://homeland.house.gov/wp-content/uploads/2024/05/2024-05-08-CTI-HRG-Testimony.pdf.

U.S. Congress. "Testimony of Christo Grozev." Homeland Security Committee, May 8, 2024, available at: https://homeland.house.gov/wp-c ontent/uploads/2024/05/2024-05-08-CTI-HRG-Testimony.pdf.

U.S. Congress. "Testimony of Greg Edgreen." Homeland Security Committee, May 8, 2024, available at: https://homeland.house.gov/wp-content/uploads/2024/05/2024-05-08-CTI-HRG-Testimony.pdf.

U.S. Congress. "Testimony of Mark Ziad, Esq." Homeland Security Committee, May 8, 2024, available at: https://homeland.house.gov/wp-content/uploads/2024/05/2024-05-08-CTI-HRG-Testimony.pdf.

U.S. Defense Intelligence Agency. "Project Sun Streak." Directorate of Science and Technology, undated, available at: https://nsarchive2.gwu.edu/NSAEBB/NSAEBB534-DIA-Declassified-Sourcebook/documents/DIA-21.pdf.

U.S. Defense Intelligence Agency. "Psychoenergetics Research." Defense Intelligence Agency Directorate of Scientific and Technical Intelligence, August 7, 1984.

U.S. Defense Intelligence Agency. "Scalar Waves." Memo, undated, available at: https://www.cia.gov/readingroom/docs/CIA-RDP96-00792R000500240001-6.pdf.

U.S. Department of Defense. "Active Denial System." *Join Intermediate Force Capabilities Office* website, https://jnlwp.defense.gov/About/Frequently-Asked-Questions/Active-Denial-System-FAQs/ (accessed July 24, 2024).

U.S. Department of Defense. "AHI Patient Registry FAQs." Military Health System, available at: https://www.health.mil/Reference-Center/Frequently-Asked-Questions/AHI-Patient-Registry?query=ahi (accessed July 30, 2024).

U.S. Department of Defense. "Bioeffects of Selected Nonlethal Weapons." Department of the Army, 1998, declassified on December 6, 2006.

U.S. Department of Defense. "Biological Effects of Electromagnetic Radiation (Radiowaves and Microwaves)." Defense Intelligence Agency, March 1976.

U.S. Department of Defense. "Controlled Offensive Behavior—USSR." Defense Intelligence Agency, July 1972.

U.S. Department of Defense. "Defense Health Program Budget." Office of the Comptroller, March 2022, available at: https://comptroller.defense.gov/Portals/45/Documents/defbudget/fy2023/budget_justification/pdfs/09_Defense_Health_Program/25-Vol_II_Sec_7-RDTE_Budget_Item_Justification_DHP_PB23.pdf.

U.S. Department of Defense. "Directed Energy Futures 2060: Visions for the Next 40 Years of U.S. Department of Defense Directed Energy Technologies." 2021, available at: https://www.afrl.af.mil/Portals/90/Documents/RD/Directed_Energy_Futures_2060_Final29June21_with_clearance_number.pdf?ver=EZ4QY5MG5UK2LDdwiuPc6Q%3D%3D.

U.S. Department of Defense. "Directive Number 3000.03E: DoD Executive Agent for Non-Lethal Weapons (NLW), and NLW Policy." April 25, 2013.

U.S. Department of Defense. "Evaluation of the DoD's Response to Anomalous Health Incidents, or 'Havana Syndrome.'" Office of the Inspector General, March 9, 2023, available at: https://media.defense.gov/2023/Mar/28/2003187716/-1/-1/1/DODIG-2023-054_REDACTED.PDF.

U.S. Department of Defense. "Memorandum for All Department of Defense Employees." Secretary of Defense, September 15, 2021, available at: https://irp.fas.org/news/2021/09/dod-ahi.pdf.

U.S. Department of Justice. "Department of Defense Non-Lethal Weapons and Equipment Review: A Research Guide for Civil Law Enforcement and Corrections." National Institute of Justice, July 2002.

U.S. Department of Justice and U.S. Department of Defense. "Joint Technology Program: Second Anniversary Report." National Institute of Justice, February 1997.

U.S. Department of State. "Cuba Accountability Review Board." *Office of the Spokesperson*, August 30, 2018, available at: https://2017-2021.state.gov/cuba-accountability-review-board/.

U.S. Department of State. "Fact Sheet: Activity at the Wuhan Institute of Virology." *Office of the Spokesperson*, January 15, 2021, available at: https://2017-2021.state.gov/fact-sheet-activity-at-the-wuhan-institute-of-virology/.
U.S. Department of State. "For Ambassador from Under Secretary Richardson." June 7, 1969.
U.S. Department of State. "Havana Cuba: Accountability Review Board." June 2018, Declassified on October 1, 2019.
U.S. Department of State. "Health Incident Response Task Force." *Deputy Secretary of State for Management and Resources*, available at: https://www.state.gov/health-incident-response-task-force/.
U.S. Department of State. "Kissinger Telephone Conversation with Ambassador Dobrynin." December 23, 1975, available at: https://nsarchive.gwu.edu/document/28818-document-10-kissinger-telephone-conversation-ambassador-dobrynin-23-december-1975.
U.S. Department of State. "Memorandum of Conversation." June 25, 1967, available at: https://nsarchive.gwu.edu/document/28809-document-1-memorandum-conversation-25-june-1967-attached-letter-ambassador-llewellyn.
U.S. Department of State. "U.S. Embassy Telegram to State Department." August 19, 1969, available at: https://nsarchive.gwu.edu/document/28811-document-3-us-embassy-moscow-telegram-4343-state-department-tums-19-august-1969.
U.S. General Accountability Office. "Science & Tech Spotlight: Directed Energy Weapons." GAO 23-106717, May 25, 2023, available at: https://www.gao.gov/assets/gao-23-106717.pdf.
U.S. Joint Chiefs of Staff. "Joint Concept for Competing." February 10, 2023, Glossary.
U.S. National Research Council. *An Assessment of Non-Lethal Weapons Science and Technology*. Washington, DC: The National Academies Press, 2003.
U.S. Navy. "Directed Energy Weapons: Counter Directed Energy Weapons and High Energy Lasers." Office of Naval Research, available at: https://www.onr.navy.mil/organization/departments/code-35/division-353/directed-energy-weapons-cdew-and-high-energy-lasers.
U.S. Office of the Director of National Intelligence. "Assessing Russian Activities and Intentions in Recent US Elections." *Intelligence Community Assessment*, January 6, 2017.
U.S. Office of the Director of National Intelligence. "IC Expert Panel on Anomalous Health Incidents Report: Executive Summary." Declassified February 1, 2022.
U.S. Office of the Director of National Intelligence. "Updated Assessment of Anomalous Health Incidents." *Intelligence Community Assessment*, March 1, 2023.
U.S. Office of the Director of National Intelligence. "Updated Assessment of COVID-19 Origins." *National Intelligence Council,* October 29, 2021, available at: https://www.dni.gov/files/ODNI/documents/assessments/Declassified-Assessment-on-COVID-19-Origins.pdf.

U.S. White House. "National Security Strategy of the United States." December 2017.

USA Today. "Victim of Suspected Health Attacks Speaks Out." *USA Today*, November 20, 2018, available at: https://www.youtube.com/watch?v=pOdXVye-4X0.

Van Creveld, Martin. *The Transformation of War*. New York: Simon & Schuster, 1991.

Verma, R., R. L. Swanson, D. Parker, A. A. Ould Ismail, R. T. Shinohara, J. A. Alapatt, and J. Doshi. "Neuroimaging Findings in U.S. Government Personnel with Possible Exposure to Directional Phenomena in Havana, Cuba." *Journal of the American Medical Association* 322, no. 4 (2019): 336–47. https://doi.org/10.1001/jama.2019.9269.

Vidal, Jacques J. "Toward Direct Brain-Computer Communication." *Annual Review of Biophysics and Bioengineering* 2, no. 1 (1973): 157–80.

Vincent, Brandi. "Army's New Brain Health Strategy to Address Anomalous Health Incidents, Havana Syndrome." *Defensescoop*, October 15, 2024, available at: https://defensescoop.com/2024/10/15/army-brain-health-strategy-address-anomalous-health-incidents-havana-syndrome/.

Vincent, Brandi. "Lawmakers Question How 'Havana Syndrome' Is Affecting DoD." *Defensescoop.com*, February 12, 2024, available at: https://defensescoop.com/2024/02/12/lawmakers-question-how-havana-syndrome-is-affecting-dod/.

Volcler, Juliette. *Extremely Loud: Sound as a Weapon*. New York: The New Press, 2013.

Wade, Nicholas. "Fischer-Spassky Charges: What Did the Russians Have in Mind?" *Science* 177, no. 4051 (1972): 778.

Walker, Mark, and Julian E. Barnes. "U.S. Refines Tools to Evaluate Havana Syndrome Cases." *New York Times*, January 13, 2022.

Wall, Judy. "PSYOPS Weaponry Used in the Persian Gulf War." *Nexus Magazine* 5, no. 6 (1998).

Wallace, Robert, and H. Keith Melton. *Spycraft: Inside the CIA's Top Secret Spy Lab*. London: Bantam Press, 2008.

Waller, J. Michael. *Big Intel: How the CIA and FBI Went from Cold War Heroes to Deep State Villains*. Washington, DC: Regnery Publishing, 2024.

Ward, Alexander, and Andrew Desiderio. "U.S. Foe or Specific Weapon Not Behind Sustained, Global Campaign Causing 'Havana Syndrome', CIA Finds." *Politico*, January 19, 2022, available at: https://www.politico.com/news/2022/01/19/havana-syndrome-cia-causes-527457.

Washington Examiner. "State Department Hopes 'New Technology' Will Identify 'Havana Syndrome.'" *Washington Examiner*, November 21, 2021, available at: https://www.washingtonexaminer.com/news/523469/state-department-hopes-new-technology-will-identify-havana-syndrome-cause/.

Wasserman, Matan. "'Even Cockroaches Won't Survive': Expert Discusses Hezbollah's New EMP Weapon." *The Jerusalem Post*, July 28, 2024, available at: https://www.jpost.com/middle-east/article-812168.

Weber, Peter. "Havana Syndrome Not Caused by Foreign Adversaries, Energy Weapons, or Aliens, U.S. Intelligence Assesses." *Newsweek*, March 2, 2023, available at: https://theweek.com/health-and-science/1021446/havana-syndrome-not-caused-by-foreign-adversaries-energy-weapons-or.

Weinberger, Sharon. "Wasted Energy: Despite 50 Years of Research on High-Power Microwaves, the US Military Has Yet to Produce a Usable Weapon." *Nature* 489, no. 7415 (2012): 198–200.

Weinberger, Sharon. "Microwave Weapons Are Real, But they Can't Explain 'Havana Syndrome.'" *Wall Street Journal*, April 6, 2024.

Weiner, Tim. "The Unanswered Question of Our Time: Is Trump an Agent of Russia?" *Washington Post*, September 21, 2020, available at: https://www.washingtonpost.com/outlook/2020/09/21/russian-agent-trump-counterintelligence/.

Wells, Jamie, and Alex Berezow. "Mystery Behind Decision to Yank Diplomats from Cuba." *USA Today*, September 29, 2017, available at: https://www.usatoday.com/story/opinion/2017/09/29/what-caused-hearing-loss-u-s-diplomats-health-mystery-alex-berezow-jamie-wells-column/698483001/.

Welsh, Cheryl. "Cold War Nonconsensual Experiments: The Threat of Neuroweapons and the Danger It Will Happen Again." *Essex Human Rights Review* 9, no. 1 (2012): 1–32.

White, Roberta F., Lea Steele, James P. O. Callaghan, Kimberly Sullivan, James H. Binns, Beatrice A. Golomb, Floyd E. Bloom, James A. Bunker, Fiona Crawford, Joel C. Graves, Anthony Hardie, Nancy Klimas, Marguerite Knox, William J. Meggs, Jack Melling, Martina A. Philbert, and Rachel Grashow. "Recent Research on Gulf War Illness and Other Health Problems in Veterans of 1991 Gulf War: Effects of Toxicant Exposures During Deployment." *Cortex* 74 (2016): 449–75.

Wilkinson, T. "Did Covert Spy Gear Cause U.S. and Canadian Diplomats in Cuba to Lose Their Hearing?" *Los Angeles Times*, August 10, 2017, available at: https://www.latimes.com/nation/la-fg-cuba-hearing-20170810-story.html.

Williams, Katie Bo, and Jeremy Herb. "US Investigating Possible Mysterious Directed Energy Attack Near White House." *CNN*, April 29, 2021.

Womac, Joyeux Noel. "Marked as Dangerous: An Investigative Analysis of No-Touch Torture on Targeted Individuals." Master Thesis, University of Purdue, 2022.

Woodley, Michael A., Jan de Nijenhuis, and Reagan Murphy. "Were the Victorians Cleverer Than Us? The Decline in General Intelligence Estimated from a Meta-Analysis of the Slowing of Simple Reaction Time." *Intelligence* 41, no. 6 (2013): 843–50.

Woodruff Swan, Betsie, Andrew Desiderio, Lara Seligman, and Erin Banco. "Pentagon Investigates Suspected Russian Directed-Energy Attacks on U.S. Troops." *Politico*, April 22, 2021, available at: https://www.politico.com/news/2021/04/22/pentagon-russia-attacks-us-troops-484150.

Woolf, Nicky. "Havana Syndrome Might Be Real and It Is Scary as Hell." *The Daily Beast*, February 2, 2023, available at: https://www.thedailybeast.com/havana-syndrome-might-be-real-and-its-scary-as-hell?ref=scroll.

Woolf, Nicky. "The Sound: Mystery of the Havana Syndrome—A Conversation with Nicky Woolf." University of Boston, November 1, 2023, available at: https://www.youtube.com/watch?v=kVZyDRBil8U.

Wright, Peter. *Spycatcher! The Candid Biography of a Senior Intelligence Officer*. New York: Viking, 1987.

Xinhua Staff. "Russia Resumes Military Presence on Cuba: Russian Lawmaker." *Xinhua News Agency*, August 3, 2008.

Yen, Amanda. "Pentagon Confirms Part of '60 Minutes' Havana Syndrome Report: A U.S. Official Had Symptoms Consistent with Havana Syndrome During a 2023 NATO Conference, the Pentagon Admitted Monday." *The Daily Beast*, April 1, 2024.

Yuste, Rafael, Jared Genser, and Stephannie Hermann. "It's Time for Neuro-Rights: New Human Rights for the Age of Neurotechnology." *Horizons* 18 (2021): 154–64.

Zimet, Elihu, and Christopher Mann. "Directed Energy Weapons—Are We There Yet? The Future of DEW Systems and Barriers to Success." Center for Technology and National Security Policy: National Defense University, May 2009.

Zimmer, Carl. "A 'Sonic Attack' on Diplomats in Cuba? These Scientists Doubt It." *New York Times*, October 5, 2017.

Index

About the Author

Armin Krishnan is associate professor and a former director of security studies at East Carolina University, where he teaches American foreign policy, international security, and intelligence studies. He has received his MA in political science, sociology, and philosophy at Ludwig-Maximilians University in Munich in 2001, MA in intelligence and international relations at the University of Salford, UK, in 2003, and PhD in security studies at the University of Salford, UK, in 2006. He has worked as a research associate at the University of Southampton, UK, before joining the University of Texas at El Paso in 2009 to teach in the Intelligence and National Security Studies program as a visiting assistant professor. In 2013, he joined the Department of Political Science of East Carolina University as a tenure-track faculty. He is the author of many journal articles and six books on different aspects of contemporary warfare, such as military service contracting, autonomous weapons systems, targeted killings, neurowarfare, paramilitary operations, and fifth-generation warfare. His current research interests include the political and military implications of blockchain technology, the Havana Syndrome, and foreign malign influence.

www.ingramcontent.com/pod-product-compliance
Ingram Content Group UK Ltd.
Pitfield, Milton Keynes, MK11 3LW, UK
UKHW020217290926
15470UKWH00001B/239